T0249004

Encyclopedia of Bladder Cancer: Biology and Basic Science

Encyclopedia of Bladder Cancer: Biology and Basic Science

Edited by **June Stewart**

New Jersey

Published by Foster Academics,
61 Van Reypen Street,
Jersey City, NJ 07306, USA
www.fosteracademics.com

Encyclopedia of Bladder Cancer: Biology and Basic Science
Edited by June Stewart

© 2015 Foster Academics

International Standard Book Number: 978-1-63242-132-6 (Hardback)

This book contains information obtained from authentic and highly regarded sources. Copyright for all individual chapters remain with the respective authors as indicated. A wide variety of references are listed. Permission and sources are indicated; for detailed attributions, please refer to the permissions page. Reasonable efforts have been made to publish reliable data and information, but the authors, editors and publisher cannot assume any responsibility for the validity of all materials or the consequences of their use.

The publisher's policy is to use permanent paper from mills that operate a sustainable forestry policy. Furthermore, the publisher ensures that the text paper and cover boards used have met acceptable environmental accreditation standards.

Trademark Notice: Registered trademark of products or corporate names are used only for explanation and identification without intent to infringe.

Printed in the United States of America.

Contents

Preface

Cancer has emerged as a prominent reason of death across the globe. This book collects a broad range of information related to the biology, epidemiology, biomarkers and predictive factors of bladder cancer. It also elucidates its clinical manifestations and diagnostic techniques. The book also studies the role of infectious agents in bladder cancer. The objective of the book is to help its readers to gain more knowledge regarding this form of cancer.

This book has been the outcome of endless efforts put in by authors and researchers on various issues and topics within the field. The book is a comprehensive collection of significant researches that are addressed in a variety of chapters. It will surely enhance the knowledge of the field among readers across the globe.

It is indeed an immense pleasure to thank our researchers and authors for their efforts to submit their piece of writing before the deadlines. Finally in the end, I would like to thank my family and colleagues who have been a great source of inspiration and support.

Editor

Part 1

Tumor Biology and Bladder Cancer

Bladder Cancer Biology

Susanne Fuessel, Doreen Kunze and Manfred P. Wirth
Department of Urology, Technical University of Dresden
Germany

1. Introduction

At present, bladder cancer (BCa) is worldwide the 9th most common tumor; in men it represents the 7th and in women 17th most common malignancy (Ploeg et al., 2009). In the European Union approximately 104,400 newly diagnosed BCa and 36,500 BCa-related deaths were estimated for the year 2006 (Ferlay et al., 2007). In the United States, approximately 70,530 new cases and 14,680 BCa-related deaths were expected for 2010 (Jemal et al., 2010). Men are three to four times more frequently affected than women (Ferlay et al., 2007; Jemal et al., 2010).

Detection of BCa is hampered due to lately emerging symptoms, such as hematuria, and the lack of specific tumor markers. Treatment options, particularly for the advanced disease, appear currently insufficient, leading together with the BCa-inherent high recurrence and progression rates to the relatively high BCa-related mortality (Ferlay et al., 2007). For the development of more specific and efficient diagnostic tools and therapeutic approaches a profound understanding of the onset and course of this disease is indispensable.

Molecular alterations that presumably lead to malignant transformation of the bladder urothelium belong to specified pathways involved in regulation of cellular homeostasis. As consequence of genetic and epigenetic alterations as well as of changes in subsequent regulatory mechanisms several major cellular processes are influenced in a manner that results in tumor development and progression. Regulation of the cell cycle, cell death and cell growth belong to these processes as well as the control of signal transduction and gene regulation. Particularly important for tumor cell spread and metastasis are changes in the regulation of interactions with stromal cells and extracellular components, of tumor cell migration and invasion and of angiogenesis (Mitra & Cote, 2009).

Interestingly, numerous associations between risk factors for the development of BCa and the affected cellular processes were identified (Mitra & Cote, 2009). For tobacco smoking or the occupational exposure to aromatic amines, polycyclic aromatic hydrocarbons and aniline dyes – the major environmental risk factors that contribute to BCa genesis – strong associations with alterations in cell cycle regulation have been reported (Bosetti et al., 2007; Golka et al., 2004; Mitra & Cote, 2009; Strope & Montie, 2008). Other factors such as use of hair dyes, several noxious substances and drugs, dietary components and urological pathologies influence with more or less evidence the control of cell cycle and the regulation of gene expression or signal transduction (Golka et al., 2004; Kelsh et al., 2008; Michaud, 2007; Mitra & Cote, 2009; Shiff et al., 2009).

Not only environmental risk factors determine the risk of BCa development, but also strong correlations with a genetic predisposition or polymorphisms in detoxification or repair genes leading to alterations in gene expression and regulation have been described (Bellmunt et al., 2007; Dong et al., 2008; Franekova et al., 2008; Garcia-Closas et al., 2006; Horikawa et al., 2008a; Kellen et al., 2007; Mitra & Cote, 2009; Sanderson et al., 2007). Several genome-wide association studies revealed the association of different single nucleotide polymorphisms (SNPs) with an altered risk of BCa. Strong associations of SNPs on the chromosomes 3q28, 4p16.3, 8q24.21 and 8q24.3 with the risk of BCa development were observed (Kiemeney et al., 2008, 2010; Rothman et al., 2010; X. Wu et al., 2009). Rothman *et al.* identified also new chromosomal regions on 2q37.1, 19q12 and 22q13.1, which are related to the susceptibility for BCa (Rothman et al., 2010).

2. Different clinical behavior due to varying genetic & molecular pathways

Clinical behavior and outcome of superficial, non muscle-invasive BCa doubtless differ from muscle-invasive BCa what is the result of varying molecular pathways characteristic for each subtype [Fig.1]. The more frequently diagnosed non muscle-invasive BCa comprise papillary Ta tumors confined to the mucosa and T1 tumors spread into submucosal layers of the bladder. In dependence on tumor grade, stage and size, the presence of concomitant *carcinoma in situ* (CIS), the occurrence of multifocal lesions and the prior recurrence rate the risk of recurrence of non muscle-invasive Ta/T1 BCa and the risk of progression to muscle-invasive BCa differ considerably (Babjuk et al., 2011; Sylvester et al., 2006). In principle, flat CIS lesions also belong to the group of non muscle-invasive BCa but are associated with a higher aggressiveness due to a completely different tumor biological behavior rather resembling muscle-invasive BCa (Kitamura & Tsukamoto, 2006; Pashos et al., 2002). It appears meaningful to regard the different types of non muscle-invasive BCa separately due to dissimilar phenotype-specific alterations in molecular and cellular pathways, which are also reflected by the varying clinical behavior. Ta tumors, which account for approximately 70% of non muscle-invasive BCa, bear a relatively high risk of local recurrence but rarely become muscle-invasive BCa (Kitamura & Tsukamoto, 2006; Pashos et al., 2002; Van Rhijn et al., 2009; Wu, 2005). The remaining non-muscle invasive BCa consist of 20% T1 tumors and about 10% primary CIS (Kitamura & Tsukamoto, 2006; Van Rhijn et al., 2009). Particularly, high grade T1 tumors (previously T1G3) have an increased propensity to progress compared to low grade T1 and Ta tumors (Emiliozzi et al., 2008; Kitamura & Tsukamoto, 2006). In contrast, CIS lesions are rather characterized by molecular alterations that are also observed in muscle-invasive BCa. Therefore, a high risk of progression of these CIS tumors seems to be implicated and leads to a poor outcome similar to that of muscle-invasive BCa (Knowles, 2008; Wu, 2005).

In low-grade papillary tumors a constitutively activated receptor tyrosine kinase/RAS pathway in consequence of activating mutations in the genes FGFR3 (*fibroblast growth factor receptor 3*) or HRAS (*Harvey rat sarcoma viral oncogene homolog*) was described (Jebar et al., 2005; Knowles, 2008; Wu, 2005). The rate of FGFR3 mutations of about 70% in Ta and in low-grade tumors is much higher than in invasive BCa with a rate of 10-20% (Bakkar et al., 2003; Billerey et al., 2001; Rieger-Christ et al., 2003; Serizawa et al., 2011).

Activating HRAS mutations are detected with an estimated overall frequency of 10-15% without a clear association with tumor grade or stage (Jebar et al., 2005; Knowles, 2008; Kompier et al., 2010a; Oxford & Theodorescu, 2003; Serizawa et al., 2011). Interestingly, mutations in FGFR3 and in RAS genes are mutually exclusive events and therefore suggested to represent alternative means to activate the MAPK (*mitogen-activated protein kinase*) pathway resulting in the same phenotype (Jebar et al., 2005; Kompier et al., 2010a). Furthermore, deletions of chromosome 9 belong to the most common genetic alterations in Ta tumors with a frequency of 36-66% (Knowles, 2008). Several putative tumor suppressor genes (TSG) located on this chromosome are affected by such deletions in combination with loss of heterozygosity (LOH) events, mutations or promoter hypermethylation (Knowles, 2008). Amongst others, the CDKN2A locus on 9p21 encoding the TSG p16^{INK4A} and p14^{ARF} is altered as well as PTCH1 (9q22.3), DBC1 (9q32-33) and TSC1 (9q34) located on the long arm of chromosome 9 (Aboulkassim et al., 2003; Berggren et al., 2003; Cairns et al., 1995; Chapman et al., 2005; Knowles, 2003, 2008; Lopez-Beltran et al., 2008; S.V. Williams et al., 2002; Williamson et al., 1995). LOH events in these chromosomal regions are associated with a high tumor grade and an elevated risk of recurrence of Ta and T1 tumors (Simoneau et al., 2000).

In principle, T1 tumors belong to the group of non-muscle-invasive BCa but obviously differ in their clinical behavior from Ta tumors since they show a higher potential for invasive growth and risk to progression. Nevertheless, dedifferentiation reflected by the tumor grade is a crucial factor for the determination of the phenotype resulting from differing molecular alterations (Kitamura & Tsukamoto, 2006). High-grade Ta tumors (TaG3) display a FGFR3 mutation frequency of 34% ranging between that of TaG1 (58-82%) and T1G3 tumors (17%) paralleling the phenotype and clinical behavior (Hernandez et al., 2005; Herr, 2000; Junker et al., 2008; Kitamura & Tsukamoto, 2006; Van Oers et al., 2007). Additionally, a high rate of homozygous deletions of the CDKN2A/INK4A gene, which was associated with an increased relative risk of recurrence, was observed in high-grade Ta tumors (Orlow et al., 1999).

Deletions or promoter hypermethylation of the CDKN2A/INK4A gene affect the expression of its gene products p14^{ARF} and p16^{INK4A} finally leading to deregulation in the p53 and RB1 (*retinoblastoma 1*) pathways. Alterations in these pathways are in fact molecular characteristics for CIS lesions and muscle-invasive BCa but can also be found in papillary tumors progressed to an invasive stage (Kitamura & Tsukamoto, 2006; Mitra & Cote, 2009; Orlow et al., 1999). Inactivation of p53 in muscle-invasive BCa is predominantly the consequence of allelic loss and mutations in this gene or of the homozygous deletion of its regulator p14^{ARF} (Mitra & Cote, 2009). Disturbed expression or uninhibited hyperphosphorylation of the tumor suppressor RB1 result in its inactivation (Mitra & Cote, 2009). Simultaneous dysfunction of p53 and RB1, the two central regulators of the cell cycle and apoptosis, is observed in more than 50% of high grade T1 tumors and in the majority of muscle-invasive BCa (Kitamura & Tsukamoto, 2006; Knowles, 2008). Furthermore, two other alterations affecting the p53 pathway are characteristic for muscle-invasive BCa: the lack of p21^{Waf1}, the *cyclin-dependent kinase inhibitor 1A* (CDKN1A), and overexpression of the p53-regulator MDM2 (*Mdm2 p53 binding protein homolog (mouse)*) (Mitra & Cote, 2009).

Muscle-invasive BCa display a high number and variety of chromosomal alterations such as loss of 5q, 6q, 8p, 9p, 9q, 10q, 11p, 11q, 17p and Y or gains of 1q, 3q, 5p, 6p, 7p, 8q, 17q, 20p and 20q (Blaveri et al., 2005; Heidenblad et al., 2008; Knowles, 2008; Richter et al., 1998; Simon et al., 2000).

The frequency of specific genomic alterations increases with tumor stage and is associated with a worse outcome (Blaveri et al., 2005; Richter et al., 1998). Several genes putatively relevant for tumor proliferation and progression are located in these altered chromosomal regions such as the transcription factors E2F3 and SOX4 on 6p22 or the supposed oncogene YWHAZ (14-3-3-zeta) on 8q22 (Heidenblad et al., 2008). Interestingly, amplification of 6p22 containing E2F3, which is involved in cell cycle regulation, and the frequently occurring homozygous deletions of CDKN2A and CDKN2B on 9p21 exist mutually exclusive indicating that they possibly play complementary roles (Feber et al., 2004; Heidenblad et al., 2008; Hurst et al., 2008; Oeggerli et al., 2004, 2006; Olsson et al., 2007).

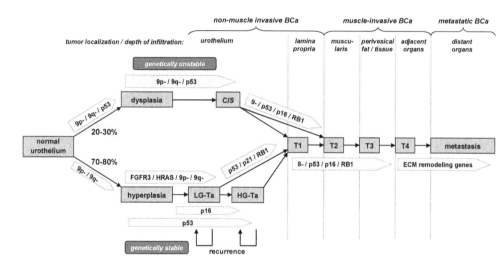

Fig. 1. Molecular pathways of BCa development and progression
Non-muscle invasive and muscle-invasive BCa fundamentally differ in their geno- and phenotypes. Varying genetic aberrations as well as the occurrence of p53 mutations in the normal urothelium are of crucial importance, which route of tumor progression will be followed. *Carcinoma in situ* (*CIS*) or muscle-invasive BCa, which may emerge from dysplasia of the urothelium, possess generally a high risk of progression. Papillary, non-muscle invasive Ta tumors, which are characterized by a high risk of recurrence and a lower risk of progression, rather develop from hyperplasia of the urothelium.
Abbreviations: 9p- / 9q- – loss of the short / long arm of chromosome 9, BCa – bladder cancer, *CIS* – *Carcinoma in situ*, ECM – extracellular matrix, HG-Ta – high grade Ta tumor, LG-Ta – low grade Ta tumor, T1 to T4 – tumor stages 1 to 4.

During progression and metastasis profound changes of regulatory networks involving the extracellular matrix (ECM), cell adhesion and migration, attraction of blood vessels and neovascularization occur, which characterize advanced tumor stages (Mitra & Cote, 2009). These processes comprise alterations in the regulation of cadherins, which are responsible for epithelial cell-cell adhesion, and *matrix metalloproteinases* (MMPs), which play an important role in the ECM-degradation as prerequisite for tumor cell migration (Mitra & Cote, 2009; Slaton et al., 2004; Wallard et al., 2006). Angiogenesis is driven by angiogenic factors such as the *vascular endothelial growth factor* (VEGF), one of the key factors responsible for tumor progression (Crew, 1999a).

3. Alterations in cell cycle regulation

Correct course of cell cycle is controlled by the p53 and RB1 pathways that are tightly linked with each other and influence regulation of apoptosis, signal transduction and gene expression [Fig.2]. The TSG p53, the central regulator of these processes, is located on chromosome 17p13.1, a region that is affected by allelic loss more frequently in BCa of higher stage and grade (Knowles, 2008; Olumi et al., 1990). Parallel to the loss of one 17p allele, frequently occurring mutations lead to the inactivation of the tumor suppressor p53 (Cordon-Cardo et al., 1994; Dalbagni et al., 1993; Sidransky et al., 1991). Mutated p53 becomes resistant to degradation and due to this longer stability detectable in the nucleus by immunohistochemistry (Dalbagni et al., 1993; Esrig et al., 1993). Such mutations were observed with a high frequency in BCa of higher stage and grade (Dalbagni et al., 1993; Esrig et al., 1993; Fujimoto et al., 1992; Puzio-Kuter et al., 2009; Serizawa et al., 2011; Sidransky et al., 1991). Therefore, the assessment of the nuclear immunoreactivity of altered p53 facilitates prognostic conclusions (Esrig et al., 1993; Kuczyk et al., 1995; Sarkis et al., 1993, 1995; Serth et al., 1995). Particularly for invasive, but still organ-confined BCa without metastasis (T1-2b N0 M0) and also for advanced BCa p53 is of prognostic importance with regard to the prediction of recurrence and cancer-specific mortality after radical cystectomy (Shariat et al., 2009a, 2009b). Nevertheless, nuclear accumulation and mutations of p53 provide differing contribution to the prediction of the outcome. Mutations and altered protein stability of p53 lead to worst prognosis compared to patients with one of these events and to patients with wild-type p53 and unchanged protein stability, who showed a more favorable outcome (George et al., 2007).

Interestingly, a study on BCa patients without evidence of distant metastases suggested that tumors harboring p53 mutations are more susceptible to adjuvant chemotherapy containing DNA-damaging agents such as e.g. cisplatin and doxorubicin (Cote et al., 1997). Possibly, these chemotherapeutics induce apoptosis in p53-mutated cells by uncoupling of the S and M cell cycle phases (Waldman et al., 1996). These observations built the basis for a large international multicenter clinical trial dealing with the assessment of response rates of high-risk patients with organ-confined invasive BCa to a chemotherapy containing DNA-damaging agents (Mitra et al., 2007). However, first data analysis did not confirm the predictive value of p53 immunohistochemistry (Stadler, 2009).

Wild-type p53 controls cell cycle progression at G1-S transition by transcriptional activation of p21^{WAF1} (CDKN1A), a cyclin-dependent kinase inhibitor (CDKI) that additionally can be regulated by p53-independent mechanisms (El-Deiry et al., 1993; Michieli et al., 1994; Parker et al., 1995; Stein et al., 1998). As potent CDKI, p21^{Waf1} inhibits the activity of cyclin-CDK2 or -CDK4 complexes, and thus functions as a regulator of cell cycle progression at G1 (Mitra et al., 2007). Loss or under-expression of p21^{Waf1} appears to have impact on tumor progression and consequently on the outcome of the patients (Stein et al., 1998). Patients with wild-type p53 and p21^{Waf1} positivity had the best prognosis whereas patients with altered p53 and maintained p21^{Waf1} expression displayed worse outcome and patients with altered p53 and lack of p21^{Waf1} showed the highest rate of recurrence and worst survival (Stein et al., 1998).

MDM2, located on chromosome 12q14.3-q15, is another component involved in the regulatory network of p53 and an indispensable factor for the feedback control of p53 stability. Transcription of MDM2 is induced by p53. In the form of an autoregulatory loop, MDM2 can build a complex with p53 and transports it to the proteasome for degradation (Mitra & Cote, 2009; Wu et al., 1993, 2005).

Degraded p53 in turn causes reduction in MDM2 levels, but this can be bypassed by MDM2 gene amplification, which is observed approximately in 5% of the BCa with an increased frequency in tumors of higher stage and grade (Simon et al., 2002). Additionally, MDM2 overexpression is a common event in BCa in strong association with p53 nuclear immunoreactivity (Lianes et al., 1994; Lu et al., 2002; Pfister et al., 1999, 2000). A combined assessment of alterations of p53, p21^{Waf1} and MDM2 revealed that patients with mutant p53 and/or p53 nuclear overexpression, loss of p21^{Waf1} and MDM2 nuclear overexpression exhibited the worst outcome (Lu et al., 2002). Furthermore, a specific SNP at nucleotide position 309 in the MDM2 promoter region was evaluated for prognostic and predictive purposes. It can predict a poor outcome particularly in conjunction with the mutation and SNP status of p53 (Horikawa et al., 2008b; Sanchez-Carbayo et al., 2007; Shinohara et al., 2009).

The chromosomal region 9q21, which is frequently lost in non-muscle invasive and in muscle-invasive BCa, harbors the gene locus CDKN2A (*cyclin-dependent kinase inhibitor 2A*) whose transcription results in two different splice variants, p14^{ARF} and p16^{INK4A} (Knowles, 2008; Quelle et al., 1995; S.G. Williams & Stein, 2004). Normally, p14^{ARF} is induced by the transcription factor E2F and can inhibit transcription of MDM2 thereby blocking the MDM2-induced p53 degradation (S.G. Williams & Stein, 2004). Thus, p14^{ARF} builds a link between the p53 and the RB1 pathways. The expression of the splice variant p14^{ARF} is predominantly reduced by homozygous deletions and also by promoter hypermethylation in BCa (Chang et al., 2003; Dominguez et al., 2003; Kawamoto et al., 2006; W.J. Kim & Quan, 2005).

The gene product of the other splice variant, p16^{INK4A}, normally functions as CDKI by blocking the cyclin D-CDK4/6-mediated phosphorylation of the RB1 protein thereby maintaining it in its active hypophosphorylated state and preventing exit from the G1 phase (Quelle et al., 1995; Serrano et al., 1993). In a study on BCa of all stages and grades homozygous deletion of p16^{INK4A} was observed in a lower frequency than of p14^{ARF} (Chang et al., 2003). In another study on non-muscle invasive BCa a higher risk of recurrence was found for homozygous deletion of the CDKN2A gene where loss of both splice variants p14^{ARF} and p16^{INK4A} correlated with clinicopathological parameters of a worse prognosis due to the potential deregulation of both the p53 and RB1 pathways (Orlow et al., 1999). Additionally, hypermethylation in the promoter region of p16^{INK4A} was reported for BCa in a range of 6-60% (Chang et al., 2003; Chapman et al., 2005; Dominguez et al., 2003; Kawamoto et al., 2006; W.J. Kim & Quan, 2005; Orlow et al., 1999). Loss of p16^{INK4A} protein expression in T1 tumors correlated significantly with a reduced progression-free survival and was an independent predictor of tumor progression (Kruger et al., 2005). In another study, aberrant p16^{INK4A} protein expression was found to be an adverse prognostic factor only in T3-T4 tumors whereas abnormal immunoreactivity of p53 and p16^{INK4A} was identified as an independent predictor of reduced survival for all muscle-invasive BCa (Korkolopoulou et al., 2001).

Concluding data on BCa, homozygous deletions in the CDKN2A gene were not associated with tumor stage or grade supporting the hypothesis that chromosomal alteration of 9p21 is an early event in bladder carcinogenesis (Berggren et al., 2003). Nevertheless, aberrant methylation of p14^{ARF} and p16^{INK4A} occurs more frequently in muscle-invasive than in non-muscle invasive BCa and seems to be associated with adverse clincopathological parameters as well as with a poor outcome (Dominguez et al., 2003; Kawamoto et al., 2006).

The CDKN2B gene located adjacent to CDKN2A on 9p21 encodes the CDKI p15[INK4B], which inhibits cyclin D1-CDK4/6 complexes similar to p16[INK4A] (Orlow et al., 1995). In contrast to p16[INK4A] no association was observed between the expression and promoter methylation status of p15[INK4B] whereas the rate of chromosomal alterations was comparable (M.W. Chan et al., 2002; Gonzalez-Zulueta et al., 1995; Le Frere-Belda et al., 2004; Orlow et al., 1995). Decreased p15[INK4B] mRNA expression was only observed in non-muscle invasive BCa; in muscle invasive BCa p15[INK4B] expression varied widely (Le Frere-Belda et al., 2001). The authors concluded that decreased p15[INK4B] expression might be an important step in early neoplastic transformation of the urothelium and could be caused by other mechanisms than deletion or promoter hypermethylation (Le Frere-Belda et al., 2001).

The potential TSG p27[Kip1] (CDKN1B) is located on chromosome 12p13.1-p12 and belongs to the Kip1 family of CDKIs. It inhibits cyclin D-CDK4/6 and cyclin E/A-CDK2 complexes consequently preventing RB1 hyperphosphorylation (Coats et al., 1996; Polyak et al., 1994). The prognostic value of p27[Kip1] was analyzed in several immunohistochemistry studies on non-muscle and muscle-invasive BCa which revealed that this factor is preferentially expressed in early stage BCa (Franke et al., 2000; Korkolopoulou et al., 2000; Rabbani et al., 2007). In non-muscle invasive BCa expression of p27[Kip1] decreased significantly with increasing grade and a significant correlation between low p27[Kip1] expression and shorter disease-free survival and overall survival was observed, facts that support the hypothesis that loss of p27[Kip1] confers a selective growth advantage to tumor cells (Kamai et al., 2001; Korkolopoulou et al., 2000; Migaldi et al., 2000; Sgambato et al., 1999). However, some studies on non-muscle invasive and/or muscle-invasive BCa did not reveal a significant association between the loss of p27[Kip1] and outcome (Doganay et al., 2003; Franke et al., 2000; Kuczyk et al., 1999), whereas other reports showed that a decreased expression of p27[Kip1] significantly correlated with worse prognosis (Kamai et al., 2001; Rabbani & Cordon-Cardo, 2000).

Another central pathway influencing cell cycle progression is the regulatory network around the nuclear phosphoprotein RB1, a TSG located on chromosome 13q14 (Cairns et al., 1991; Mitra et al., 2007; Takahashi et al., 1991; S.G. Williams & Stein, 2004). RB1 in its physiological active, hypophosphorylated form inhibits cell cycle progression at the G1-S checkpoint by sequestering transcription factors of the E2F family (Chellappan et al., 1991; Fung et al., 1987; Hiebert et al., 1992; Mihara et al., 1989). Hyperphosphorylation of RB1 abolishes its cell cycle-inhibitory activity by the release of E2F transcription factors leading to transcription of genes involved in DNA synthesis and progression through mitosis (Degregori et al., 1995; Hernando et al., 2004; Mitra et al., 2007). RB1 becomes hyperphosphorylated by different cyclin-CDK complexes, such as cyclin D1-CDK4/6 and cyclin E-CDK2, which in turn can be inhibited by specific CDKIs, such as p16[INK4A], p21[Waf1] and p27[Kip1]. The phosphorylation-mediated inactivation of RB1 can be the consequence of the already described loss of different CDKIs (Mitra et al., 2007).

In addition, mutations and LOH events in the RB1 gene can also lead to loss of RB1 expression and consequently to unregulated cellular proliferation (Miyamoto et al., 1995; Wada et al., 2000; Xu et al., 1993). Therefore, both aberrant RB1 down-regulation and dominance of the hyperphosphorylated inactive RB1 can be associated with tumor progression (Cote et al., 1998). For BCa, the proportion of RB1 alterations due to loss or inactivation was reported to increase with tumor stage and grade (Cairns et al., 1991; Ishikawa et al., 1991; Wada et al., 2000; Xu et al., 1993).

Particularly muscle-invasive, advanced BCa with an altered RB1 expression had a more aggressive behavior reflected by significantly decreased survival (Cordon-Cardo et al., 1992; Cote et al., 1998; Logothetis et al., 1992).

Regarding both p53 and RB1 – the key players of cell cycle regulation – as well as the other components of this regulatory network, a combined analysis of multiple factors seems to be reasonable. Therefore, a multitude of comprehensive immunohistochemical analyses of different cell cycle regulators such as p53, RB1, MDM2, cyclin D1 and E, p14ARF, p16INK4A, p21Waf1, p27Kip1, Ki67 and PCNA (*proliferating cell nuclear antigen*) were performed on tissue specimens originating from non-muscle invasive and muscle-invasive BCa (Brunner et al., 2008; Cordon-Cardo et al., 1997; Cote et al., 1998; Grossman et al., 1998; Hitchings et al., 2004; Kamai et al., 2001; Korkolopoulou et al., 2000; Lu et al., 2002; Migaldi et al., 2000; Niehans et al., 1999; Pfister et al., 1999, 2000; Sarkar et al., 2000; Shariat et al., 2004, 2006, 2007a, 2007b, 2007c; 2007d, 2009a; Tut et al., 2001).

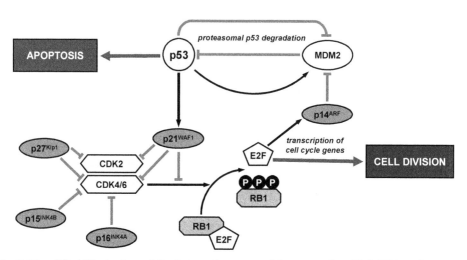

Fig. 2. Simplified illustration of the interactive network between the p53 & RB1 pathways Transcription of MDM2 is induced by p53. In the form of an autoregulatory loop, MDM2 conveys p53 by ubiquitination to proteasomal degradation. Degraded p53 in turn causes reduction in MDM2 levels. Wild-type p53 can induce transcription of the CDKI p21WAF1, which inhibits the activity of cyclin-CDK2 or -CDK4 complexes similar to the CDKI p15INK4B, p16INK4A and p27Kip1. When RB1 gets hyperphosphorylated by different cyclin-CDK complexes bound E2F transcription factors are released leading to the induction of cell cycle-promoting genes, but also to transcription of p14ARF, which can inhibit MDM2. Abbreviations: CDK – cyclin-dependent kinase, CDKI – cyclin-dependent kinase inhibitor, E2F – E2F transcription factors, MDM2 – *Mdm2 p53 binding protein homolog (mouse)*, p14ARF and p16 INK4A – splice variants of the *cyclin-dependent kinase inhibitor 2A* gene, p15INK4B – *cyclin-dependent kinase inhibitor 2B*, p27Kip1 – *cyclin-dependent kinase inhibitor 1B*, RB1 – *retinoblastoma 1*.

The bottom line of most of these studies is that changes in gene expression, which can be caused by chromosomal alterations, promoter hypermethylation or altered regulation of transcriptional induction, as well as alterations of stability, modification and activity of the different involved factors contribute to deregulation of the complex processes during cell cycle progression. The number of altered components correlates with the severity of dysfunction and deregulation finally leading to increased aggressiveness of the tumor and to worse prognosis. Most promising candidates, when analyzed in parallel with regard to prediction of the outcome of BCa patients, seem to be p53, RB1, p16^{INK4A}, p21^{Waf1}, p27^{Kip1} and the proliferation marker Ki67. This prognostic information can support the stratification of the tumors according to their aggressiveness and the selection of adapted treatment options (Grossman et al., 1998).

4. Deregulation of cell death pathways

Course of development, cell differentiation and homeostasis is normally regulated by the tight control of cell death pathways [Fig.3]. This programmed cell death, the apoptosis, is usually induced by a variety of extra- and intracellular stimuli and is mediated by a complex arrangement of sensors, regulators and effectors whose interactions are frequently perturbed in tumor cells. Failure of apoptosis permits mutated cells to continue progression through the cell cycle, to accumulate mutations and to increase molecular deregulations. The resulting unrestricted propagation of active oncogenes and defective TSG finally leads to the uncontrolled proliferation and spread of these abnormal cells (Bryan et al., 2005a; Duggan et al., 2001; Mcknight et al., 2005). Defects and deregulation in the extrinsic and in the intrinsic apoptotic pathways contribute to development and progression of many tumors including BCa and are also the main reason for therapeutic failure. Particularly, defective p53 fails as detector of DNA damage and main inductor of apoptosis, when DNA repair was not achieved (Duggan et al., 2001).

The extrinsic apoptotic pathway is induced through the stimulation of cell surface death receptors by their corresponding ligands while the intrinsic pathway is switched on by the disruption of mitochondrial membranes. There is a cross-talk between both routes that finally lead to the cleavage of cellular proteins by caspases and subsequently to the degradation of the cells by gradual destruction of cellular components (Mcknight et al., 2005).

Transmembrane death receptors, such as FAS (CD95, APO-1), TNFR1, TRAILR1 or TRAILR2, belong to the *tumor necrosis factor* (TNF) receptor superfamily and contain an intracellular death domain. After binding of the respective ligands, such as FAS ligand, TNFα or TRAIL, extracellular death signals are transmitted via these domains by formation of a death-inducing signaling complex that activates the initiator caspases 8 and 10 (Mcknight et al., 2005; Mitra & Cote, 2009). Impairment of this processes was reported in BCa e.g. for FAS-mediated apoptosis that might be caused by mutation or decreased expression of FAS, which is associated with disease progression and poor outcome (Lee et al., 1999; Mcknight et al., 2005; Yamana et al., 2005). An alternative splice variant of FAS results in circulating soluble FAS that can capture the respective ligands and consequently prevent the normal death signal transduction. Soluble FAS, which was detected in serum and also in urine samples from BCa patients, could serve as predictor of recurrence and progression of BCa (Mizutani et al., 2001; Svatek et al., 2006).

The intrinsic or mitochondrial induced apoptotic pathway can be initiated by DNA damage or different cellular stress signals (Mcknight et al., 2005). The BCL2 (*B-cell CLL/lymphoma 2*) family, which plays a crucial role in the intrinsic apoptotic pathway, consists of anti-apoptotic members, such as BCL2 and BCLXL (*BCL2-like 1*), as well as of pro-apoptotic members, such as BAX (*BCL2-associated X protein*), BID (*BH3 interacting domain death agonist*) and BAD (*BCL2-associated agonist of cell death*). BCL2 is an integral protein of the outer mitochondrial membrane that is involved in the control of ion channels, inhibition of cytochrome c release from the mitochondria or modulation of caspase activation (Mcknight et al., 2005; Mitra & Cote, 2009).

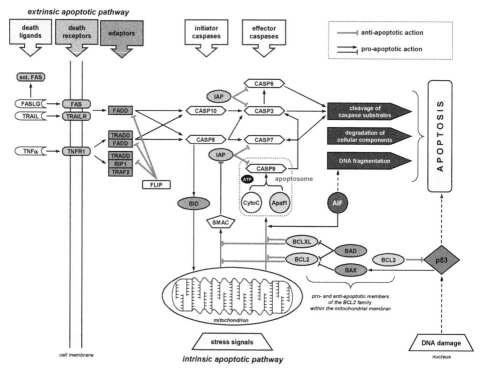

Fig. 3. Simplified illustration of the apoptotic cell death pathways
The extrinsic apoptotic pathway is induced through stimulation of cell surface death receptors by their corresponding ligands. The intrinsic mitochondrial route of apoptosis is initiated by DNA damage and cellular stress signals. Both pathways are interconnected and lead to the caspase-mediated cleavage of cellular proteins and consequently to the gradual degradation of further cellular components and cellular destruction.
Abbreviations: AIF – *apoptosis-inducing factor*, APAF1 – *apoptotic peptidase activating factor 1*, ATP – adenosine-5'-triphosphate, BAD – *BCL2-associated agonist of cell death*, BAX – *BCL2-associated X protein*, BCL2 – *B-cell CLL/lymphoma 2*, BCLXL – *BCL2-like 1*, BID – *BH3 interacting domain death agonist*, CASP – *caspase*, Cyto C – *cytochrome c*, DNA – deoxyribonucleic acid, FADD – *Fas-associated via death domain*, FAS – *Fas (TNF receptor superfamily, member 6)*, FASLG – *Fas ligand*, FLIP – *FLICE-inhibitory protein*, IAP – inhibitors of apoptosis, RIP1 – *receptor interacting protein 1*, SMAC – *second mitochondria-derived activator of caspase*, TNFR – *tumor necrosis factor receptor*, TRADD – *TNFR1-associated death domain protein*, TRAF2 – *TNF receptor-associated factor 2*, TRAIL – *TNF-related apoptosis inducing ligand*.

The export of cytochrome c into the cytoplasm and its binding to APAF1 (*apoptotic peptidase activating factor 1*) together with ATP induces the formation of apoptosomes that can cleave and activate pro-caspase 9. Subsequently, caspase 9 activates the effector caspases 3 and 7, which can be alternatively activated in the extrinsic pathway by the initiator caspases 8 and 10 as mentioned above. This caspase cascade finally commits the cell to apoptosis by gradual degradation of cellular proteins (Mcknight et al., 2005; Mitra & Cote, 2009). BCL2 can block the apoptotic death and thereby trigger tumor recurrence and progression as well as mediate resistance to chemotherapy and radiation (Duggan et al., 2001). Different studies on non-muscle invasive and muscle-invasive BCa showed, that BCL2 was up-regulated in a varying number of the analyzed cases ranging from 41 to 63% (Cooke et al., 2000; Korkolopoulou et al., 2002; Liukkonen et al., 1997; Maluf et al., 2006; Ong et al., 2001). This BCL2 up-regulation correlated only partially with tumor stage and grade, but was frequently indicative for patients with poor prognosis after chemo- and/or radiotherapy (Cooke et al., 2000; Hussain et al., 2003; Ong et al., 2001; Pollack et al., 1997). Expression analyses of BCL2 together with other prognostic markers such as p53 and MDM2 revealed their usefulness as complementary predictors of survival of patients with non-muscle invasive and muscle-invasive BCa (Gonzalez-Campora et al., 2007; Maluf et al., 2006; Ong et al., 2001; Wolf et al., 2001).

Furthermore, the ratio between the anti-apoptotic factor BCL2 and the pro-apoptotic factor BAX seems to act as a cellular rheostat that might be predictive for a cell's response toward life or death after an apoptotic stimulus (Gazzaniga et al., 1996). BAX can be activated by BID that in turn can be induced by the initiator caspase 8. BAX forms a heterodimer with BCL2 and functions as an apoptotic activator by increasing the opening of the mitochondrial *voltage-dependent anion channel* (VDAC), which leads to the loss in membrane potential and the release of cytochrome c. The predominant expression of BCL2 over that of BAX correlated with a worse outcome and shorter time to relapse in low grade and non-muscle invasive BCa (Gazzaniga et al., 1996, 2003).

Apoptotic cell death can also be hampered by members of the IAP (inhibitor of apoptosis proteins) family that are also known as *baculoviral IAP repeat-containing* (BIRC) proteins. With regard to BCa, survivin (BIRC5) is the most interesting IAP since it can serve as diagnostic, prognostic and predictive marker (Margulis et al., 2008). Survivin inhibits apoptosis, promotes cell proliferation and enhances angiogenesis leading to its prominent role for tumor onset and progression in general and in particular for BCa (Margulis et al., 2008). For this tumor entity, high survivin expression at mRNA and protein levels is associated with advanced tumor grade and stage as well as with affection of lymph nodes (Karam et al., 2007a; I.J. Schultz et al., 2003; Shariat et al., 2007a; Swana et al., 1999; Weikert et al., 2005a). Survivin may serve either alone or together with other markers, such as p53, BCL2 and caspase 3, as a significant predictor of disease recurrence, progression and/or mortality after transurethral resection or radical cystectomy (Gonzalez et al., 2008; Karam et al., 2007a; 2007b; Ku et al., 2004; Shariat et al., 2007a). Response to chemo- and radiotherapy could also be estimated by the use of survivin as a predictive marker in BCa patients (Hausladen et al., 2003; Weiss et al., 2009).

For XIAP (*X-linked inhibitor of apoptosis* / BIRC4), which can directly inhibit the action of caspase 3, 7 and 9 and also interfere with the TNFR-associated cell death signaling, an up-regulation and association with an earlier recurrence was described in non-muscle invasive BCa (Dubrez-Daloz et al., 2008; Li et al., 2007).

Another IAP – cIAP2 (BIRC3) – that regulates apoptosis by binding to the TNFR-associated factors TRAF1 and TRAF2, has been shown to provoke chemoresistance when overexpressed in BCa cell lines (Jonsson et al., 2003). In expression analyses of livin (BIRC7) in tissue specimens from non-muscle invasive BCa only its anti-apoptotic isoform α was detected which was significantly associated with BCa relapse (Gazzaniga et al., 2003; Liu et al., 2009).

5. Immortalization of tumor cells – importance of the human telomerase

Activation of the human telomerase represents a very early event during the development of malignant tumors that leads to immortalization and as a consequence to the capability for unlimited division of tumor cells (Hiyama & Hiyama, 2002). Telomeres, the ends of eukaryotic chromosomes, normally get truncated during each cell division until they reach a critical length. This results in a severe impairment of the division capability leading to senescence of the cells (Harley, 1991). This senescence and the consequential cell death can be bypassed through activation of the telomerase ribonucleoprotein complex, since its catalytic subunit TERT (*telomerase reverse transcriptase*) supports the continuous prolongation of telomeres (Blackburn, 2005). Most of the differentiated somatic cells do not possess telomerase activity, whereas germline and stem cells as well as tumor cells frequently are telomerase-positive (Hiyama & Hiyama, 2002; N.W. Kim et al., 1994).

Several studies proved that TERT as well as the *telomerase RNA component* (TERC) represent essential subunits of the telomerase complex, but only TERT is specifically induced in cancer and functions as limiting factor of the enzymatic telomerase activity (Ito et al., 1998; Meyerson et al., 1997). Nevertheless, TERT protects the chromosomal ends also independently from its catalytic activity through its so-called capping function thereby providing tumor cells with further survival benefit (Blackburn, 2005; Blasco, 2002; S.W. Chan & Blackburn, 2002).

For most tumors it remains unclear whether TERT expression originates from telomerase-positive tumor stem cells or from the activation of the gene during tumorigenesis. A number of transcription factors, tumor suppressors, cell cycle inhibitors, hormones, cytokines and oncogenes have been implicated in the control of TERT expression but without providing a clear explanation for the tumor-specific TERT activity so far (Ducrest et al., 2002; Kyo et al., 2008).

Definitely, a tumor-specific activation of the telomerase complex is detectable in the majority of BCa. In contrast to telomerase-negative normal urothelium cells, > 90% of the analyzed BCa tissue specimens displayed a high expression and activity of telomerase (de Kok et al., 2000a; Heine et al., 1998; Hiyama & Hiyama, 2002; Ito et al., 1998; Lin et al., 1996; Muller, 2002). Therefore, the detection of TERT expression or the determination of telomerase activity in tissue or urine samples from patients suspected of having BCa is very useful for tumor detection (Alvarez & Lokeshwar, 2007; Glas et al., 2003; Muller, 2002; Weikert et al., 2005b). Possibly, quantitative determination of the TERT transcript levels in urine or bladder washings can support the prediction of recurrent BCa (Brems-Eskildsen et al., 2010; de Kok et al., 2000b).

6. Alterations in cell growth signaling

Cell growth signaling is transduced from the cell surface to the nucleus by different signaling cascades which can be altered and disturbed in tumor cells at different levels eading to uncontrolled cell growth and proliferation [Fig.4]. In principle, peptide growth factors bind to their corresponding growth factor receptors on the cell surface leading to receptor activation and via several signal transduction events to the activation of downstream factors (RAS and RAF1). Through the subsequent activation of the MAPK pathway several transcription factors, such as MYC (*v-myc myelocytomatosis viral oncogene homolog (avian)*) or ELK1 (*ETS-like transcription factor 1*), are induced, which finally regulate the expression of growth-promoting genes. Transmission of extracellular growth signals can be altered in tumor cells at different levels of these cascades, e.g. by an abnormally increased supply of growth factors or by amplification, mutation or alternative up-regulation of the growth factor receptors leading to their constitutive, excessive and uncontrolled activity (Hanahan & Weinberg, 2000). Mutations or other regulatory alterations affecting downstream targets, such as members of the RAS family, can additionally provide tumor cells with an increased growth potential (Jebar et al., 2005; Knowles, 2008).

FGFR3, one of the four members of the FGFR family, is constitutively activated by different mutations, which are found in approximately 70% of low-grade Ta and to a much lower extent of 10-20% in muscle-invasive BCa (Bakkar et al., 2003; Billerey et al., 2001; Hernandez et al., 2006; Jebar et al., 2005; Junker et al., 2008; Knowles, 2008; Kompier et al., 2010a; Rieger-Christ et al., 2003; Van Oers et al., 2007; Van Rhijn et al., 2004). The most frequent mutations lead to amino acid substitutions to cysteine residues which can build covalent disulfide bonds mimicking dimerization and thereby activation of the receptor (Kompier et al., 2010b). Mutated FGFR3 correlates with favorable disease parameters and improved survival (Kompier et al., 2010b; Van Oers et al., 2007, 2009; Van Rhijn et al., 2001, 2004, 2010). In a recent multicenter study, the so called molecular grade, a combination of the FGFR3 mutation status and the proliferation marker Ki67, could improve the predictive accuracy of the EORTC (European Organisation for Research and Treatment of Cancer) risk scores for progression (Van Rhijn et al., 2010).

Mutated FGFR3 leads to the activation of the RAS-MAPK-pathway and consequently to an augmented transduction of growth signals. RAS mutations are found in BCa with an overall frequency of approximately 10-15% and do not depend on tumor grade or stage, (Jebar et al., 2005; Knowles, 2008; Kompier et al., 2010a; Oxford & Theodorescu, 2003; Serizawa et al., 2011). Such mutations occur in all three RAS genes (HRAS, NRAS and KRAS) whereby HRAS is affected most frequently (Jebar et al., 2005). Interestingly, simultaneous mutations in FGFR3 and RAS, both resulting in the activation of the same pathway, are very uncommon and rather occur mutually exclusive (Jebar et al., 2005). Thus, low grade and Ta tumors harbor mutations either of FGFR3 or HRAS in more than 80% of the cases reflecting the necessity of constitutive activation of the MAPK pathway for non muscle-invasive BCa (Jebar et al., 2005; Knowles, 2008).

Additionally, the up-regulation of FGFs can contribute to the pathogenesis of cancer (Bryan et al., 2005a). Levels of FGF1 (acidic FGF) in urine samples correlated with tumor stage (Chopin et al., 1993). An association with an increased tumor stage and early local recurrence was shown for the expression of FGF2 (basic FGF) (Bryan et al., 2005a; Gazzaniga et al., 1999).

The *epidermal growth factor* (EGF) receptor family comprising EGFR (ERBB1), ERBB2 (HER-2/neu), ERBB3 (HER3) and ERBB4 (HER4) represents another tyrosine kinase receptor family involved in growth signaling in BCa cells that can also transduce extracelluar growth signals via the RAS-MAPK pathway or alternatively via the *phosphatidylinositol 3-kinase* (PIK3)-Akt pathway (Bryan et al., 2005a; Mitra & Cote, 2009). Expression at mRNA and protein level of all members of the EGFR family was observed in BCa specimens but with varying patterns of coexpression and differing prognostic impact possibly depending on the size and composition of the patients cohorts and the detection techniques used in the different studies (Amsellem-Ouazana et al., 2006; Chow et al., 2001; Chow et al., 1997b; Forster et al., 2011; Junttila et al., 2003; Kassouf et al., 2008; Memon et al., 2006; Rotterud et al., 2005). Increased expression of EGFR and ERBB2 has been observed in a number of studies (Black & Dinney, 2008; Mitra & Cote, 2009). Many of these analyses revealed a correlation between increased levels of these two receptors and parameters of high risk tumors or of a poor prognosis for BCa patients (Black & Dinney, 2008; Mitra & Cote, 2009).

Several studies analyzed the BCa-related impact of growth factors activating EGFR, which comprise EGF, TGFα (*transforming growth factor alpha*), HB-EGF (*heparin-binding EGF-like growth factor*), epiregulin and others. Levels of TGFα in tissue samples and urine specimens from BCa patients correlated strongly with poor prognosis (Gazzaniga et al., 1998; Ravery et al., 1997; Thogersen et al., 2001; Turkeri et al., 1998). An association with tumor recurrence was also observed for EGF in BCa tissues, but not for urinary EGF (Chow et al., 1997a; Turkeri et al., 1998). Further studies revealed also an inverse correlation between the expression of epiregulin or nuclear HB-EGF and the survival of BCa patients (Adam et al., 2003; Kramer et al., 2007; Thogersen et al., 2001).

Another growth signaling pathway profoundly altered in many tumor entities including BCa is that of VEGF. This pathway is predominantly involved in the regulation of angiogenesis through the attraction and direction of blood vessels to the tumor by VEGF, which is secreted by tumor cells (Sato et al., 1998). Additionally, an autocrine function of VEGF in direct activation of the tumor cells themselves is assumed due to the observed up-regulation of different VEGF receptors such as FLT1 (VEGFR1) and KDR (VEGFR2 = FLK1) in BCa (Black & Dinney, 2008; Sato et al., 1998; Xia et al., 2006). An increased expression of KDR in BCa patients correlated with higher disease stage, muscle invasion and lymph node metastasis (Mitra et al., 2006; Xia et al., 2006).

PIK3CA (*phosphoinositide-3-kinase catalytic subunit alpha*) is part of the Akt signaling pathway and in this way also involved in the transformation of extracellular growth signals into an increased potential of cell proliferation and survival. PIK3CA mutations with an overall frequency of 13-25% seem to be a common event that occurs early in bladder carcinogenesis (Kompier et al., 2010a; Lopez-Knowles et al., 2006; Platt et al., 2009; Serizawa et al., 2011). A correlation with low stage and grade was observed in several studies (Lopez-Knowles et al., 2006; Serizawa et al., 2011). Interestingly, PIK3CA mutations were shown to be strongly associated with FGFR3 mutations possibly indicating cooperative oncogenic effects (Castillo-Martin et al., 2010; Kompier et al., 2010a; Lopez-Knowles et al., 2006; Serizawa et al., 2011). However, PIK3CA mutations showed no correlation with progression or disease-specific survival (Kompier et al., 2010a).

PTEN (*phosphatase and tensin homolog*), which is a phosphatidylinositol-3,4,5-trisphosphate 3-phosphatase and as such a negative regulator of the PIK3/Akt signaling pathway, acts by this way as a TSG. The PTEN gene located on 10q23.3 is frequently inactivated by chromosomal loss and mutations in a number of malignant tumors including BCa (Aveyard et al., 1999; Cairns et al., 1998; Knowles et al., 2009; Platt et al., 2009; Teng et al., 1997). The rate of LOH events and allelic imbalances in a chromosomal region including the PTEN gene is with 23-32% in muscle-invasive BCa notably higher than in non-muscle invasive BCa (Aveyard et al., 1999; Cappellen et al., 1997; Knowles et al., 2009). Nevertheless, mutations in the retained PTEN allele or homozygous deletions do not occur very frequently indicating the existence of further mechanisms of PTEN inactivation (Aveyard et al., 1999; Cairns et al., 1998; Platt et al., 2009). A reduction in PTEN protein levels in BCa tissue specimens was observed in several studies and correlated with higher grade and/or higher stage (Harris et al., 2008; Platt et al., 2009; Puzio-Kuter et al., 2009; L. Schultz et al., 2010; Sun et al., 2011; Tsuruta et al., 2006). Interestingly, a reduced PTEN expression was related to poor outcome in BCa patients, particularly in those displaying alterations of p53 and PTEN (Puzio-Kuter et al., 2009).

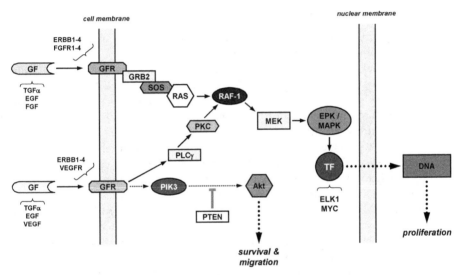

Fig. 4. Simplified illustration of the principles of growth factor signaling
Growth factors bind to their corresponding receptors at the cell surface thereby starting signaling cascades which transduce the signal through cytoplasmatic factors into the nucleus. There, genes supporting survival, proliferation and migration of the tumor cells are induced as final consequence. For BCa, the RAS/RAF/MEK/ERK- and the PIK3/AKT-pathways are of particular importance.
Abbreviations: Akt – *v-akt murine thymoma viral oncogene homolog 1*, DNA – deoxyribonucleic acid, EGF – *epidermal growth factor*, ELK – *member of ETS oncogene family*, ERBB – EGF receptor family member, ERK = MAPK1 – *mitogen-activated protein kinase 1*, FGF – *fibroblast growth factor*, FGFR – FGF receptor family member, GF – growth factor, GFR – growth factor receptor, GRB2 – *growth factor receptor-bound protein 2*, MEK – *mitogen-activated protein kinase kinase*, MYC – *v-myc myelocytomatosis viral oncogene homolog*, PIK3 – *phosphoinositide-3-kinase*, PKC – *protein kinase C*, PLCγ – *phospholipase C gamma*,
PTEN – *phosphatase and tensin homolog*, RAF-1 – *v-raf-1 murine leukemia viral oncogene homolog 1*, RAS – *rat sarcoma viral oncogene homolog*, SOS – *son of sevenless homolog*,
TF – transcription factor, VEGF – *vascular endothelial growth factor*, VEGFR – VEGF receptor family member.

The activation of the PIK3 pathway leads to transmission of extracellular growth signals via the phosphorylation of the serine-threonine protein kinase Akt (*v-akt murine thymoma viral oncogene homolog 1*) to the activation of several downstream signaling routes resulting in an increased proliferation, survival or migration of tumor cells (Wu et al., 2004). Elevated levels of phosphorylated Akt (pAkt) compared to normal bladder tissue were observed in different immunohistochemical studies on BCa tissue specimens (L. Schultz et al., 2010; Wu et al., 2004). Increased detection rates of pAkt correlated significantly with high-grade and advanced stage BCa as well as with a poor clinical outcome and survival (Sun et al., 2011). Furthermore, Askham *et al.* reported the detection of a transforming Akt mutation (G49A / E17K) in 2.7% of 184 analyzed BCa samples (Askham et al., 2010).

7. Tumor angiogenesis and metastasis

Angiogenesis comprises the recruitment and accelerated formation of new blood vessels from the surrounding vasculature. After proteolytic degradation of the adjacent ECM activated endothelial cells become able to migrate and invade as well as to maturate to coalescent, water-tight blood tubules (S.G. Williams & Stein, 2004). This essential physiologic process that occurs during development, reproduction and repair is tightly controlled by stimulatory and inhibitory regulators. During tumor genesis and progression this balance is disturbed by the up-regulation of angiogenic inducers and/or loss of anti-angiogenic factors which can be secreted by the tumor cells themselves, by neighboring tumor-associated stromal cells or by tumor-infiltrating inflammatory cells (S.G. Williams & Stein, 2004). Newly formed blood vessels provide the tumor cells with oxygen and nutrients, which is an essential prerequisite for rapid tumor growth and also for tumor cell spread during metastasis (Mitra & Cote, 2009). A high microvessel density (MVD) in the tumor as reflector of angiogenic processes is a strong predictor of a poor outcome of BCa patients (Bochner et al., 1995; Canoglu et al., 2004; Chaudhary et al., 1999; Dickinson et al., 1994; Hawke et al., 1998; Jaeger et al., 1995; Philp et al., 1996).

Hypoxia, which is frequently occurring in growing tumors, results in elevated levels of the hypoxia-inducible transcription factors HIF-1 and HIF-2. Stability of the HIF-1 subunit α is regulated by the cellular oxygen concentration via the inhibition of its oxygen-dependent degradation. HIF-1α (HIF1A) can induce transcription of VEGF which in turn stimulates tumor vascularization (Mitra & Cote, 2009). In BCa specimens, a significant positive correlation between HIF-1α, VEGF and MVD was observed (Chai et al., 2008; Theodoropoulos et al., 2004). Similar to MVD and VEGF, HIF-1α can serve as indicator of a high recurrence rate and short survival of patients with non-muscle invasive and muscle-invasive BCa (Chai et al., 2008; Palit et al., 2005; Theodoropoulos et al., 2004). Focused on non-muscle invasive BCa, HIF-1α overexpression combined with aberrant nuclear p53 accumulation seemed to indicate an aggressive phenotype with a high risk of progression (Theodoropoulos et al., 2005).

High mRNA expression of VEGF in non-muscle invasive BCa correlated with high recurrence and progression rates, particularly in combination with aberrant p53 staining (Crew et al., 1997). Elevated VEGF protein levels in urine samples from patients with non-muscle invasive BCa showed a significant association with tumor recurrence (Crew et al., 1999b).

Elevated VEGF serum levels were observed in BCa patients with high tumor grade and stage, with vascular invasion, CIS tumors or distant metastases and correlated with a shorter disease-free survival (Bernardini et al., 2001). Furthermore, VEGF expression and MVD in biopsy specimens taken prior to therapy were significant predictors of recurrence of muscle-invasive BCa after neoadjuvant chemotherapy and radical cystectomy (Inoue et al., 2000). Increased VEGF levels in tissue samples from patients with locally advanced BCa treated by radical cystectomy and chemotherapy (MVAC) were strongly related to poor disease-specific survival (Slaton et al., 2004).

Thrombospondin-1 (TSP-1) is an ECM component glycoprotein that functions as potent inhibitor of angiogenesis. Expression analyses of this putative tumor suppressor in tissue specimens from patients with muscle-invasive BCa who underwent radical cystectomy revealed a significant association between low TSP-1 levels and increased recurrence rates as well as with a decreased overall survival (Grossfeld et al., 1997). In non-muscle invasive BCa a reduced perivascular TSP-1 staining served as independent predictor of progression to muscle-invasive or metastatic disease (Goddard et al., 2002). Furthermore, expression of *angiopoietin 2* (ANG-2), an angiogenic modulator that potentiates angiogenesis in presence of VEGF, was identified as a strong and independent predictor of tumor recurrence of non-muscle invasive BCa (Szarvas et al., 2008).

The scaffolding ECM serves to maintain endothelial cell function and its degradation is mediated amongst others by MMPs. Additionally, MMPs activate the basic and acidic FGF (FGF1 and FGF2) as well as the *scatter factor* (SF; identical to HGF = *hepatocyte growth factor*) – all regulators which promote migration and invasion of endothelial cells as well as of tumor cells thereby supporting angiogenesis and metastasis (Mitra & Cote, 2009). These factors are also stimulated by plasmin that is proteolytically generated by the *urokinase-type plasminogen activator* (uPA = PLAU = *plasminogen activator, urokinase*). uPA, which can be induced by VEGF, as well as its receptor uPAR (PLAUR= *plasminogen activator, urokinase receptor*) are also involved in ECM degradation, adhesion and migration of tumor cells (Mitra & Cote, 2009). Determination of the FGF1 and FGF2 levels in urine samples of patients with BCa revealed their prognostic value as indicators of increased disease stage and high rates of local recurrence (Chopin et al., 1993; Gazzaniga et al., 1999; Gravas et al., 2004; Nguyen et al., 1993). SF/HGF levels in urine and serum samples were elevated in BCa patients and related particularly to higher tumor stages as well as to metastasis and worse survival (Gohji et al., 2000; Joseph et al., 1995; Rosen et al., 1997; Wang et al., 2007). The receptor of SF/HFG, the *met proto-oncogene* (MET), was also detected in BCa tissue specimens. Its up-regulation correlated with disease progression and poor long-term survival (Cheng et al., 2002, 2005; Joseph et al., 1995; Miyata et al., 2009).

A significant association between the expression of uPA and uPAR was observed in BCa tissues; both factors were higher in muscle-invasive than in non-muscle invasive BCa and correlated with a worse outcome (Champelovier et al., 2002; Hasui et al., 1994; Seddighzadeh et al., 2002). Elevated levels of uPA and uPAR were also detected in urine and plasma samples from BCa patients compared to controls without BCa (Casella et al., 2002; Shariat et al., 2003). Furthermore, increased preoperative uPA plasma levels in BCa patients were shown to be indicators of a poor outcome after radical cystectomy (Shariat et al., 2003).

Metastasis is initiated by the ability of the tumor to degrade the ECM and to invade the basement membrane followed by the invasion of tumor cells into blood and lymphatic vessels, the path for tumor cell to spread into regional lymph nodes and secondary organs (Gontero et al., 2004; Mitra & Cote, 2009). Several key mediators are involved in metastatic spread such as cadherins which are located at adherens junctions and desmosomes between neighboring cells. Particularly, E-cadherin plays an important role in epithelial cell-cell contacts which is mediated by homodimerization and anchoring to the actin cytoskeleton via binding to catenins (Bryan et al., 2005b). In BCa patients, a reduced expression of E-cadherin was associated with an increased aggressiveness and a higher risk of tumor recurrence and progression as well as with a shorter survival (Bringuier et al., 1993; Byrne et al., 2001; Mahnken et al., 2005; Mhawech-Fauceglia et al., 2006; Nakopoulou et al., 2000; Popov et al., 2000). Immunohistochemical analyses of E-cadherin, α- and β-catenin revealed that loss of these factors can indicate a poor survival of BCa patients (Clairotte et al., 2006; Garcia Del Muro et al., 2000; Kashibuchi et al., 2007; Mialhe et al., 1997; Shimazui et al., 1996).

In addition, integrins are involved in the regulation of processes linked to tumor cell invasion and migration consequently leading to metastasis. Integrins are heterodimeric transmembrane glycoproteins on the surface of tumor cells that function as receptors of ECM proteins such as laminin and collagen. Thereby, integrins serve as molecular links between the ECM and the intracellular actin cytoskeleton and are in this way involved in the maintenance of normal tissue architecture (Gontero et al., 2004). Among the numerous members of the integrin family $\alpha6\beta4$ integrin, which closely interacts with collagen VII and laminin thereby restricting cell migration, is one of the best studied integrins in BCa patients (Gontero et al., 2004). Altered expression of $\alpha6\beta4$ integrin was observed in superficial BCa; in muscle-invasive BCa loss of $\alpha6\beta4$ integrin and/or collagen VII or lack of their co-localization was reported (Liebert et al., 1994). BCa patients with weak $\alpha6\beta4$ integrin immunoreactivity showed a better outcome than those with either no or strong expression (Grossman et al., 2000).

MMPs and members of the uPA system are proteases involved not only in invasion processes of endothelial cells, they are also key factors triggering the invasion of tumor cells by degradation of ECM and the basement membrane (Gontero et al., 2004). MMPs are frequently overexpressed and secreted in human tumors (Bryan et al., 2005b; Wallard et al., 2006). Additionally, members of the ADAM (*a disintegrin and metalloproteinase domain*) family have been implicated in cancer progression (Frohlich et al., 2006). An imbalance between MMPs and their natural counterparts, the *tissue inhibitors of metalloproteases* (TIMPs), which is frequently observed in tumors, is also assumed to support tumor cell invasion and metastasis (Gontero et al., 2004). TIMPs might be paradoxically up-regulated in response to the elevation of MMPs levels (Gontero et al., 2004).

For BCa, MMP-2 and MMP-9 are of particular prognostic importance since increase in their tissue levels correlated with higher tumor grade and/or stage (Davies et al., 1993; Kanayama et al., 1998; Papathoma et al., 2000). Overexpression of MMP-2 and MMP-9 in BCa tissues was associated with disease progression and poor survival (Durkan et al., 2003; Vasala et al., 2003). The ratio of the MMP-9 to E-cadherin levels in BCa tissue specimens was also useful for prediction of the disease-specific survival of patients with locally advanced BCa (Slaton et al., 2004).

Additionally, poor outcome was reported for BCa patients with high levels of TIMP-2 in tumor and/or stromal cells and for patients with increased tissue expression of MMP-2 and TIMP-2 or MMP-9 and TIMP-2 (Gakiopoulou et al., 2003; Grignon et al., 1996; Hara et al., 2001; Kanayama et al., 1998).

Higher recurrence rates and poor prognosis were observed in BCa patients with high serum levels of MMP-2, MMP-3 or with high ratios of the serum levels of MMP-2 to TIMP-2 (Gohji et al., 1996a, 1996b, 1998). MMP-1, MMP-2, MMP-9 and TIMP-1 were also detectable in urine samples from BCa patients and correlated with increasing grade and/or stage (Durkan et al., 2003; Durkan et al., 2001; Gerhards et al., 2001; Nutt et al., 1998, 2003; Sier et al., 2000). Urinary MMP-1 was associated with higher rates of disease progression and death from cancer (Durkan et al., 2001).

ADAM12, a disintegrin and metalloproteinase, that was shown to be up-regulated in BCa tissues in association with disease stage, could also be detected in urine samples, where it might serve as biomarker reflecting presence of BCa (Frohlich et al., 2006).

8. Conclusion

On the basis of specific genetic and molecular patterns two clearly distinguishable types of BCa can be defined, which differ in their phenotype and clinical behavior. They mainly diverge in the genetic stability and in the presence of alterations in the genes p53 and FGFR3. The knowledge of BCa-related genetic and molecular processes provides the basis for the development of new diagnostic and therapeutic approaches. Molecular-diagnostic assays can be designed for BCa subtypes, e.g. for low grade and low stage tumors, which are poorly detectable by the currently used techniques. Furthermore, new BCa subtype-selective therapeutics will provide more specific and effective treatment options leading to the reduction of tumor recurrence and progression. After successful implementation, both aspects will improve clinical outcome of BCa patients and save costs for diagnosis and therapy for this tumor type, which are huge compared to other tumor entities.

9. References

Aboulkassim, T.O.; LaRue, H.; Lemieux, P.; Rousseau, F. & Fradet, Y. (2003). Alteration of the PATCHED locus in superficial bladder cancer. *Oncogene*, Vol.22, No.19, pp. 2967-2971

Adam, R.M.; Danciu, T.; McLellan, D.L.; Borer, J.G.; Lin, J.; Zurakowski, D.; Weinstein, M.H.; Rajjayabun, P.H.; Mellon, J.K. & Freeman, M.R. (2003). A nuclear form of the heparin-binding epidermal growth factor-like growth factor precursor is a feature of aggressive transitional cell carcinoma. *Cancer Res*, Vol.63, No.2, pp. 484-490

Alvarez, A. & Lokeshwar, V.B. (2007). Bladder cancer biomarkers: current developments and future implementation. *Curr Opin Urol*, Vol.17, No.5, pp. 341-346

Amsellem-Ouazana, D.; Bieche, I.; Tozlu, S.; Botto, H.; Debre, B. & Lidereau, R. (2006). Gene expression profiling of ERBB receptors and ligands in human transitional cell carcinoma of the bladder. *J Urol*, Vol.175, No.3 Pt 1, pp. 1127-1132

Askham, J.M.; Platt, F.; Chambers, P.A.; Snowden, H.; Taylor, C.F. & Knowles, M.A. (2010). AKT1 mutations in bladder cancer: identification of a novel oncogenic mutation that can co-operate with E17K. *Oncogene*, Vol.29, No.1, pp. 150-155

Aveyard, J.S.; Skilleter, A.; Habuchi, T. & Knowles, M.A. (1999). Somatic mutation of PTEN in bladder carcinoma. *Br J Cancer*, Vol.80, No.5-6, pp. 904-908

Babjuk, M.; Oosterlinck, W.; Sylvester, R.; Kaasinen, E.; Bohle, A.; Palou-Redorta, J. & Roupret, M. (2011). EAU guidelines on non-muscle-invasive urothelial carcinoma of the bladder, the 2011 update. *Eur Urol*, Vol.59, No.6, pp. 997-1008

Bakkar, A.A.; Wallerand, H.; Radvanyi, F.; Lahaye, J.B.; Pissard, S.; Lecerf, L.; Kouyoumdjian, J.C.; Abbou, C.C.; Pairon, J.C.; Jaurand, M.C.; Thiery, J.P.; Chopin, D.K. & de Medina, S.G. (2003). FGFR3 and TP53 gene mutations define two distinct pathways in urothelial cell carcinoma of the bladder. *Cancer Res*, Vol.63, No.23, pp. 8108-8112

Bellmunt, J.; Paz-Ares, L.; Cuello, M.; Cecere, F.L.; Albiol, S.; Guillem, V.; Gallardo, E.; Carles, J.; Mendez, P.; de la Cruz, J.J.; Taron, M.; Rosell, R. & Baselga, J. (2007). Gene expression of ERCC1 as a novel prognostic marker in advanced bladder cancer patients receiving cisplatin-based chemotherapy. *Ann Oncol*, Vol.18, No.3, pp. 522-528

Berggren, P.; Kumar, R.; Sakano, S.; Hemminki, L.; Wada, T.; Steineck, G.; Adolfsson, J.; Larsson, P.; Norming, U.; Wijkstrom, H. & Hemminki, K. (2003). Detecting homozygous deletions in the CDKN2A(p16(INK4a))/ARF(p14(ARF)) gene in urinary bladder cancer using real-time quantitative PCR. *Clin Cancer Res*, Vol.9, No.1, pp. 235-242

Bernardini, S.; Fauconnet, S.; Chabannes, E.; Henry, P.C.; Adessi, G. & Bittard, H. (2001). Serum levels of vascular endothelial growth factor as a prognostic factor in bladder cancer. *J Urol*, Vol.166, No.4, pp. 1275-1279

Billerey, C.; Chopin, D.; Aubriot-Lorton, M.H.; Ricol, D.; Gil Diez de Medina, S.; Van Rhijn, B.; Bralet, M.P.; Lefrere-Belda, M.A.; Lahaye, J.B.; Abbou, C.C.; Bonaventure, J.; Zafrani, E.S.; van der Kwast, T.; Thiery, J.P. & Radvanyi, F. (2001). Frequent FGFR3 mutations in papillary non-invasive bladder (pTa) tumors. *Am J Pathol*, Vol.158, No.6, pp. 1955-1959

Black, P.C. & Dinney, C.P. (2008). Growth factors and receptors as prognostic markers in urothelial carcinoma. *Curr Urol Rep*, Vol.9, No.1, pp. 55-61

Blackburn, E.H. (2005). Telomeres and telomerase: their mechanisms of action and the effects of altering their functions. *FEBS Lett*, Vol.579, No.4, pp. 859-862

Blasco, M.A. (2002). Telomerase beyond telomeres. *Nat Rev Cancer*, Vol.2, No.8, pp. 627-633

Blaveri, E.; Brewer, J.L.; Roydasgupta, R.; Fridlyand, J.; DeVries, S.; Koppie, T.; Pejavar, S.; Mehta, K.; Carroll, P.; Simko, J.P. & Waldman, F.M. (2005). Bladder cancer stage and outcome by array-based comparative genomic hybridization. *Clin Cancer Res*, Vol.11, No.19 Pt 1, pp. 7012-7022

Bochner, B.H.; Cote, R.J.; Weidner, N.; Groshen, S.; Chen, S.C.; Skinner, D.G. & Nichols, P.W. (1995). Angiogenesis in bladder cancer: relationship between microvessel density and tumor prognosis. *J Natl Cancer Inst*, Vol.87, No.21, pp. 1603-1612

Bosetti, C.; Boffetta, P. & La Vecchia, C. (2007). Occupational exposures to polycyclic aromatic hydrocarbons, and respiratory and urinary tract cancers: a quantitative review to 2005. *Ann Oncol*, Vol.18, No.3, pp. 431-446

Brems-Eskildsen, A.S.; Zieger, K.; Toldbod, H.; Holcomb, C.; Higuchi, R.; Mansilla, F.; Munksgaard, P.P.; Borre, M.; Orntoft, T.F. & Dyrskjot, L. (2010). Prediction and diagnosis of bladder cancer recurrence based on urinary content of hTERT, SENP1, PPP1CA, and MCM5 transcripts. *BMC Cancer*, Vol.10, pp. 646

Bringuier, P.P.; Umbas, R.; Schaafsma, H.E.; Karthaus, H.F.; Debruyne, F.M. & Schalken, J.A. (1993). Decreased E-cadherin immunoreactivity correlates with poor survival in patients with bladder tumors. *Cancer Res*, Vol.53, No.14, pp. 3241-3245

Brunner, A.; Verdorfer, I.; Prelog, M.; Mayerl, C.; Mikuz, G. & Tzankov, A. (2008). Large-scale analysis of cell cycle regulators in urothelial bladder cancer identifies p16 and p27 as potentially useful prognostic markers. *Pathobiology*, Vol.75, No.1, pp. 25-33

Bryan, R.T.; Hussain, S.A.; James, N.D.; Jankowski, J.A. & Wallace, D.M. (2005a). Molecular pathways in bladder cancer: part 1. *BJU Int*, Vol.95, No.4, pp. 485-490

Bryan, R.T.; Hussain, S.A.; James, N.D.; Jankowski, J.A. & Wallace, D.M. (2005b). Molecular pathways in bladder cancer: part 2. *BJU Int*, Vol.95, No.4, pp. 491-496

Byrne, R.R.; Shariat, S.F.; Brown, R.; Kattan, M.W.; Morton, R.J.; Wheeler, T.M. & Lerner, S.P. (2001). E-cadherin immunostaining of bladder transitional cell carcinoma, carcinoma in situ and lymph node metastases with long-term followup. *J Urol*, Vol.165, No.5, pp. 1473-1479

Cairns, P.; Proctor, A.J. & Knowles, M.A. (1991). Loss of heterozygosity at the RB locus is frequent and correlates with muscle invasion in bladder carcinoma. *Oncogene*, Vol.6, No.12, pp. 2305-2309

Cairns, P.; Polascik, T.J.; Eby, Y.; Tokino, K.; Califano, J.; Merlo, A.; Mao, L.; Herath, J.; Jenkins, R.; Westra, W. & et al. (1995). Frequency of homozygous deletion at p16/CDKN2 in primary human tumours. *Nat Genet*, Vol.11, No.2, pp. 210-212

Cairns, P.; Evron, E.; Okami, K.; Halachmi, N.; Esteller, M.; Herman, J.G.; Bose, S.; Wang, S.I.; Parsons, R. & Sidransky, D. (1998). Point mutation and homozygous deletion of PTEN/MMAC1 in primary bladder cancers. *Oncogene*, Vol.16, No.24, pp. 3215-3218

Canoglu, A.; Gogus, C.; Beduk, Y.; Orhan, D.; Tulunay, O. & Baltaci, S. (2004). Microvessel density as a prognostic marker in bladder carcinoma: correlation with tumor grade, stage and prognosis. *Int Urol Nephrol*, Vol.36, No.3, pp. 401-405

Cappellen, D.; Gil Diez de Medina, S.; Chopin, D.; Thiery, J.P. & Radvanyi, F. (1997). Frequent loss of heterozygosity on chromosome 10q in muscle-invasive transitional cell carcinomas of the bladder. *Oncogene*, Vol.14, No.25, pp. 3059-3066

Casella, R.; Shariat, S.F.; Monoski, M.A. & Lerner, S.P. (2002). Urinary levels of urokinase-type plasminogen activator and its receptor in the detection of bladder carcinoma. *Cancer*, Vol.95, No.12, pp. 2494-2499

Castillo-Martin, M.; Domingo-Domenech, J.; Karni-Schmidt, O.; Matos, T. & Cordon-Cardo, C. (2010). Molecular pathways of urothelial development and bladder tumorigenesis. *Urol Oncol*, Vol.28, No.4, pp. 401-408

Chai, C.Y.; Chen, W.T.; Hung, W.C.; Kang, W.Y.; Huang, Y.C.; Su, Y.C. & Yang, C.H. (2008). Hypoxia-inducible factor-1alpha expression correlates with focal macrophage infiltration, angiogenesis and unfavourable prognosis in urothelial carcinoma. *J Clin Pathol*, Vol.61, No.5, pp. 658-664

Champelovier, P.; Boucard, N.; Levacher, G.; Simon, A.; Seigneurin, D. & Praloran, V. (2002). Plasminogen- and colony-stimulating factor-1-associated markers in bladder carcinoma: diagnostic value of urokinase plasminogen activator receptor and plasminogen activator inhibitor type-2 using immunocytochemical analysis. *Urol Res*, Vol.30, No.5, pp. 301-309

Chan, M.W.; Chan, L.W.; Tang, N.L.; Tong, J.H.; Lo, K.W.; Lee, T.L.; Cheung, H.Y.; Wong, W.S.; Chan, P.S.; Lai, F.M. & To, K.F. (2002). Hypermethylation of multiple genes in tumor tissues and voided urine in urinary bladder cancer patients. *Clin Cancer Res*, Vol.8, No.2, pp. 464-470

Chan, S.W. & Blackburn, E.H. (2002). New ways not to make ends meet: telomerase, DNA damage proteins and heterochromatin. *Oncogene*, Vol.21, No.4, pp. 553-563

Chang, L.L.; Yeh, W.T.; Yang, S.Y.; Wu, W.J. & Huang, C.H. (2003). Genetic alterations of p16INK4a and p14ARF genes in human bladder cancer. *J Urol*, Vol.170, No.2 Pt 1, pp. 595-600

Chapman, E.J.; Harnden, P.; Chambers, P.; Johnston, C. & Knowles, M.A. (2005). Comprehensive analysis of CDKN2A status in microdissected urothelial cell carcinoma reveals potential haploinsufficiency, a high frequency of homozygous co-deletion and associations with clinical phenotype. *Clin Cancer Res*, Vol.11, No.16, pp. 5740-5747

Chaudhary, R.; Bromley, M.; Clarke, N.W.; Betts, C.D.; Barnard, R.J.; Ryder, W.D. & Kumar, S. (1999). Prognostic relevance of micro-vessel density in cancer of the urinary bladder. *Anticancer Res*, Vol.19, No.4C, pp. 3479-3484

Chellappan, S.P.; Hiebert, S.; Mudryj, M.; Horowitz, J.M. & Nevins, J.R. (1991). The E2F transcription factor is a cellular target for the RB protein. *Cell*, Vol.65, No.6, pp. 1053-1061

Cheng, H.L.; Trink, B.; Tzai, T.S.; Liu, H.S.; Chan, S.H.; Ho, C.L.; Sidransky, D. & Chow, N.H. (2002). Overexpression of c-met as a prognostic indicator for transitional cell carcinoma of the urinary bladder: a comparison with p53 nuclear accumulation. *J Clin Oncol*, Vol.20, No.6, pp. 1544-1550

Cheng, H.L.; Liu, H.S.; Lin, Y.J.; Chen, H.H.; Hsu, P.Y.; Chang, T.Y.; Ho, C.L.; Tzai, T.S. & Chow, N.H. (2005). Co-expression of RON and MET is a prognostic indicator for patients with transitional-cell carcinoma of the bladder. *Br J Cancer*, Vol.92, No.10, pp. 1906-1914

Chopin, D.K.; Caruelle, J.P.; Colombel, M.; Palcy, S.; Ravery, V.; Caruelle, D.; Abbou, C.C. & Barritault, D. (1993). Increased immunodetection of acidic fibroblast growth factor in bladder cancer, detectable in urine. *J Urol*, Vol.150, No.4, pp. 1126-1130

Chow, N.H.; Liu, H.S.; Lee, E.I.; Chang, C.J.; Chan, S.H.; Cheng, H.L.; Tzai, T.S. & Lin, J.S. (1997a). Significance of urinary epidermal growth factor and its receptor expression in human bladder cancer. *Anticancer Res*, Vol.17, No.2B, pp. 1293-1296

Chow, N.H.; Liu, H.S.; Yang, H.B.; Chan, S.H. & Su, I.J. (1997b). Expression patterns of erbB receptor family in normal urothelium and transitional cell carcinoma. An immunohistochemical study. *Virchows Arch*, Vol.430, No.6, pp. 461-466

Chow, N.H.; Chan, S.H.; Tzai, T.S.; Ho, C.L. & Liu, H.S. (2001). Expression profiles of ErbB family receptors and prognosis in primary transitional cell carcinoma of the urinary bladder. *Clin Cancer Res*, Vol.7, No.7, pp. 1957-1962

Clairotte, A.; Lascombe, I.; Fauconnet, S.; Mauny, F.; Felix, S.; Algros, M.P.; Bittard, H. & Kantelip, B. (2006). Expression of E-cadherin and alpha-, beta-, gamma-catenins in patients with bladder cancer: identification of gamma-catenin as a new prognostic marker of neoplastic progression in T1 superficial urothelial tumors. *Am J Clin Pathol*, Vol.125, No.1, pp. 119-126

Coats, S.; Flanagan, W.M.; Nourse, J. & Roberts, J.M. (1996). Requirement of p27Kip1 for restriction point control of the fibroblast cell cycle. *Science*, Vol.272, No.5263, pp. 877-880

Cooke, P.W.; James, N.D.; Ganesan, R.; Burton, A.; Young, L.S. & Wallace, D.M. (2000). Bcl-2 expression identifies patients with advanced bladder cancer treated by radiotherapy who benefit from neoadjuvant chemotherapy. *BJU Int*, Vol.85, No.7, pp. 829-835

Cordon-Cardo, C.; Wartinger, D.; Petrylak, D.; Dalbagni, G.; Fair, W.R.; Fuks, Z. & Reuter, V.E. (1992). Altered expression of the retinoblastoma gene product: prognostic indicator in bladder cancer. *J Natl Cancer Inst*, Vol.84, No.16, pp. 1251-1256

Cordon-Cardo, C.; Dalbagni, G.; Saez, G.T.; Oliva, M.R.; Zhang, Z.F.; Rosai, J.; Reuter, V.E. & Pellicer, A. (1994). p53 mutations in human bladder cancer: genotypic versus phenotypic patterns. *Int J Cancer*, Vol.56, No.3, pp. 347-353

Cordon-Cardo, C.; Zhang, Z.F.; Dalbagni, G.; Drobnjak, M.; Charytonowicz, E.; Hu, S.X.; Xu, H.J.; Reuter, V.E. & Benedict, W.F. (1997). Cooperative effects of p53 and pRB alterations in primary superficial bladder tumors. *Cancer Res*, Vol.57, No.7, pp. 1217-1221

Cote, R.J.; Esrig, D.; Groshen, S.; Jones, P.A. & Skinner, D.G. (1997). p53 and treatment of bladder cancer. *Nature*, Vol.385, No.6612, pp. 123-125

Cote, R.J.; Dunn, M.D.; Chatterjee, S.J.; Stein, J.P.; Shi, S.R.; Tran, Q.C.; Hu, S.X.; Xu, H.J.; Groshen, S.; Taylor, C.R.; Skinner, D.G. & Benedict, W.F. (1998). Elevated and absent pRb expression is associated with bladder cancer progression and has cooperative effects with p53. *Cancer Res*, Vol.58, No.6, pp. 1090-1094

Crew, J.P.; O'Brien, T.; Bradburn, M.; Fuggle, S.; Bicknell, R.; Cranston, D. & Harris, A.L. (1997). Vascular endothelial growth factor is a predictor of relapse and stage progression in superficial bladder cancer. *Cancer Res*, Vol.57, No.23, pp. 5281-5285

Crew, J.P. (1999a). Vascular endothelial growth factor: an important angiogenic mediator in bladder cancer. *Eur Urol*, Vol.35, No.1, pp. 2-8

Crew, J.P.; O'Brien, T.; Bicknell, R.; Fuggle, S.; Cranston, D. & Harris, A.L. (1999b). Urinary vascular endothelial growth factor and its correlation with bladder cancer recurrence rates. *J Urol*, Vol.161, No.3, pp. 799-804

Dalbagni, G.; Presti, J.C., Jr.; Reuter, V.E.; Zhang, Z.F.; Sarkis, A.S.; Fair, W.R. & Cordon-Cardo, C. (1993). Molecular genetic alterations of chromosome 17 and p53 nuclear overexpression in human bladder cancer. *Diagn Mol Pathol*, Vol.2, No.1, pp. 4-13

Davies, B.; Waxman, J.; Wasan, H.; Abel, P.; Williams, G.; Krausz, T.; Neal, D.; Thomas, D.; Hanby, A. & Balkwill, F. (1993). Levels of matrix metalloproteases in bladder cancer correlate with tumor grade and invasion. *Cancer Res*, Vol.53, No.22, pp. 5365-5369

de Kok, J.B.; Schalken, J.A.; Aalders, T.W.; Ruers, T.J.; Willems, H.L. & Swinkels, D.W. (2000a). Quantitative measurement of telomerase reverse transcriptase (hTERT) mRNA in urothelial cell carcinomas. *Int J Cancer*, Vol.87, No.2, pp. 217-220

de Kok, J.B.; van Balken, M.R.; Roelofs, R.W.; van Aarssen, Y.A.; Swinkels, D.W. & Klein Gunnewiek, J.M. (2000b). Quantification of hTERT mRNA and telomerase activity in bladder washings of patients with recurrent urothelial cell carcinomas. *Clin Chem*, Vol.46, No.12, pp. 2003-2007

DeGregori, J.; Kowalik, T. & Nevins, J.R. (1995). Cellular targets for activation by the E2F1 transcription factor include DNA synthesis- and G1/S-regulatory genes. *Mol Cell Biol*, Vol.15, No.8, pp. 4215-4224

Dickinson, A.J.; Fox, S.B.; Persad, R.A.; Hollyer, J.; Sibley, G.N. & Harris, A.L. (1994). Quantification of angiogenesis as an independent predictor of prognosis in invasive bladder carcinomas. *Br J Urol*, Vol.74, No.6, pp. 762-766

Doganay, L.; Altaner, S.; Bilgi, S.; Kaya, E.; Ekuklu, G. & Kutlu, K. (2003). Expression of the cyclin-dependent kinase inhibitor p27 in transitional cell bladder cancers: is it a good predictor for tumor behavior? *Int Urol Nephrol*, Vol.35, No.2, pp. 181-188

Dominguez, G.; Silva, J.; Garcia, J.M.; Silva, J.M.; Rodriguez, R.; Munoz, C.; Chacon, I.; Sanchez, R.; Carballido, J.; Colas, A.; Espana, P. & Bonilla, F. (2003). Prevalence of aberrant methylation of p14ARF over p16INK4a in some human primary tumors. *Mutat Res*, Vol.530, No.1-2, pp. 9-17

Dong, L.M.; Potter, J.D.; White, E.; Ulrich, C.M.; Cardon, L.R. & Peters, U. (2008). Genetic susceptibility to cancer: the role of polymorphisms in candidate genes. *Jama*, Vol.299, No.20, pp. 2423-2436

Dubrez-Daloz, L.; Dupoux, A. & Cartier, J. (2008). IAPs: more than just inhibitors of apoptosis proteins. *Cell Cycle*, Vol.7, No.8, pp. 1036-1046

Ducrest, A.L.; Szutorisz, H.; Lingner, J. & Nabholz, M. (2002). Regulation of the human telomerase reverse transcriptase gene. *Oncogene*, Vol.21, No.4, pp. 541-552

Duggan, B.J.; Kelly, J.D.; Keane, P.F. & Johnston, S.R. (2001). Molecular targets for the therapeutic manipulation of apoptosis in bladder cancer. *J Urol*, Vol.165, No.3, pp. 946-954

Durkan, G.C.; Nutt, J.E.; Rajjayabun, P.H.; Neal, D.E.; Lunec, J. & Mellon, J.K. (2001). Prognostic significance of matrix metalloproteinase-1 and tissue inhibitor of metalloproteinase-1 in voided urine samples from patients with transitional cell carcinoma of the bladder. *Clin Cancer Res*, Vol.7, No.11, pp. 3450-3456

Durkan, G.C.; Nutt, J.E.; Marsh, C.; Rajjayabun, P.H.; Robinson, M.C.; Neal, D.E.; Lunec, J. & Mellon, J.K. (2003). Alteration in urinary matrix metalloproteinase-9 to tissue inhibitor of metalloproteinase-1 ratio predicts recurrence in nonmuscle-invasive bladder cancer. *Clin Cancer Res*, Vol.9, No.7, pp. 2576-2582

el-Deiry, W.S.; Tokino, T.; Velculescu, V.E.; Levy, D.B.; Parsons, R.; Trent, J.M.; Lin, D.; Mercer, W.E.; Kinzler, K.W. & Vogelstein, B. (1993). WAF1, a potential mediator of p53 tumor suppression. *Cell*, Vol.75, No.4, pp. 817-825

Emiliozzi, P.; Pansadoro, A. & Pansadoro, V. (2008). The optimal management of T1G3 bladder cancer. *BJU Int*, Vol.102, No.9 Pt B, pp. 1265-1273

Esrig, D.; Spruck, C.H., 3rd; Nichols, P.W.; Chaiwun, B.; Steven, K.; Groshen, S.; Chen, S.C.; Skinner, D.G.; Jones, P.A. & Cote, R.J. (1993). p53 nuclear protein accumulation correlates with mutations in the p53 gene, tumor grade, and stage in bladder cancer. *Am J Pathol*, Vol.143, No.5, pp. 1389-1397

Feber, A.; Clark, J.; Goodwin, G.; Dodson, A.R.; Smith, P.H.; Fletcher, A.; Edwards, S.; Flohr, P.; Falconer, A.; Roe, T.; Kovacs, G.; Dennis, N.; Fisher, C.; Wooster, R.; Huddart, R.; Foster, C.S. & Cooper, C.S. (2004). Amplification and overexpression of E2F3 in human bladder cancer. *Oncogene*, Vol.23, No.8, pp. 1627-1630

Ferlay, J.; Autier, P.; Boniol, M.; Heanue, M.; Colombet, M. & Boyle, P. (2007). Estimates of the cancer incidence and mortality in Europe in 2006. *Ann Oncol*, Vol.18, No.3, pp. 581-592

Forster, J.A.; Paul, A.B.; Harnden, P. & Knowles, M.A. (2011). Expression of NRG1 and its receptors in human bladder cancer. *Br J Cancer*, Vol.104, No.7, pp. 1135-1143

Franekova, M.; Halasova, E.; Bukovska, E.; Luptak, J. & Dobrota, D. (2008). Gene polymorphisms in bladder cancer. *Urol Oncol*, Vol.26, No.1, pp. 1-8

Franke, K.H.; Miklosi, M.; Goebell, P.; Clasen, S.; Steinhoff, C.; Anastasiadis, A.G.; Gerharz, C. & Schulz, W.A. (2000). Cyclin-dependent kinase inhibitor P27(KIP1) is expressed preferentially in early stages of urothelial carcinoma. *Urology*, Vol.56, No.4, pp. 689-695

Frohlich, C.; Albrechtsen, R.; Dyrskjot, L.; Rudkjaer, L.; Orntoft, T.F. & Wewer, U.M. (2006). Molecular profiling of ADAM12 in human bladder cancer. *Clin Cancer Res*, Vol.12, No.24, pp. 7359-7368

Fujimoto, K.; Yamada, Y.; Okajima, E.; Kakizoe, T.; Sasaki, H.; Sugimura, T. & Terada, M. (1992). Frequent association of p53 gene mutation in invasive bladder cancer. *Cancer Res*, Vol.52, No.6, pp. 1393-1398

Fung, Y.K.; Murphree, A.L.; T'Ang, A.; Qian, J.; Hinrichs, S.H. & Benedict, W.F. (1987). Structural evidence for the authenticity of the human retinoblastoma gene. *Science*, Vol.236, No.4809, pp. 1657-1661

Gakiopoulou, H.; Nakopoulou, L.; Siatelis, A.; Mavrommatis, I.; Panayotopoulou, E.G.; Tsirmpa, I.; Stravodimos, C. & Giannopoulos, A. (2003). Tissue inhibitor of metalloproteinase-2 as a multifunctional molecule of which the expression is associated with adverse prognosis of patients with urothelial bladder carcinomas. *Clin Cancer Res*, Vol.9, No.15, pp. 5573-5581

Garcia-Closas, M.; Malats, N.; Real, F.X.; Welch, R.; Kogevinas, M.; Chatterjee, N.; Pfeiffer, R.; Silverman, D.; Dosemeci, M.; Tardon, A.; Serra, C.; Carrato, A.; Garcia-Closas, R.; Castano-Vinyals, G.; Chanock, S.; Yeager, M. & Rothman, N. (2006). Genetic variation in the nucleotide excision repair pathway and bladder cancer risk. *Cancer Epidemiol Biomarkers Prev*, Vol.15, No.3, pp. 536-542

Garcia del Muro, X.; Torregrosa, A.; Munoz, J.; Castellsague, X.; Condom, E.; Vigues, F.; Arance, A.; Fabra, A. & Germa, J.R. (2000). Prognostic value of the expression of E-cadherin and beta-catenin in bladder cancer. *Eur J Cancer*, Vol.36, No.3, pp. 357-362

Gazzaniga, P.; Gradilone, A.; Vercillo, R.; Gandini, O.; Silvestri, I.; Napolitano, M.; Albonici, L.; Vincenzoni, A.; Gallucci, M.; Frati, L. & Agliano, A.M. (1996). Bcl-2/bax mRNA expression ratio as prognostic factor in low-grade urinary bladder cancer. *Int J Cancer*, Vol.69, No.2, pp. 100-104

Gazzaniga, P.; Gradilone, A.; Silvestri, I.; Gandini, O.; Napolitano, M.; Vercillo, R.; Vincenzoni, A.; Gallucci, M.; Frati, L. & Agliano, A.M. (1998). High levels of transforming growth factor-alpha (TGF-alpha) mRNA may predict local relapses in early stage urinary bladder cancer. *Eur J Cancer*, Vol.34, No.6, pp. 934-936

Gazzaniga, P.; Gandini, O.; Gradilone, A.; Silvestri, I.; Giuliani, L.; Magnanti, M.; Gallucci, M.; Saccani, G.; Frati, L. & Agliano, A.M. (1999). Detection of basic fibroblast growth factor mRNA in urinary bladder cancer: correlation with local relapses. *Int J Oncol*, Vol.14, No.6, pp. 1123-1127

Gazzaniga, P.; Gradilone, A.; Giuliani, L.; Gandini, O.; Silvestri, I.; Nofroni, I.; Saccani, G.; Frati, L. & Agliano, A.M. (2003). Expression and prognostic significance of LIVIN, SURVIVIN and other apoptosis-related genes in the progression of superficial bladder cancer. *Ann Oncol*, Vol.14, No.1, pp. 85-90

George, B.; Datar, R.H.; Wu, L.; Cai, J.; Patten, N.; Beil, S.J.; Groshen, S.; Stein, J.; Skinner, D.; Jones, P.A. & Cote, R.J. (2007). p53 gene and protein status: the role of p53 alterations in predicting outcome in patients with bladder cancer. *J Clin Oncol*, Vol.25, No.34, pp. 5352-5358

Gerhards, S.; Jung, K.; Koenig, F.; Daniltchenko, D.; Hauptmann, S.; Schnorr, D. & Loening, S.A. (2001). Excretion of matrix metalloproteinases 2 and 9 in urine is associated with a high stage and grade of bladder carcinoma. *Urology*, Vol.57, No.4, pp. 675-679

Glas, A.S.; Roos, D.; Deutekom, M.; Zwinderman, A.H.; Bossuyt, P.M. & Kurth, K.H. (2003).
    Tumor markers in the diagnosis of primary bladder cancer. A systematic review. *J*
    Urol, Vol.169, No.6, pp. 1975-1982

Goddard, J.C.; Sutton, C.D.; Jones, J.L.; O'Byrne, K.J. & Kockelbergh, R.C. (2002). Reduced
    thrombospondin-1 at presentation predicts disease progression in superficial
    bladder cancer. *Eur Urol*, Vol.42, No.5, pp. 464-468

Gohji, K.; Fujimoto, N.; Fujii, A.; Komiyama, T.; Okawa, J. & Nakajima, M. (1996a).
    Prognostic significance of circulating matrix metalloproteinase-2 to tissue inhibitor
    of metalloproteinases-2 ratio in recurrence of urothelial cancer after complete
    resection. *Cancer Res*, Vol.56, No.14, pp. 3196-3198

Gohji, K.; Fujimoto, N.; Komiyama, T.; Fujii, A.; Ohkawa, J.; Kamidono, S. & Nakajima, M.
    (1996b). Elevation of serum levels of matrix metalloproteinase-2 and -3 as new
    predictors of recurrence in patients with urothelial carcinoma. *Cancer*, Vol.78,
    No.11, pp. 2379-2387

Gohji, K.; Fujimoto, N.; Ohkawa, J.; Fujii, A. & Nakajima, M. (1998). Imbalance between
    serum matrix metalloproteinase-2 and its inhibitor as a predictor of recurrence of
    urothelial cancer. *Br J Cancer*, Vol.77, No.4, pp. 650-655

Gohji, K.; Nomi, M.; Niitani, Y.; Kitazawa, S.; Fujii, A.; Katsuoka, Y. & Nakajima, M. (2000).
    Independent prognostic value of serum hepatocyte growth factor in bladder cancer.
    J Clin Oncol, Vol.18, No.16, pp. 2963-2971

Golka, K.; Wiese, A.; Assennato, G. & Bolt, H.M. (2004). Occupational exposure and
    urological cancer. *World J Urol*, Vol.21, No.6, pp. 382-391

Gontero, P.; Banisadr, S.; Frea, B. & Brausi, M. (2004). Metastasis markers in bladder cancer:
    a review of the literature and clinical considerations. *Eur Urol*, Vol.46, No.3, pp.
    296-311

Gonzalez-Campora, R.; Davalos-Casanova, G.; Beato-Moreno, A.; Garcia-Escudero, A.;
    Pareja Megia, M.J.; Montironi, R. & Lopez-Beltran, A. (2007). BCL-2, TP53 and BAX
    protein expression in superficial urothelial bladder carcinoma. *Cancer Lett*, Vol.250,
    No.2, pp. 292-299

Gonzalez-Zulueta, M.; Bender, C.M.; Yang, A.S.; Nguyen, T.; Beart, R.W.; Van Tornout, J.M.
    & Jones, P.A. (1995). Methylation of the 5' CpG island of the p16/CDKN2 tumor
    suppressor gene in normal and transformed human tissues correlates with gene
    silencing. *Cancer Res*, Vol.55, No.20, pp. 4531-4535

Gonzalez, S.; Aubert, S.; Kerdraon, O.; Haddad, O.; Fantoni, J.C.; Biserte, J. & Leroy, X.
    (2008). Prognostic value of combined p53 and survivin in pT1G3 urothelial
    carcinoma of the bladder. *Am J Clin Pathol*, Vol.129, No.2, pp. 232-237

Gravas, S.; Bosinakou, I.; Kehayas, P. & Giannopoulos, A. (2004). Urinary basic fibroblast
    growth factor in bladder cancer patients. Histopathological correlation and clinical
    potential. *Urol Int*, Vol.73, No.2, pp. 173-177

Grignon, D.J.; Sakr, W.; Toth, M.; Ravery, V.; Angulo, J.; Shamsa, F.; Pontes, J.E.; Crissman,
    J.C. & Fridman, R. (1996). High levels of tissue inhibitor of metalloproteinase-2
    (TIMP-2) expression are associated with poor outcome in invasive bladder cancer.
    Cancer Res, Vol.56, No.7, pp. 1654-1659

Grossfeld, G.D.; Ginsberg, D.A.; Stein, J.P.; Bochner, B.H.; Esrig, D.; Groshen, S.; Dunn, M.;
    Nichols, P.W.; Taylor, C.R.; Skinner, D.G. & Cote, R.J. (1997). Thrombospondin-1
    expression in bladder cancer: association with p53 alterations, tumor angiogenesis,
    and tumor progression. *J Natl Cancer Inst*, Vol.89, No.3, pp. 219-227

Grossman, H.B.; Liebert, M.; Antelo, M.; Dinney, C.P.; Hu, S.X.; Palmer, J.L. & Benedict, W.F. (1998). p53 and RB expression predict progression in T1 bladder cancer. *Clin Cancer Res*, Vol.4, No.4, pp. 829-834

Grossman, H.B.; Lee, C.; Bromberg, J. & Liebert, M. (2000). Expression of the alpha6beta4 integrin provides prognostic information in bladder cancer. *Oncol Rep*, Vol.7, No.1, pp. 13-16

Hanahan, D. & Weinberg, R.A. (2000). The hallmarks of cancer. *Cell*, Vol.100, No.1, pp. 57-70

Hara, I.; Miyake, H.; Hara, S.; Arakawa, S. & Kamidono, S. (2001). Significance of matrix metalloproteinases and tissue inhibitors of metalloproteinase expression in the recurrence of superficial transitional cell carcinoma of the bladder. *J Urol*, Vol.165, No.5, pp. 1769-1772

Harley, C.B. (1991). Telomere loss: mitotic clock or genetic time bomb? *Mutat Res*, Vol.256, No.2-6, pp. 271-282

Harris, L.D.; De La Cerda, J.; Tuziak, T.; Rosen, D.; Xiao, L.; Shen, Y.; Sabichi, A.L.; Czerniak, B. & Grossman, H.B. (2008). Analysis of the expression of biomarkers in urinary bladder cancer using a tissue microarray. *Mol Carcinog*, Vol.47, No.9, pp. 678-685

Hasui, Y.; Marutsuka, K.; Nishi, S.; Kitada, S.; Osada, Y. & Sumiyoshi, A. (1994). The content of urokinase-type plasminogen activator and tumor recurrence in superficial bladder cancer. *J Urol*, Vol.151, No.1, pp. 16-19;

Hausladen, D.A.; Wheeler, M.A.; Altieri, D.C.; Colberg, J.W. & Weiss, R.M. (2003). Effect of intravesical treatment of transitional cell carcinoma with bacillus Calmette-Guerin and mitomycin C on urinary survivin levels and outcome. *J Urol*, Vol.170, No.1, pp. 230-234

Hawke, C.K.; Delahunt, B. & Davidson, P.J. (1998). Microvessel density as a prognostic marker for transitional cell carcinoma of the bladder. *Br J Urol*, Vol.81, No.4, pp. 585-590

Heidenblad, M.; Lindgren, D.; Jonson, T.; Liedberg, F.; Veerla, S.; Chebil, G.; Gudjonsson, S.; Borg, A.; Mansson, W. & Hoglund, M. (2008). Tiling resolution array CGH and high density expression profiling of urothelial carcinomas delineate genomic amplicons and candidate target genes specific for advanced tumors. *BMC Med Genomics*, Vol.1, pp. 3

Heine, B.; Hummel, M.; Muller, M.; Heicappell, R.; Miller, K. & Stein, H. (1998). Non-radioactive measurement of telomerase activity in human bladder cancer, bladder washings, and in urine. *J Pathol*, Vol.184, No.1, pp. 71-76

Hernandez, S.; Lopez-Knowles, E.; Lloreta, J.; Kogevinas, M.; Jaramillo, R.; Amoros, A.; Tardon, A.; Garcia-Closas, R.; Serra, C.; Carrato, A.; Malats, N. & Real, F.X. (2005). FGFR3 and Tp53 mutations in T1G3 transitional bladder carcinomas: independent distribution and lack of association with prognosis. *Clin Cancer Res*, Vol.11, No.15, pp. 5444-5450

Hernandez, S.; Lopez-Knowles, E.; Lloreta, J.; Kogevinas, M.; Amoros, A.; Tardon, A.; Carrato, A.; Serra, C.; Malats, N. & Real, F.X. (2006). Prospective study of FGFR3 mutations as a prognostic factor in nonmuscle invasive urothelial bladder carcinomas. *J Clin Oncol*, Vol.24, No.22, pp. 3664-3671

Hernando, E.; Nahle, Z.; Juan, G.; Diaz-Rodriguez, E.; Alaminos, M.; Hemann, M.; Michel, L.; Mittal, V.; Gerald, W.; Benezra, R.; Lowe, S.W. & Cordon-Cardo, C. (2004). Rb inactivation promotes genomic instability by uncoupling cell cycle progression from mitotic control. *Nature*, Vol.430, No.7001, pp. 797-802

Herr, H.W. (2000). Tumor progression and survival of patients with high grade, noninvasive papillary (TaG3) bladder tumors: 15-year outcome. *J Urol*, Vol.163, No.1, pp. 60-61;

Hiebert, S.W.; Chellappan, S.P.; Horowitz, J.M. & Nevins, J.R. (1992). The interaction of RB with E2F coincides with an inhibition of the transcriptional activity of E2F. *Genes Dev*, Vol.6, No.2, pp. 177-185

Hitchings, A.W.; Kumar, M.; Jordan, S.; Nargund, V.; Martin, J. & Berney, D.M. (2004). Prediction of progression in pTa and pT1 bladder carcinomas with p53, p16 and pRb. *Br J Cancer*, Vol.91, No.3, pp. 552-557

Hiyama, E. & Hiyama, K. (2002). Clinical utility of telomerase in cancer. *Oncogene*, Vol.21, No.4, pp. 643-649

Horikawa, Y.; Gu, J. & Wu, X. (2008a). Genetic susceptibility to bladder cancer with an emphasis on gene-gene and gene-environmental interactions. *Curr Opin Urol*, Vol.18, No.5, pp. 493-498

Horikawa, Y.; Nadaoka, J.; Saito, M.; Kumazawa, T.; Inoue, T.; Yuasa, T.; Tsuchiya, N.; Nishiyama, H.; Ogawa, O. & Habuchi, T. (2008b). Clinical implications of the MDM2 SNP309 and p53 Arg72Pro polymorphisms in transitional cell carcinoma of the bladder. *Oncol Rep*, Vol.20, No.1, pp. 49-55

Hurst, C.D.; Tomlinson, D.C.; Williams, S.V.; Platt, F.M. & Knowles, M.A. (2008). Inactivation of the Rb pathway and overexpression of both isoforms of E2F3 are obligate events in bladder tumours with 6p22 amplification. *Oncogene*, Vol.27, No.19, pp. 2716-2727

Hussain, S.A.; Ganesan, R.; Hiller, L.; Cooke, P.W.; Murray, P.; Young, L.S. & James, N.D. (2003). BCL2 expression predicts survival in patients receiving synchronous chemoradiotherapy in advanced transitional cell carcinoma of the bladder. *Oncol Rep*, Vol.10, No.3, pp. 571-576

Inoue, K.; Slaton, J.W.; Karashima, T.; Yoshikawa, C.; Shuin, T.; Sweeney, P.; Millikan, R. & Dinney, C.P. (2000). The prognostic value of angiogenesis factor expression for predicting recurrence and metastasis of bladder cancer after neoadjuvant chemotherapy and radical cystectomy. *Clin Cancer Res*, Vol.6, No.12, pp. 4866-4873

Ishikawa, J.; Xu, H.J.; Hu, S.X.; Yandell, D.W.; Maeda, S.; Kamidono, S.; Benedict, W.F. & Takahashi, R. (1991). Inactivation of the retinoblastoma gene in human bladder and renal cell carcinomas. *Cancer Res*, Vol.51, No.20, pp. 5736-5743

Ito, H.; Kyo, S.; Kanaya, T.; Takakura, M.; Inoue, M. & Namiki, M. (1998). Expression of human telomerase subunits and correlation with telomerase activity in urothelial cancer. *Clin Cancer Res*, Vol.4, No.7, pp. 1603-1608

Jaeger, T.M.; Weidner, N.; Chew, K.; Moore, D.H.; Kerschmann, R.L.; Waldman, F.M. & Carroll, P.R. (1995). Tumor angiogenesis correlates with lymph node metastases in invasive bladder cancer. *J Urol*, Vol.154, No.1, pp. 69-71

Jebar, A.H.; Hurst, C.D.; Tomlinson, D.C.; Johnston, C.; Taylor, C.F. & Knowles, M.A. (2005). FGFR3 and Ras gene mutations are mutually exclusive genetic events in urothelial cell carcinoma. *Oncogene*, Vol.24, No.33, pp. 5218-5225

Jemal, A.; Siegel, R.; Xu, J. & Ward, E. (2010). Cancer statistics, 2010. *CA Cancer J Clin*, Vol.60, No.5, pp. 277-300

Jonsson, G.; Paulie, S. & Grandien, A. (2003). cIAP-2 block apoptotic events in bladder cancer cells. *Anticancer Res*, Vol.23, No.4, pp. 3311-3316

Joseph, A.; Weiss, G.H.; Jin, L.; Fuchs, A.; Chowdhury, S.; O'Shaugnessy, P.; Goldberg, I.D. & Rosen, E.M. (1995). Expression of scatter factor in human bladder carcinoma. *J Natl Cancer Inst*, Vol.87, No.5, pp. 372-377

Junker, K.; van Oers, J.M.; Zwarthoff, E.C.; Kania, I.; Schubert, J. & Hartmann, A. (2008). Fibroblast growth factor receptor 3 mutations in bladder tumors correlate with low frequency of chromosome alterations. *Neoplasia*, Vol.10, No.1, pp. 1-7

Junttila, T.T.; Laato, M.; Vahlberg, T.; Soderstrom, K.O.; Visakorpi, T.; Isola, J. & Elenius, K. (2003). Identification of patients with transitional cell carcinoma of the bladder overexpressing ErbB2, ErbB3, or specific ErbB4 isoforms: real-time reverse transcription-PCR analysis in estimation of ErbB receptor status from cancer patients. *Clin Cancer Res*, Vol.9, No.14, pp. 5346-5357

Kamai, T.; Takagi, K.; Asami, H.; Ito, Y.; Oshima, H. & Yoshida, K.I. (2001). Decreasing of p27(Kip1)and cyclin E protein levels is associated with progression from superficial into invasive bladder cancer. *Br J Cancer*, Vol.84, No.9, pp. 1242-1251

Kanayama, H.; Yokota, K.; Kurokawa, Y.; Murakami, Y.; Nishitani, M. & Kagawa, S. (1998). Prognostic values of matrix metalloproteinase-2 and tissue inhibitor of metalloproteinase-2 expression in bladder cancer. *Cancer*, Vol.82, No.7, pp. 1359-1366

Karam, J.A.; Lotan, Y.; Ashfaq, R.; Sagalowsky, A.I. & Shariat, S.F. (2007a). Survivin expression in patients with non-muscle-invasive urothelial cell carcinoma of the bladder. *Urology*, Vol.70, No.3, pp. 482-486

Karam, J.A.; Lotan, Y.; Karakiewicz, P.I.; Ashfaq, R.; Sagalowsky, A.I.; Roehrborn, C.G. & Shariat, S.F. (2007b). Use of combined apoptosis biomarkers for prediction of bladder cancer recurrence and mortality after radical cystectomy. *Lancet Oncol*, Vol.8, No.2, pp. 128-136

Kashibuchi, K.; Tomita, K.; Schalken, J.A.; Kume, H.; Takeuchi, T. & Kitamura, T. (2007). The prognostic value of E-cadherin, alpha-, beta- and gamma-catenin in bladder cancer patients who underwent radical cystectomy. *Int J Urol*, Vol.14, No.9, pp. 789-794

Kassouf, W.; Black, P.C.; Tuziak, T.; Bondaruk, J.; Lee, S.; Brown, G.A.; Adam, L.; Wei, C.; Baggerly, K.; Bar-Eli, M.; McConkey, D.; Czerniak, B. & Dinney, C.P. (2008). Distinctive expression pattern of ErbB family receptors signifies an aggressive variant of bladder cancer. *J Urol*, Vol.179, No.1, pp. 353-358

Kawamoto, K.; Enokida, H.; Gotanda, T.; Kubo, H.; Nishiyama, K.; Kawahara, M. & Nakagawa, M. (2006). p16INK4a and p14ARF methylation as a potential biomarker for human bladder cancer. *Biochem Biophys Res Commun*, Vol.339, No.3, pp. 790-796

Kellen, E.; Hemelt, M.; Broberg, K.; Golka, K.; Kristensen, V.N.; Hung, R.J.; Matullo, G.; Mittal, R.D.; Porru, S.; Povey, A.; Schulz, W.A.; Shen, J.; Buntinx, F.; Zeegers, M.P. & Taioli, E. (2007). Pooled analysis and meta-analysis of the glutathione S-transferase P1 Ile 105Val polymorphism and bladder cancer: a HuGE-GSEC review. *Am J Epidemiol*, Vol.165, No.11, pp. 1221-1230

Kelsh, M.A.; Alexander, D.D.; Kalmes, R.M. & Buffler, P.A. (2008). Personal use of hair dyes and risk of bladder cancer: a meta-analysis of epidemiologic data. *Cancer Causes Control*, Vol.19, No.6, pp. 549-558

Kiemeney, L.A.; Thorlacius, S.; Sulem, P.; Geller, F.; Aben, K.K.; Stacey, S.N.; Gudmundsson, J.; Jakobsdottir, M.; Bergthorsson, J.T.; Sigurdsson, A.; Blondal, T.; Witjes, J.A.; Vermeulen, S.H.; Hulsbergen-van de Kaa, C.A.; Swinkels, D.W.; Ploeg, M.; Cornel, E.B.; Vergunst, H.; Thorgeirsson, T.E.; Gudbjartsson, D.; Gudjonsson, S.A.;

Thorleifsson, G.; Kristinsson, K.T.; Mouy, M.; Snorradottir, S.; Placidi, D.; Campagna, M.; Arici, C.; Koppova, K.; Gurzau, E.; Rudnai, P.; Kellen, E.; Polidoro, S.; Guarrera, S.; Sacerdote, C.; Sanchez, M.; Saez, B.; Valdivia, G.; Ryk, C.; de Verdier, P.; Lindblom, A.; Golka, K.; Bishop, D.T.; Knowles, M.A.; Nikulasson, S.; Petursdottir, V.; Jonsson, E.; Geirsson, G.; Kristjansson, B.; Mayordomo, J.I.; Steineck, G.; Porru, S.; Buntinx, F.; Zeegers, M.P.; Fletcher, T.; Kumar, R.; Matullo, G.; Vineis, P.; Kiltie, A.E.; Gulcher, J.R.; Thorsteinsdottir, U.; Kong, A.; Rafnar, T. & Stefansson, K. (2008). Sequence variant on 8q24 confers susceptibility to urinary bladder cancer. *Nat Genet*, Vol.40, No.11, pp. 1307-1312

Kiemeney, L.A.; Sulem, P.; Besenbacher, S.; Vermeulen, S.H.; Sigurdsson, A.; Thorleifsson, G.; Gudbjartsson, D.F.; Stacey, S.N.; Gudmundsson, J.; Zanon, C.; Kostic, J.; Masson, G.; Bjarnason, H.; Palsson, S.T.; Skarphedinsson, O.B.; Gudjonsson, S.A.; Witjes, J.A.; Grotenhuis, A.J.; Verhaegh, G.W.; Bishop, D.T.; Sak, S.C.; Choudhury, A.; Elliott, F.; Barrett, J.H.; Hurst, C.D.; de Verdier, P.J.; Ryk, C.; Rudnai, P.; Gurzau, E.; Koppova, K.; Vineis, P.; Polidoro, S.; Guarrera, S.; Sacerdote, C.; Campagna, M.; Placidi, D.; Arici, C.; Zeegers, M.P.; Kellen, E.; Gutierrez, B.S.; Sanz-Velez, J.I.; Sanchez-Zalabardo, M.; Valdivia, G.; Garcia-Prats, M.D.; Hengstler, J.G.; Blaszkewicz, M.; Dietrich, H.; Ophoff, R.A.; van den Berg, L.H.; Alexiusdottir, K.; Kristjansson, K.; Geirsson, G.; Nikulasson, S.; Petursdottir, V.; Kong, A.; Thorgeirsson, T.; Mungan, N.A.; Lindblom, A.; van Es, M.A.; Porru, S.; Buntinx, F.; Golka, K.; Mayordomo, J.I.; Kumar, R.; Matullo, G.; Steineck, G.; Kiltie, A.E.; Aben, K.K.; Jonsson, E.; Thorsteinsdottir, U.; Knowles, M.A.; Rafnar, T. & Stefansson, K. (2010). A sequence variant at 4p16.3 confers susceptibility to urinary bladder cancer. *Nat Genet*, Vol.42, No.5, pp. 415-419

Kim, N.W.; Piatyszek, M.A.; Prowse, K.R.; Harley, C.B.; West, M.D.; Ho, P.L.; Coviello, G.M.; Wright, W.E.; Weinrich, S.L. & Shay, J.W. (1994). Specific association of human telomerase activity with immortal cells and cancer. *Science*, Vol.266, No.5193, pp. 2011-2015

Kim, W.J. & Quan, C. (2005). Genetic and epigenetic aspects of bladder cancer. *J Cell Biochem*, Vol.95, No.1, pp. 24-33

Kitamura, H. & Tsukamoto, T. (2006). Early bladder cancer: concept, diagnosis, and management. *Int J Clin Oncol*, Vol.11, No.1, pp. 28-37

Knowles, M.A.; Habuchi, T.; Kennedy, W. & Cuthbert-Heavens, D. (2003). Mutation spectrum of the 9q34 tuberous sclerosis gene TSC1 in transitional cell carcinoma of the bladder. *Cancer Res*, Vol.63, No.22, pp. 7652-7656

Knowles, M.A. (2008). Molecular pathogenesis of bladder cancer. *Int J Clin Oncol*, Vol.13, No.4, pp. 287-297

Knowles, M.A.; Platt, F.M.; Ross, R.L. & Hurst, C.D. (2009). Phosphatidylinositol 3-kinase (PI3K) pathway activation in bladder cancer. *Cancer Metastasis Rev*, Vol.28, No.3-4, pp. 305-316

Kompier, L.C.; Lurkin, I.; van der Aa, M.N.; van Rhijn, B.W.; van der Kwast, T.H. & Zwarthoff, E.C. (2010a). FGFR3, HRAS, KRAS, NRAS and PIK3CA mutations in bladder cancer and their potential as biomarkers for surveillance and therapy. *PLoS One*, Vol.5, No.11, pp. e13821

Kompier, L.C.; van Tilborg, A.A. & Zwarthoff, E.C. (2010b). Bladder cancer: novel molecular characteristics, diagnostic, and therapeutic implications. *Urol Oncol*, Vol.28, No.1, pp. 91-96

Korkolopoulou, P.; Christodoulou, P.; Konstantinidou, A.E.; Thomas-Tsagli, E.; Kapralos, P. & Davaris, P. (2000). Cell cycle regulators in bladder cancer: a multivariate survival study with emphasis on p27Kip1. *Hum Pathol*, Vol.31, No.6, pp. 751-760

Korkolopoulou, P.; Christodoulou, P.; Lazaris, A.; Thomas-Tsagli, E.; Kapralos, P.; Papanikolaou, A.; Kalliteraki, I. & Davaris, P. (2001). Prognostic implications of aberrations in p16/pRb pathway in urothelial bladder carcinomas: a multivariate analysis including p53 expression and proliferation markers. *Eur Urol*, Vol.39, No.2, pp. 167-177

Korkolopoulou, P.; Lazaris, A.; Konstantinidou, A.E.; Kavantzas, N.; Patsouris, E.; Christodoulou, P.; Thomas-Tsagli, E. & Davaris, P. (2002). Differential expression of bcl-2 family proteins in bladder carcinomas. Relationship with apoptotic rate and survival. *Eur Urol*, Vol.41, No.3, pp. 274-283

Kramer, C.; Klasmeyer, K.; Bojar, H.; Schulz, W.A.; Ackermann, R. & Grimm, M.O. (2007). Heparin-binding epidermal growth factor-like growth factor isoforms and epidermal growth factor receptor/ErbB1 expression in bladder cancer and their relation to clinical outcome. *Cancer*, Vol.109, No.10, pp. 2016-2024

Kruger, S.; Mahnken, A.; Kausch, I. & Feller, A.C. (2005). P16 immunoreactivity is an independent predictor of tumor progression in minimally invasive urothelial bladder carcinoma. *Eur Urol*, Vol.47, No.4, pp. 463-467

Ku, J.H.; Kwak, C.; Lee, H.S.; Park, H.K.; Lee, E. & Lee, S.E. (2004). Expression of survivin, a novel inhibitor of apoptosis, in superficial transitional cell carcinoma of the bladder. *J Urol*, Vol.171, No.2 Pt 1, pp. 631-635

Kuczyk, M.A.; Bokemeyer, C.; Serth, J.; Hervatin, C.; Oelke, M.; Hofner, K.; Tan, H.K. & Jonas, U. (1995). p53 overexpression as a prognostic factor for advanced stage bladder cancer. *Eur J Cancer*, Vol.31A, No.13-14, pp. 2243-2247

Kuczyk, M.A.; Machtens, S.; Bokemeyer, C.; Hradil, K.; Macheel, I.; Jetscho, V.; Hartmann, J.; Thon, W.F.; Jonas, U. & Serth, J. (1999). Prognostic value of p27Kip1 and p21WAF/Cip protein expression in muscle invasive bladder cancer. *Oncol Rep*, Vol.6, No.3, pp. 687-693

Kyo, S.; Takakura, M.; Fujiwara, T. & Inoue, M. (2008). Understanding and exploiting hTERT promoter regulation for diagnosis and treatment of human cancers. *Cancer Sci*, Vol.99, No.8, pp. 1528-1538

Le Frere-Belda, M.A.; Cappellen, D.; Daher, A.; Gil-Diez-de-Medina, S.; Besse, F.; Abbou, C.C.; Thiery, J.P.; Zafrani, E.S.; Chopin, D.K. & Radvanyi, F. (2001). p15(INK4b) in bladder carcinomas: decreased expression in superficial tumours. *Br J Cancer*, Vol.85, No.10, pp. 1515-1521

Le Frere-Belda, M.A.; Gil Diez de Medina, S.; Daher, A.; Martin, N.; Albaud, B.; Heudes, D.; Abbou, C.C.; Thiery, J.P.; Zafrani, E.S.; Radvanyi, F. & Chopin, D. (2004). Profiles of the 2 INK4a gene products, p16 and p14ARF, in human reference urothelium and bladder carcinomas, according to pRb and p53 protein status. *Hum Pathol*, Vol.35, No.7, pp. 817-824

Lee, S.H.; Shin, M.S.; Park, W.S.; Kim, S.Y.; Dong, S.M.; Pi, J.H.; Lee, H.K.; Kim, H.S.; Jang, J.J.; Kim, C.S.; Kim, S.H.; Lee, J.Y. & Yoo, N.J. (1999). Alterations of Fas (APO-1/CD95) gene in transitional cell carcinomas of urinary bladder. *Cancer Res*, Vol.59, No.13, pp. 3068-3072

Li, M.; Song, T.; Yin, Z.F. & Na, Y.Q. (2007). XIAP as a prognostic marker of early recurrence of nonmuscular invasive bladder cancer. *Chin Med J (Engl)*, Vol.120, No.6, pp. 469-473

Lianes, P.; Orlow, I.; Zhang, Z.F.; Oliva, M.R.; Sarkis, A.S.; Reuter, V.E. & Cordon-Cardo, C. (1994). Altered patterns of MDM2 and TP53 expression in human bladder cancer. *J Natl Cancer Inst*, Vol.86, No.17, pp. 1325-1330

Liebert, M.; Washington, R.; Wedemeyer, G.; Carey, T.E. & Grossman, H.B. (1994). Loss of co-localization of alpha 6 beta 4 integrin and collagen VII in bladder cancer. *Am J Pathol*, Vol.144, No.4, pp. 787-795

Lin, Y.; Miyamoto, H.; Fujinami, K.; Uemura, H.; Hosaka, M.; Iwasaki, Y. & Kubota, Y. (1996). Telomerase activity in human bladder cancer. *Clin Cancer Res*, Vol.2, No.6, pp. 929-932

Liu, H.B.; Kong, C.Z.; Zeng, Y.; Liu, X.K.; Bi, J.B.; Jiang, Y.J. & Han, S. (2009). Livin may serve as a marker for prognosis of bladder cancer relapse and a target of bladder cancer treatment. *Urol Oncol*, Vol.27, No.3, pp. 277-283

Liukkonen, T.J.; Lipponen, P.K.; Helle, M. & Jauhiainen, K.E. (1997). Immunoreactivity of bcl-2, p53 and EGFr is associated with tumor stage, grade and cell proliferation in superficial bladder cancer. Finnbladder III Group. *Urol Res*, Vol.25, No.1, pp. 1-7

Logothetis, C.J.; Xu, H.J.; Ro, J.Y.; Hu, S.X.; Sahin, A.; Ordonez, N. & Benedict, W.F. (1992). Altered expression of retinoblastoma protein and known prognostic variables in locally advanced bladder cancer. *J Natl Cancer Inst*, Vol.84, No.16, pp. 1256-1261

Lopez-Beltran, A.; Alvarez-Kindelan, J.; Luque, R.J.; Blanca, A.; Quintero, A.; Montironi, R.; Cheng, L.; Gonzalez-Campora, R. & Requena, M.J. (2008). Loss of heterozygosity at 9q32-33 (DBC1 locus) in primary non-invasive papillary urothelial neoplasm of low malignant potential and low-grade urothelial carcinoma of the bladder and their associated normal urothelium. *J Pathol*, Vol.215, No.3, pp. 263-272

Lopez-Knowles, E.; Hernandez, S.; Malats, N.; Kogevinas, M.; Lloreta, J.; Carrato, A.; Tardon, A.; Serra, C. & Real, F.X. (2006). PIK3CA mutations are an early genetic alteration associated with FGFR3 mutations in superficial papillary bladder tumors. *Cancer Res*, Vol.66, No.15, pp. 7401-7404

Lu, M.L.; Wikman, F.; Orntoft, T.F.; Charytonowicz, E.; Rabbani, F.; Zhang, Z.; Dalbagni, G.; Pohar, K.S.; Yu, G. & Cordon-Cardo, C. (2002). Impact of alterations affecting the p53 pathway in bladder cancer on clinical outcome, assessed by conventional and array-based methods. *Clin Cancer Res*, Vol.8, No.1, pp. 171-179

Mahnken, A.; Kausch, I.; Feller, A.C. & Kruger, S. (2005). E-cadherin immunoreactivity correlates with recurrence and progression of minimally invasive transitional cell carcinomas of the urinary bladder. *Oncol Rep*, Vol.14, No.4, pp. 1065-1070

Maluf, F.C.; Cordon-Cardo, C.; Verbel, D.A.; Satagopan, J.M.; Boyle, M.G.; Herr, H. & Bajorin, D.F. (2006). Assessing interactions between mdm-2, p53, and bcl-2 as prognostic variables in muscle-invasive bladder cancer treated with neo-adjuvant chemotherapy followed by locoregional surgical treatment. *Ann Oncol*, Vol.17, No.11, pp. 1677-1686

Margulis, V.; Lotan, Y. & Shariat, S.F. (2008). Survivin: a promising biomarker for detection and prognosis of bladder cancer. *World J Urol*, Vol.26, No.1, pp. 59-65

McKnight, J.J.; Gray, S.B.; O'Kane, H.F.; Johnston, S.R. & Williamson, K.E. (2005). Apoptosis and chemotherapy for bladder cancer. *J Urol*, Vol.173, No.3, pp. 683-690

Memon, A.A.; Sorensen, B.S.; Meldgaard, P.; Fokdal, L.; Thykjaer, T. & Nexo, E. (2006). The relation between survival and expression of HER1 and HER2 depends on the expression of HER3 and HER4: a study in bladder cancer patients. *Br J Cancer*, Vol.94, No.11, pp. 1703-1709

Meyerson, M.; Counter, C.M.; Eaton, E.N.; Ellisen, L.W.; Steiner, P.; Caddle, S.D.; Ziaugra, L.; Beijersbergen, R.L.; Davidoff, M.J.; Liu, Q.; Bacchetti, S.; Haber, D.A. & Weinberg, R.A. (1997). hEST2, the putative human telomerase catalytic subunit gene, is up-regulated in tumor cells and during immortalization. *Cell*, Vol.90, No.4, pp. 785-795

Mhawech-Fauceglia, P.; Cheney, R.T. & Schwaller, J. (2006). Genetic alterations in urothelial bladder carcinoma: an updated review. *Cancer*, Vol.106, No.6, pp. 1205-1216

Mialhe, A.; Louis, J.; Montlevier, S.; Peoch, M.; Pasquier, D.; Bosson, J.L.; Rambeaud, J.J. & Seigneurin, D. (1997). Expression of E-cadherin and alpha-,beta- and gamma-catenins in human bladder carcinomas: are they good prognostic factors? *Invasion Metastasis*, Vol.17, No.3, pp. 124-137

Michaud, D.S. (2007). Chronic inflammation and bladder cancer. *Urol Oncol*, Vol.25, No.3, pp. 260-268

Michieli, P.; Chedid, M.; Lin, D.; Pierce, J.H.; Mercer, W.E. & Givol, D. (1994). Induction of WAF1/CIP1 by a p53-independent pathway. *Cancer Res*, Vol.54, No.13, pp. 3391-3395

Migaldi, M.; Sgambato, A.; Garagnani, L.; Ardito, R.; Ferrari, P.; De Gaetani, C.; Cittadini, A. & Trentini, G.P. (2000). Loss of p21Waf1 expression is a strong predictor of reduced survival in primary superficial bladder cancers. *Clin Cancer Res*, Vol.6, No.8, pp. 3131-3138

Mihara, K.; Cao, X.R.; Yen, A.; Chandler, S.; Driscoll, B.; Murphree, A.L.; T'Ang, A. & Fung, Y.K. (1989). Cell cycle-dependent regulation of phosphorylation of the human retinoblastoma gene product. *Science*, Vol.246, No.4935, pp. 1300-1303

Mitra, A.P.; Datar, R.H. & Cote, R.J. (2006). Molecular pathways in invasive bladder cancer: new insights into mechanisms, progression, and target identification. *J Clin Oncol*, Vol.24, No.35, pp. 5552-5564

Mitra, A.P.; Birkhahn, M. & Cote, R.J. (2007). p53 and retinoblastoma pathways in bladder cancer. *World J Urol*, Vol.25, No.6, pp. 563-571

Mitra, A.P. & Cote, R.J. (2009). Molecular pathogenesis and diagnostics of bladder cancer. *Annu Rev Pathol*, Vol.4, pp. 251-285

Miyamoto, H.; Shuin, T.; Torigoe, S.; Iwasaki, Y. & Kubota, Y. (1995). Retinoblastoma gene mutations in primary human bladder cancer. *Br J Cancer*, Vol.71, No.4, pp. 831-835

Miyata, Y.; Sagara, Y.; Kanda, S.; Hayashi, T. & Kanetake, H. (2009). Phosphorylated hepatocyte growth factor receptor/c-Met is associated with tumor growth and prognosis in patients with bladder cancer: correlation with matrix metalloproteinase-2 and -7 and E-cadherin. *Hum Pathol*, Vol.40, No.4, pp. 496-504

Mizutani, Y.; Hongo, F.; Sato, N.; Ogawa, O.; Yoshida, O. & Miki, T. (2001). Significance of serum soluble Fas ligand in patients with bladder carcinoma. *Cancer*, Vol.92, No.2, pp. 287-293

Muller, M. (2002). Telomerase: its clinical relevance in the diagnosis of bladder cancer. *Oncogene*, Vol.21, No.4, pp. 650-655

Nakopoulou, L.; Zervas, A.; Gakiopoulou-Givalou, H.; Constantinides, C.; Doumanis, G.; Davaris, P. & Dimopoulos, C. (2000). Prognostic value of E-cadherin, beta-catenin,

P120ctn in patients with transitional cell bladder cancer. *Anticancer Res*, Vol.20, No.6B, pp. 4571-4578

Nguyen, M.; Watanabe, H.; Budson, A.E.; Richie, J.P. & Folkman, J. (1993). Elevated levels of the angiogenic peptide basic fibroblast growth factor in urine of bladder cancer patients. *J Natl Cancer Inst*, Vol.85, No.3, pp. 241-242

Niehans, G.A.; Kratzke, R.A.; Froberg, M.K.; Aeppli, D.M.; Nguyen, P.L. & Geradts, J. (1999). G1 checkpoint protein and p53 abnormalities occur in most invasive transitional cell carcinomas of the urinary bladder. *Br J Cancer*, Vol.80, No.8, pp. 1175-1184

Nutt, J.E.; Mellon, J.K.; Qureshi, K. & Lunec, J. (1998). Matrix metalloproteinase-1 is induced by epidermal growth factor in human bladder tumour cell lines and is detectable in urine of patients with bladder tumours. *Br J Cancer*, Vol.78, No.2, pp. 215-220

Nutt, J.E.; Durkan, G.C.; Mellon, J.K. & Lunec, J. (2003). Matrix metalloproteinases (MMPs) in bladder cancer: the induction of MMP9 by epidermal growth factor and its detection in urine. *BJU Int*, Vol.91, No.1, pp. 99-104

Oeggerli, M.; Tomovska, S.; Schraml, P.; Calvano-Forte, D.; Schafroth, S.; Simon, R.; Gasser, T.; Mihatsch, M.J. & Sauter, G. (2004). E2F3 amplification and overexpression is associated with invasive tumor growth and rapid tumor cell proliferation in urinary bladder cancer. *Oncogene*, Vol.23, No.33, pp. 5616-5623

Oeggerli, M.; Schraml, P.; Ruiz, C.; Bloch, M.; Novotny, H.; Mirlacher, M.; Sauter, G. & Simon, R. (2006). E2F3 is the main target gene of the 6p22 amplicon with high specificity for human bladder cancer. *Oncogene*, Vol.25, No.49, pp. 6538-6543

Olsson, A.Y.; Feber, A.; Edwards, S.; Te Poele, R.; Giddings, I.; Merson, S. & Cooper, C.S. (2007). Role of E2F3 expression in modulating cellular proliferation rate in human bladder and prostate cancer cells. *Oncogene*, Vol.26, No.7, pp. 1028-1037

Olumi, A.F.; Tsai, Y.C.; Nichols, P.W.; Skinner, D.G.; Cain, D.R.; Bender, L.I. & Jones, P.A. (1990). Allelic loss of chromosome 17p distinguishes high grade from low grade transitional cell carcinomas of the bladder. *Cancer Res*, Vol.50, No.21, pp. 7081-7083

Ong, F.; Moonen, L.M.; Gallee, M.P.; ten Bosch, C.; Zerp, S.F.; Hart, A.A.; Bartelink, H. & Verheij, M. (2001). Prognostic factors in transitional cell cancer of the bladder: an emerging role for Bcl-2 and p53. *Radiother Oncol*, Vol.61, No.2, pp. 169-175

Orlow, I.; Lacombe, L.; Hannon, G.J.; Serrano, M.; Pellicer, I.; Dalbagni, G.; Reuter, V.E.; Zhang, Z.F.; Beach, D. & Cordon-Cardo, C. (1995). Deletion of the p16 and p15 genes in human bladder tumors. *J Natl Cancer Inst*, Vol.87, No.20, pp. 1524-1529

Orlow, I.; LaRue, H.; Osman, I.; Lacombe, L.; Moore, L.; Rabbani, F.; Meyer, F.; Fradet, Y. & Cordon-Cardo, C. (1999). Deletions of the INK4A gene in superficial bladder tumors. Association with recurrence. *Am J Pathol*, Vol.155, No.1, pp. 105-113

Oxford, G. & Theodorescu, D. (2003). The role of Ras superfamily proteins in bladder cancer progression. *J Urol*, Vol.170, No.5, pp. 1987-1993

Palit, V.; Phillips, R.M.; Puri, R.; Shah, T. & Bibby, M.C. (2005). Expression of HIF-1alpha and Glut-1 in human bladder cancer. *Oncol Rep*, Vol.14, No.4, pp. 909-913

Papathoma, A.S.; Petraki, C.; Grigorakis, A.; Papakonstantinou, H.; Karavana, V.; Stefanakis, S.; Sotsiou, F. & Pintzas, A. (2000). Prognostic significance of matrix metalloproteinases 2 and 9 in bladder cancer. *Anticancer Res*, Vol.20, No.3B, pp. 2009-2013

Parker, S.B.; Eichele, G.; Zhang, P.; Rawls, A.; Sands, A.T.; Bradley, A.; Olson, E.N.; Harper, J.W. & Elledge, S.J. (1995). p53-independent expression of p21Cip1 in muscle and other terminally differentiating cells. *Science*, Vol.267, No.5200, pp. 1024-1027

Pashos, C.L.; Botteman, M.F.; Laskin, B.L. & Redaelli, A. (2002). Bladder cancer: epidemiology, diagnosis, and management. *Cancer Pract*, Vol.10, No.6, pp. 311-322

Pfister, C.; Moore, L.; Allard, P.; Larue, H.; Lacombe, L.; Tetu, B.; Meyer, F. & Fradet, Y. (1999). Predictive value of cell cycle markers p53, MDM2, p21, and Ki-67 in superficial bladder tumor recurrence. *Clin Cancer Res*, Vol.5, No.12, pp. 4079-4084

Pfister, C.; Larue, H.; Moore, L.; Lacombe, L.; Veilleux, C.; Tetu, B.; Meyer, F. & Fradet, Y. (2000). Tumorigenic pathways in low-stage bladder cancer based on p53, MDM2 and p21 phenotypes. *Int J Cancer*, Vol.89, No.1, pp. 100-104

Philp, E.A.; Stephenson, T.J. & Reed, M.W. (1996). Prognostic significance of angiogenesis in transitional cell carcinoma of the human urinary bladder. *Br J Urol*, Vol.77, No.3, pp. 352-357

Platt, F.M.; Hurst, C.D.; Taylor, C.F.; Gregory, W.M.; Harnden, P. & Knowles, M.A. (2009). Spectrum of phosphatidylinositol 3-kinase pathway gene alterations in bladder cancer. *Clin Cancer Res*, Vol.15, No.19, pp. 6008-6017

Ploeg, M.; Aben, K.K. & Kiemeney, L.A. (2009). The present and future burden of urinary bladder cancer in the world. *World J Urol*, Vol.27, No.3, pp. 289-293

Pollack, A.; Wu, C.S.; Czerniak, B.; Zagars, G.K.; Benedict, W.F. & McDonnell, T.J. (1997). Abnormal bcl-2 and pRb expression are independent correlates of radiation response in muscle-invasive bladder cancer. *Clin Cancer Res*, Vol.3, No.10, pp. 1823-1829

Polyak, K.; Lee, M.H.; Erdjument-Bromage, H.; Koff, A.; Roberts, J.M.; Tempst, P. & Massague, J. (1994). Cloning of p27Kip1, a cyclin-dependent kinase inhibitor and a potential mediator of extracellular antimitogenic signals. *Cell*, Vol.78, No.1, pp. 59-66

Popov, Z.; Gil-Diez de Medina, S.; Lefrere-Belda, M.A.; Hoznek, A.; Bastuji-Garin, S.; Abbou, C.C.; Thiery, J.P.; Radvanyi, F. & Chopin, D.K. (2000). Low E-cadherin expression in bladder cancer at the transcriptional and protein level provides prognostic information. *Br J Cancer*, Vol.83, No.2, pp. 209-214

Puzio-Kuter, A.M.; Castillo-Martin, M.; Kinkade, C.W.; Wang, X.; Shen, T.H.; Matos, T.; Shen, M.M.; Cordon-Cardo, C. & Abate-Shen, C. (2009). Inactivation of p53 and Pten promotes invasive bladder cancer. *Genes Dev*, Vol.23, No.6, pp. 675-680

Quelle, D.E.; Zindy, F.; Ashmun, R.A. & Sherr, C.J. (1995). Alternative reading frames of the INK4a tumor suppressor gene encode two unrelated proteins capable of inducing cell cycle arrest. *Cell*, Vol.83, No.6, pp. 993-1000

Rabbani, F. & Cordon-Cardo, C. (2000). Mutation of cell cycle regulators and their impact on superficial bladder cancer. *Urol Clin North Am*, Vol.27, No.1, pp. 83-102,

Rabbani, F.; Koppie, T.M.; Charytonowicz, E.; Drobnjak, M.; Bochner, B.H. & Cordon-Cardo, C. (2007). Prognostic significance of p27Kip1 expression in bladder cancer. *BJU Int*, Vol.100, No.2, pp. 259-263

Ravery, V.; Grignon, D.; Angulo, J.; Pontes, E.; Montie, J.; Crissman, J. & Chopin, D. (1997). Evaluation of epidermal growth factor receptor, transforming growth factor alpha, epidermal growth factor and c-erbB2 in the progression of invasive bladder cancer. *Urol Res*, Vol.25, No.1, pp. 9-17

Richter, J.; Beffa, L.; Wagner, U.; Schraml, P.; Gasser, T.C.; Moch, H.; Mihatsch, M.J. & Sauter, G. (1998). Patterns of chromosomal imbalances in advanced urinary bladder cancer detected by comparative genomic hybridization. *Am J Pathol*, Vol.153, No.5, pp. 1615-1621

Rieger-Christ, K.M.; Mourtzinos, A.; Lee, P.J.; Zagha, R.M.; Cain, J.; Silverman, M.; Libertino, J.A. & Summerhayes, I.C. (2003). Identification of fibroblast growth factor receptor 3 mutations in urine sediment DNA samples complements cytology in bladder tumor detection. *Cancer*, Vol.98, No.4, pp. 737-744

Rosen, E.M.; Joseph, A.; Jin, L.; Yao, Y.; Chau, M.H.; Fuchs, A.; Gomella, L.; Hastings, H.; Goldberg, I.D. & Weiss, G.H. (1997). Urinary and tissue levels of scatter factor in transitional cell carcinoma of bladder. *J Urol*, Vol.157, No.1, pp. 72-78

Rothman, N.; Garcia-Closas, M.; Chatterjee, N.; Malats, N.; Wu, X.; Figueroa, J.D.; Real, F.X.; Van Den Berg, D.; Matullo, G.; Baris, D.; Thun, M.; Kiemeney, L.A.; Vineis, P.; De Vivo, I.; Albanes, D.; Purdue, M.P.; Rafnar, T.; Hildebrandt, M.A.; Kiltie, A.E.; Cussenot, O.; Golka, K.; Kumar, R.; Taylor, J.A.; Mayordomo, J.I.; Jacobs, K.B.; Kogevinas, M.; Hutchinson, A.; Wang, Z.; Fu, Y.P.; Prokunina-Olsson, L.; Burdett, L.; Yeager, M.; Wheeler, W.; Tardon, A.; Serra, C.; Carrato, A.; Garcia-Closas, R.; Lloreta, J.; Johnson, A.; Schwenn, M.; Karagas, M.R.; Schned, A.; Andriole, G., Jr.; Grubb, R., 3rd; Black, A.; Jacobs, E.J.; Diver, W.R.; Gapstur, S.M.; Weinstein, S.J.; Virtamo, J.; Cortessis, V.K.; Gago-Dominguez, M.; Pike, M.C.; Stern, M.C.; Yuan, J.M.; Hunter, D.J.; McGrath, M.; Dinney, C.P.; Czerniak, B.; Chen, M.; Yang, H.; Vermeulen, S.H.; Aben, K.K.; Witjes, J.A.; Makkinje, R.R.; Sulem, P.; Besenbacher, S.; Stefansson, K.; Riboli, E.; Brennan, P.; Panico, S.; Navarro, C.; Allen, N.E.; Bueno-de-Mesquita, H.B.; Trichopoulos, D.; Caporaso, N.; Landi, M.T.; Canzian, F.; Ljungberg, B.; Tjonneland, A.; Clavel-Chapelon, F.; Bishop, D.T.; Teo, M.T.; Knowles, M.A.; Guarrera, S.; Polidoro, S.; Ricceri, F.; Sacerdote, C.; Allione, A.; Cancel-Tassin, G.; Selinski, S.; Hengstler, J.G.; Dietrich, H.; Fletcher, T.; Rudnai, P.; Gurzau, E.; Koppova, K.; Bolick, S.C.; Godfrey, A.; Xu, Z.; Sanz-Velez, J.I.; M, D.G.-P.; Sanchez, M.; Valdivia, G.; Porru, S.; Benhamou, S.; Hoover, R.N.; Fraumeni, J.F., Jr.; Silverman, D.T. & Chanock, S.J. (2010). A multi-stage genome-wide association study of bladder cancer identifies multiple susceptibility loci. *Nat Genet*, Vol.42, No.11, pp. 978-984

Rotterud, R.; Nesland, J.M.; Berner, A. & Fossa, S.D. (2005). Expression of the epidermal growth factor receptor family in normal and malignant urothelium. *BJU Int*, Vol.95, No.9, pp. 1344-1350

Sanchez-Carbayo, M.; Socci, N.D.; Kirchoff, T.; Erill, N.; Offit, K.; Bochner, B.H. & Cordon-Cardo, C. (2007). A polymorphism in HDM2 (SNP309) associates with early onset in superficial tumors, TP53 mutations, and poor outcome in invasive bladder cancer. *Clin Cancer Res*, Vol.13, No.11, pp. 3215-3220

Sanderson, S.; Salanti, G. & Higgins, J. (2007). Joint effects of the N-acetyltransferase 1 and 2 (NAT1 and NAT2) genes and smoking on bladder carcinogenesis: a literature-based systematic HuGE review and evidence synthesis. *Am J Epidemiol*, Vol.166, No.7, pp. 741-751

Sarkar, S.; Julicher, K.P.; Burger, M.S.; Della Valle, V.; Larsen, C.J.; Yeager, T.R.; Grossman, T.B.; Nickells, R.W.; Protzel, C.; Jarrard, D.F. & Reznikoff, C.A. (2000). Different combinations of genetic/epigenetic alterations inactivate the p53 and pRb pathways in invasive human bladder cancers. *Cancer Res*, Vol.60, No.14, pp. 3862-3871

Sarkis, A.S.; Dalbagni, G.; Cordon-Cardo, C.; Zhang, Z.F.; Sheinfeld, J.; Fair, W.R.; Herr, H.W. & Reuter, V.E. (1993). Nuclear overexpression of p53 protein in transitional cell bladder carcinoma: a marker for disease progression. *J Natl Cancer Inst*, Vol.85, No.1, pp. 53-59

Sarkis, A.S.; Bajorin, D.F.; Reuter, V.E.; Herr, H.W.; Netto, G.; Zhang, Z.F.; Schultz, P.K.; Cordon-Cardo, C. & Scher, H.I. (1995). Prognostic value of p53 nuclear overexpression in patients with invasive bladder cancer treated with neoadjuvant MVAC. *J Clin Oncol*, Vol.13, No.6, pp. 1384-1390

Sato, K.; Sasaki, R.; Ogura, Y.; Shimoda, N.; Togashi, H.; Terada, K.; Sugiyama, T.; Kakinuma, H.; Ogawa, O. & Kato, T. (1998). Expression of vascular endothelial growth factor gene and its receptor (flt-1) gene in urinary bladder cancer. *Tohoku J Exp Med*, Vol.185, No.3, pp. 173-184

Schultz, I.J.; Kiemeney, L.A.; Witjes, J.A.; Schalken, J.A.; Willems, J.L.; Swinkels, D.W. & de Kok, J.B. (2003). Survivin mRNA expression is elevated in malignant urothelial cell carcinomas and predicts time to recurrence. *Anticancer Res*, Vol.23, No.4, pp. 3327-3331

Schultz, L.; Albadine, R.; Hicks, J.; Jadallah, S.; DeMarzo, A.M.; Chen, Y.B.; Neilsen, M.E.; Gonzalgo, M.L.; Sidransky, D.; Schoenberg, M. & Netto, G.J. (2010). Expression status and prognostic significance of mammalian target of rapamycin pathway members in urothelial carcinoma of urinary bladder after cystectomy. *Cancer*, Vol.116, No.23, pp. 5517-5526

Seddighzadeh, M.; Steineck, G.; Larsson, P.; Wijkstrom, H.; Norming, U.; Onelov, E. & Linder, S. (2002). Expression of UPA and UPAR is associated with the clinical course of urinary bladder neoplasms. *Int J Cancer*, Vol.99, No.5, pp. 721-726

Serizawa, R.R.; Ralfkiaer, U.; Steven, K.; Lam, G.W.; Schmiedel, S.; Schuz, J.; Hansen, A.B.; Horn, T. & Guldberg, P. (2011). Integrated genetic and epigenetic analysis of bladder cancer reveals an additive diagnostic value of FGFR3 mutations and hypermethylation events. *Int J Cancer*, Vol.129, No.1, pp. 78-87

Serrano, M.; Hannon, G.J. & Beach, D. (1993). A new regulatory motif in cell-cycle control causing specific inhibition of cyclin D/CDK4. *Nature*, Vol.366, No.6456, pp. 704-707

Serth, J.; Kuczyk, M.A.; Bokemeyer, C.; Hervatin, C.; Nafe, R.; Tan, H.K. & Jonas, U. (1995). p53 immunohistochemistry as an independent prognostic factor for superficial transitional cell carcinoma of the bladder. *Br J Cancer*, Vol.71, No.1, pp. 201-205

Sgambato, A.; Migaldi, M.; Faraglia, B.; Garagnani, L.; Romano, G.; De Gaetani, C.; Ferrari, P.; Capelli, G.; Trentini, G.P. & Cittadini, A. (1999). Loss of P27Kip1 expression correlates with tumor grade and with reduced disease-free survival in primary superficial bladder cancers. *Cancer Res*, Vol.59, No.13, pp. 3245-3250

Shariat, S.F.; Monoski, M.A.; Andrews, B.; Wheeler, T.M.; Lerner, S.P. & Slawin, K.M. (2003). Association of plasma urokinase-type plasminogen activator and its receptor with clinical outcome in patients undergoing radical cystectomy for transitional cell carcinoma of the bladder. *Urology*, Vol.61, No.5, pp. 1053-1058

Shariat, S.F.; Tokunaga, H.; Zhou, J.; Kim, J.; Ayala, G.E.; Benedict, W.F. & Lerner, S.P. (2004). p53, p21, pRB, and p16 expression predict clinical outcome in cystectomy with bladder cancer. *J Clin Oncol*, Vol.22, No.6, pp. 1014-1024

Shariat, S.F.; Ashfaq, R.; Sagalowsky, A.I. & Lotan, Y. (2006). Correlation of cyclin D1 and E1 expression with bladder cancer presence, invasion, progression, and metastasis. *Hum Pathol*, Vol.37, No.12, pp. 1568-1576

Shariat, S.F.; Ashfaq, R.; Karakiewicz, P.I.; Saeedi, O.; Sagalowsky, A.I. & Lotan, Y. (2007a).
    Survivin expression is associated with bladder cancer presence, stage, progression,
    and mortality. *Cancer*, Vol.109, No.6, pp. 1106-1113
Shariat, S.F.; Ashfaq, R.; Sagalowsky, A.I. & Lotan, Y. (2007b). Association of cyclin D1 and
    E1 expression with disease progression and biomarkers in patients with
    nonmuscle-invasive urothelial cell carcinoma of the bladder. *Urol Oncol*, Vol.25,
    No.6, pp. 468-475
Shariat, S.F.; Ashfaq, R.; Sagalowsky, A.I. & Lotan, Y. (2007c). Predictive value of cell cycle
    biomarkers in nonmuscle invasive bladder transitional cell carcinoma. *J Urol*,
    Vol.177, No.2, pp. 481-487;
Shariat, S.F.; Zlotta, A.R.; Ashfaq, R.; Sagalowsky, A.I. & Lotan, Y. (2007d). Cooperative
    effect of cell-cycle regulators expression on bladder cancer development and
    biologic aggressiveness. *Mod Pathol*, Vol.20, No.4, pp. 445-459
Shariat, S.F.; Bolenz, C.; Godoy, G.; Fradet, Y.; Ashfaq, R.; Karakiewicz, P.I.; Isbarn, H.;
    Jeldres, C.; Rigaud, J.; Sagalowsky, A.I. & Lotan, Y. (2009a). Predictive value of
    combined immunohistochemical markers in patients with pT1 urothelial carcinoma
    at radical cystectomy. *J Urol*, Vol.182, No.1, pp. 78-84;
Shariat, S.F.; Lotan, Y.; Karakiewicz, P.I.; Ashfaq, R.; Isbarn, H.; Fradet, Y.; Bastian, P.J.;
    Nielsen, M.E.; Capitanio, U.; Jeldres, C.; Montorsi, F.; Muller, S.C.; Karam, J.A.;
    Heukamp, L.C.; Netto, G.; Lerner, S.P.; Sagalowsky, A.I. & Cote, R.J. (2009b). p53
    predictive value for pT1-2 N0 disease at radical cystectomy. *J Urol*, Vol.182, No.3,
    pp. 907-913
Shiff, C.; Naples, J.M.; Isharwal, S.; Bosompem, K.M. & Veltri, R.W. (2010). Non-invasive
    methods to detect schistosome-based bladder cancer: is the association sufficient
    for epidemiological use? *Trans R Soc Trop Med Hyg*, *Vol.104, No.1, pp. 3-5*
Shimazui, T.; Schalken, J.A.; Giroldi, L.A.; Jansen, C.F.; Akaza, H.; Koiso, K.; Debruyne, F.M.
    & Bringuier, P.P. (1996). Prognostic value of cadherin-associated molecules (alpha-,
    beta-, and gamma-catenins and p120cas) in bladder tumors. *Cancer Res*, Vol.56,
    No.18, pp. 4154-4158
Shinohara, A.; Sakano, S.; Hinoda, Y.; Nishijima, J.; Kawai, Y.; Misumi, T.; Nagao, K.; Hara,
    T. & Matsuyama, H. (2009). Association of TP53 and MDM2 polymorphisms with
    survival in bladder cancer patients treated with chemoradiotherapy. *Cancer Sci*,
    Vol.100, No.12, pp. 2376-2382
Sidransky, D.; Von Eschenbach, A.; Tsai, Y.C.; Jones, P.; Summerhayes, I.; Marshall, F.; Paul,
    M.; Green, P.; Hamilton, S.R.; Frost, P. & et al. (1991). Identification of p53 gene
    mutations in bladder cancers and urine samples. *Science*, Vol.252, No.5006, pp. 706-
    709
Sier, C.F.; Casetta, G.; Verheijen, J.H.; Tizzani, A.; Agape, V.; Kos, J.; Blasi, F. & Hanemaaijer,
    R. (2000). Enhanced urinary gelatinase activities (matrix metalloproteinases 2 and
    9) are associated with early-stage bladder carcinoma: a comparison with clinically
    used tumor markers. *Clin Cancer Res*, Vol.6, No.6, pp. 2333-2340
Simon, R.; Burger, H.; Semjonow, A.; Hertle, L.; Terpe, H.J. & Bocker, W. (2000). Patterns of
    chromosomal imbalances in muscle invasive bladder cancer. *Int J Oncol*, Vol.17,
    No.5, pp. 1025-1029
Simon, R.; Struckmann, K.; Schraml, P.; Wagner, U.; Forster, T.; Moch, H.; Fijan, A.;
    Bruderer, J.; Wilber, K.; Mihatsch, M.J.; Gasser, T. & Sauter, G. (2002). Amplification

pattern of 12q13-q15 genes (MDM2, CDK4, GLI) in urinary bladder cancer. *Oncogene*, Vol.21, No.16, pp. 2476-2483

Simoneau, M.; LaRue, H.; Aboulkassim, T.O.; Meyer, F.; Moore, L. & Fradet, Y. (2000). Chromosome 9 deletions and recurrence of superficial bladder cancer: identification of four regions of prognostic interest. *Oncogene*, Vol.19, No.54, pp. 6317-6323

Slaton, J.W.; Millikan, R.; Inoue, K.; Karashima, T.; Czerniak, B.; Shen, Y.; Yang, Y.; Benedict, W.F. & Dinney, C.P. (2004). Correlation of metastasis related gene expression and relapse-free survival in patients with locally advanced bladder cancer treated with cystectomy and chemotherapy. *J Urol*, Vol.171, No.2 Pt 1, pp. 570-574

Stadler, W.M. (2009). Randomized trial of p53 targeted adjuvant therapy for patients (pts) with organ- confined node-negative urothelial bladder cancer (UBC). *J Clin Oncol*, Vol.27, No.15s, abstract 5017

Stein, J.P.; Ginsberg, D.A.; Grossfeld, G.D.; Chatterjee, S.J.; Esrig, D.; Dickinson, M.G.; Groshen, S.; Taylor, C.R.; Jones, P.A.; Skinner, D.G. & Cote, R.J. (1998). Effect of p21WAF1/CIP1 expression on tumor progression in bladder cancer. *J Natl Cancer Inst*, Vol.90, No.14, pp. 1072-1079

Strope, S.A. & Montie, J.E. (2008). The causal role of cigarette smoking in bladder cancer initiation and progression, and the role of urologists in smoking cessation. *J Urol*, Vol.180, No.1, pp. 31-37;

Sun, C.H.; Chang, Y.H. & Pan, C.C. (2011). Activation of the PI3K/Akt/mTOR pathway correlates with tumour progression and reduced survival in patients with urothelial carcinoma of the urinary bladder. *Histopathology*, Vol.58, No.7, pp. 1054-1063

Svatek, R.S.; Herman, M.P.; Lotan, Y.; Casella, R.; Hsieh, J.T.; Sagalowsky, A.I. & Shariat, S.F. (2006). Soluble Fas--a promising novel urinary marker for the detection of recurrent superficial bladder cancer. *Cancer*, Vol.106, No.8, pp. 1701-1707

Swana, H.S.; Grossman, D.; Anthony, J.N.; Weiss, R.M. & Altieri, D.C. (1999). Tumor content of the antiapoptosis molecule survivin and recurrence of bladder cancer. *N Engl J Med*, Vol.341, No.6, pp. 452-453

Sylvester, R.J.; van der Meijden, A.P.; Oosterlinck, W.; Witjes, J.A.; Bouffioux, C.; Denis, L.; Newling, D.W. & Kurth, K. (2006). Predicting recurrence and progression in individual patients with stage Ta T1 bladder cancer using EORTC risk tables: a combined analysis of 2596 patients from seven EORTC trials. *Eur Urol*, Vol.49, No.3, pp. 466-465; discussion 475-467

Szarvas, T.; Jager, T.; Totsch, M.; vom Dorp, F.; Kempkensteffen, C.; Kovalszky, I.; Romics, I.; Ergun, S. & Rubben, H. (2008). Angiogenic switch of angiopietins-Tie2 system and its prognostic value in bladder cancer. *Clin Cancer Res*, Vol.14, No.24, pp. 8253-8262

Takahashi, R.; Hashimoto, T.; Xu, H.J.; Hu, S.X.; Matsui, T.; Miki, T.; Bigo-Marshall, H.; Aaronson, S.A. & Benedict, W.F. (1991). The retinoblastoma gene functions as a growth and tumor suppressor in human bladder carcinoma cells. *Proc Natl Acad Sci U S A*, Vol.88, No.12, pp. 5257-5261

Teng, D.H.; Hu, R.; Lin, H.; Davis, T.; Iliev, D.; Frye, C.; Swedlund, B.; Hansen, K.L.; Vinson, V.L.; Gumpper, K.L.; Ellis, L.; El-Naggar, A.; Frazier, M.; Jasser, S.; Langford, L.A.; Lee, J.; Mills, G.B.; Pershouse, M.A.; Pollack, R.E.; Tornos, C.; Troncoso, P.; Yung, W.K.; Fujii, G.; Berson, A.; Steck, P.A. & et al. (1997). MMAC1/PTEN mutations in primary tumor specimens and tumor cell lines. *Cancer Res*, Vol.57, No.23, pp. 5221-5225

Theodoropoulos, V.E.; Lazaris, A.; Sofras, F.; Gerzelis, I.; Tsoukala, V.; Ghikonti, I.; Manikas, K. & Kastriotis, I. (2004). Hypoxia-inducible factor 1 alpha expression correlates with angiogenesis and unfavorable prognosis in bladder cancer. *Eur Urol*, Vol.46, No.2, pp. 200-208

Theodoropoulos, V.E.; Lazaris, A.C.; Kastriotis, I.; Spiliadi, C.; Theodoropoulos, G.E.; Tsoukala, V.; Patsouris, E. & Sofras, F. (2005). Evaluation of hypoxia-inducible factor 1alpha overexpression as a predictor of tumour recurrence and progression in superficial urothelial bladder carcinoma. *BJU Int*, Vol.95, No.3, pp. 425-431

Thogersen, V.B.; Sorensen, B.S.; Poulsen, S.S.; Orntoft, T.F.; Wolf, H. & Nexo, E. (2001). A subclass of HER1 ligands are prognostic markers for survival in bladder cancer patients. *Cancer Res*, Vol.61, No.16, pp. 6227-6233

Tsuruta, H.; Kishimoto, H.; Sasaki, T.; Horie, Y.; Natsui, M.; Shibata, Y.; Hamada, K.; Yajima, N.; Kawahara, K.; Sasaki, M.; Tsuchiya, N.; Enomoto, K.; Mak, T.W.; Nakano, T.; Habuchi, T. & Suzuki, A. (2006). Hyperplasia and carcinomas in Pten-deficient mice and reduced PTEN protein in human bladder cancer patients. *Cancer Res*, Vol.66, No.17, pp. 8389-8396

Turkeri, L.N.; Erton, M.L.; Cevik, I. & Akdas, A. (1998). Impact of the expression of epidermal growth factor, transforming growth factor alpha, and epidermal growth factor receptor on the prognosis of superficial bladder cancer. *Urology*, Vol.51, No.4, pp. 645-649

Tut, V.M.; Braithwaite, K.L.; Angus, B.; Neal, D.E.; Lunec, J. & Mellon, J.K. (2001). Cyclin D1 expression in transitional cell carcinoma of the bladder: correlation with p53, waf1, pRb and Ki67. *Br J Cancer*, Vol.84, No.2, pp. 270-275

van Oers, J.M.; Wild, P.J.; Burger, M.; Denzinger, S.; Stoehr, R.; Rosskopf, E.; Hofstaedter, F.; Steyerberg, E.W.; Klinkhammer-Schalke, M.; Zwarthoff, E.C.; van der Kwast, T.H. & Hartmann, A. (2007). FGFR3 mutations and a normal CK20 staining pattern define low-grade noninvasive urothelial bladder tumours. *Eur Urol*, Vol.52, No.3, pp. 760-768

van Oers, J.M.; Zwarthoff, E.C.; Rehman, I.; Azzouzi, A.R.; Cussenot, O.; Meuth, M.; Hamdy, F.C. & Catto, J.W. (2009). FGFR3 mutations indicate better survival in invasive upper urinary tract and bladder tumours. *Eur Urol*, Vol.55, No.3, pp. 650-657

van Rhijn, B.W.; Lurkin, I.; Radvanyi, F.; Kirkels, W.J.; van der Kwast, T.H. & Zwarthoff, E.C. (2001). The fibroblast growth factor receptor 3 (FGFR3) mutation is a strong indicator of superficial bladder cancer with low recurrence rate. *Cancer Res*, Vol.61, No.4, pp. 1265-1268

van Rhijn, B.W.; van der Kwast, T.H.; Vis, A.N.; Kirkels, W.J.; Boeve, E.R.; Jobsis, A.C. & Zwarthoff, E.C. (2004). FGFR3 and P53 characterize alternative genetic pathways in the pathogenesis of urothelial cell carcinoma. *Cancer Res*, Vol.64, No.6, pp. 1911-1914

van Rhijn, B.W.; Burger, M.; Lotan, Y.; Solsona, E.; Stief, C.G.; Sylvester, R.J.; Witjes, J.A. & Zlotta, A.R. (2009). Recurrence and Progression of Disease in Non-Muscle-Invasive Bladder Cancer: From Epidemiology to Treatment Strategy. *Eur Urol*, *Vol.56, No.3, pp. 430-442*

van Rhijn, B.W.; Zuiverloon, T.C.; Vis, A.N.; Radvanyi, F.; van Leenders, G.J.; Ooms, B.C.; Kirkels, W.J.; Lockwood, G.A.; Boeve, E.R.; Jobsis, A.C.; Zwarthoff, E.C. & van der

Kwast, T.H. (2010). Molecular grade (FGFR3/MIB-1) and EORTC risk scores are predictive in primary non-muscle-invasive bladder cancer. *Eur Urol*, Vol.58, No.3, pp. 433-441

Vasala, K.; Paakko, P. & Turpeenniemi-Hujanen, T. (2003). Matrix metalloproteinase-2 immunoreactive protein as a prognostic marker in bladder cancer. *Urology*, Vol.62, No.5, pp. 952-957

Wada, T.; Louhelainen, J.; Hemminki, K.; Adolfsson, J.; Wijkstrom, H.; Norming, U.; Borgstrom, E.; Hansson, J.; Sandstedt, B. & Steineck, G. (2000). Bladder cancer: allelic deletions at and around the retinoblastoma tumor suppressor gene in relation to stage and grade. *Clin Cancer Res*, Vol.6, No.2, pp. 610-615

Waldman, T.; Lengauer, C.; Kinzler, K.W. & Vogelstein, B. (1996). Uncoupling of S phase and mitosis induced by anticancer agents in cells lacking p21. *Nature*, Vol.381, No.6584, pp. 713-716

Wallard, M.J.; Pennington, C.J.; Veerakumarasivam, A.; Burtt, G.; Mills, I.G.; Warren, A.; Leung, H.Y.; Murphy, G.; Edwards, D.R.; Neal, D.E. & Kelly, J.D. (2006). Comprehensive profiling and localisation of the matrix metalloproteinases in urothelial carcinoma. *Br J Cancer*, Vol.94, No.4, pp. 569-577

Wang, P.; Nishitani, M.A.; Tanimoto, S.; Kishimoto, T.; Fukumori, T.; Takahashi, M. & Kanayama, H.O. (2007). Bladder cancer cell invasion is enhanced by cross-talk with fibroblasts through hepatocyte growth factor. *Urology*, Vol.69, No.4, pp. 780-784

Weikert, S.; Christoph, F.; Schrader, M.; Krause, H.; Miller, K. & Muller, M. (2005a). Quantitative analysis of survivin mRNA expression in urine and tumor tissue of bladder cancer patients and its potential relevance for disease detection and prognosis. *Int J Cancer*, Vol.116, No.1, pp. 100-104

Weikert, S.; Krause, H.; Wolff, I.; Christoph, F.; Schrader, M.; Emrich, T.; Miller, K. & Muller, M. (2005b). Quantitative evaluation of telomerase subunits in urine as biomarkers for noninvasive detection of bladder cancer. *Int J Cancer*, Vol.117, No.2, pp. 274-280

Weiss, C.; von Romer, F.; Capalbo, G.; Ott, O.J.; Wittlinger, M.; Krause, S.F.; Sauer, R.; Rodel, C. & Rodel, F. (2009). Survivin expression as a predictive marker for local control in patients with high-risk T1 bladder cancer treated with transurethral resection and radiochemotherapy. *Int J Radiat Oncol Biol Phys*, Vol.74, No.5, pp. 1455-1460

Williams, S.G. & Stein, J.P. (2004). Molecular pathways in bladder cancer. *Urol Res*, Vol.32, No.6, pp. 373-385

Williams, S.V.; Sibley, K.D.; Davies, A.M.; Nishiyama, H.; Hornigold, N.; Coulter, J.; Kennedy, W.J.; Skilleter, A.; Habuchi, T. & Knowles, M.A. (2002). Molecular genetic analysis of chromosome 9 candidate tumor-suppressor loci in bladder cancer cell lines. *Genes Chromosomes Cancer*, Vol.34, No.1, pp. 86-96

Williamson, M.P.; Elder, P.A.; Shaw, M.E.; Devlin, J. & Knowles, M.A. (1995). p16 (CDKN2) is a major deletion target at 9p21 in bladder cancer. *Hum Mol Genet*, Vol.4, No.9, pp. 1569-1577

Wolf, H.K.; Stober, C.; Hohenfellner, R. & Leissner, J. (2001). Prognostic value of p53, p21/WAF1, Bcl-2, Bax, Bak and Ki-67 immunoreactivity in pT1 G3 urothelial bladder carcinomas. *Tumour Biol*, Vol.22, No.5, pp. 328-336

Wu, X.; Bayle, J.H.; Olson, D. & Levine, A.J. (1993). The p53-mdm-2 autoregulatory feedback loop. *Genes Dev*, Vol.7, No.7A, pp. 1126-1132

Wu, X.; Obata, T.; Khan, Q.; Highshaw, R.A.; De Vere White, R. & Sweeney, C. (2004). The phosphatidylinositol-3 kinase pathway regulates bladder cancer cell invasion. *BJU Int*, Vol.93, No.1, pp. 143-150

Wu, X. (2005). Urothelial tumorigenesis: a tale of divergent pathways. *Nat Rev Cancer*, Vol.5, No.9, pp. 713-725

Wu, X.; Ye, Y.; Kiemeney, L.A.; Sulem, P.; Rafnar, T.; Matullo, G.; Seminara, D.; Yoshida, T.; Saeki, N.; Andrew, A.S.; Dinney, C.P.; Czerniak, B.; Zhang, Z.F.; Kiltie, A.E.; Bishop, D.T.; Vineis, P.; Porru, S.; Buntinx, F.; Kellen, E.; Zeegers, M.P.; Kumar, R.; Rudnai, P.; Gurzau, E.; Koppova, K.; Mayordomo, J.I.; Sanchez, M.; Saez, B.; Lindblom, A.; de Verdier, P.; Steineck, G.; Mills, G.B.; Schned, A.; Guarrera, S.; Polidoro, S.; Chang, S.C.; Lin, J.; Chang, D.W.; Hale, K.S.; Majewski, T.; Grossman, H.B.; Thorlacius, S.; Thorsteinsdottir, U.; Aben, K.K.; Witjes, J.A.; Stefansson, K.; Amos, C.I.; Karagas, M.R. & Gu, J. (2009). Genetic variation in the prostate stem cell antigen gene PSCA confers susceptibility to urinary bladder cancer. *Nat Genet*, Vol.41, No.9, pp. 991-995

Xia, G.; Kumar, S.R.; Hawes, D.; Cai, J.; Hassanieh, L.; Groshen, S.; Zhu, S.; Masood, R.; Quinn, D.I.; Broek, D.; Stein, J.P. & Gill, P.S. (2006). Expression and significance of vascular endothelial growth factor receptor 2 in bladder cancer. *J Urol*, Vol.175, No.4, pp. 1245-1252

Xu, H.J.; Cairns, P.; Hu, S.X.; Knowles, M.A. & Benedict, W.F. (1993). Loss of RB protein expression in primary bladder cancer correlates with loss of heterozygosity at the RB locus and tumor progression. *Int J Cancer*, Vol.53, No.5, pp. 781-784

Yamana, K.; Bilim, V.; Hara, N.; Kasahara, T.; Itoi, T.; Maruyama, R.; Nishiyama, T.; Takahashi, K. & Tomita, Y. (2005). Prognostic impact of FAS/CD95/APO-1 in urothelial cancers: decreased expression of Fas is associated with disease progression. *Br J Cancer*, Vol.93, No.5, pp. 544-551

Part 2

Epidemiology, Biomarkers and Prognostic Factors

2

Epigenetic Biomarkers in Bladder Cancer

Daniela Zimbardi, Mariana Bisarro dos Reis,
Érika da Costa Prando and Cláudia Aparecida Rainho
Department of Genetics, Institute of Biosciences, Sao Paulo State University – UNESP,
Botucatu – SP,
Brazil

1. Introduction

1.1 Epigenetics and cancer: An overview

Genetic and epigenetic alterations are hallmarks of human cancer. In the last few decades, it has been well established that epigenetic changes are important events in human cancer development and progression in addition to genetic alterations (such as chromosomal rearrangements, aneuploidies and point mutations). Epigenetics refers to the study of changes in gene expression that are determined by mechanisms other than changes in the DNA sequence. Epigenetic phenomena include X-chromosome inactivation, genomic imprinting, cellular differentiation and the maintenance of cell identity. These events are mediated by several molecular mechanisms, including DNA methylation, post-translational histone modifications and various RNA-mediated processes. Many studies in the field of epigenetics have focused on the effects of histone modifications and DNA methylation in the transcription process because these mechanisms are often linked and interdependent (Ballestar, 2011). A variety of methods are currently being applied to detect epigenetic changes, and the past two decades have shown an exponential increase in novel approaches aimed at elucidating the molecular basis of epigenetic inheritance.

DNA methylation is the most well studied epigenetic modification in human diseases (Fernandez et al., 2011). It involves the addition of a methyl group to the 5 carbon of a cytosine that is immediately followed by one guanine; i.e., DNA methylation typically occurs in a CpG dinucleotide context. CpG dinucleotides are generally underrepresented in the genome due to the increased mutation frequencies of the methylcytosines that are spontaneously converted to thymines. However, within the regions that are known as CpG islands, these dinucleotides are found at higher frequencies than is expected. It is believed that the human genome is comprised of approximately 38,000 CpG islands, and a large proportion of them (~37%) are located in the 5′ gene regulatory regions (promoters). The aberrant content of DNA methylation (global genome hypomethylation) and patterns of cytosine methylation, especially hypermethylation in promoter-associated CpG islands, are known to be associated with cancer. Gene-specific promoter hypermethylation causes the breakdown of normal cell physiology by silencing tumor suppressor genes, while DNA hypomethylation can reactivate oncogenes and repetitive sequences of the genome and lead to chromosomal instability (Sawan et al., 2008).

Histones (H2A, H2B, H3 and H4) are the main protein components of chromatin that package and order DNA into structural units that are called nucleosomes. The histone code consists of post-translational covalent changes of specific amino acid residues that are located at histone tails (NH_2 terminal regions). These modifications include methylation, acetylation, phosphorylation, poly-ADP ribosylation, ubiquitinylation, sumoylation, carbonylation and glycosylation (Kouzarides, 2007). The histone code and DNA methylation interact to promote the regulation of specific gene activity and mediate chromatin accessibility and compaction by changing the local chromatin structure, as has been reported to occur during the silencing of tumor suppressor genes. In cancer cells, the hypermethylation of CpG islands in the promoter regions of tumor suppressor genes was associated with a specific profile of histone markers such as the loss of acetylation of histones H3 and H4, loss of H3K4 trimethylation, and gains of methylation in lysine residues of histone H3 (such as H3K9 and H3K27) (Portela & Esteller, 2010).

The most recently discovered epigenetic modification is mediated by a small class of RNAs that are also known as microRNAs (miRNAs). These molecules promote the silencing of target genes by associating with the 3' untranslated region of messenger RNA (mRNA), which culminates in endonucleolytic cleavage, mRNA degradation by deadenylation or the inhibition of mRNA translation (Valeri et al., 2009). It is estimated that at least 30% of all human genes are regulated by miRNAs. Similar to the protein-coding genes, the down-regulation of miRNAs in cancer cells has been correlated with the presence of DNA hypermethylation in the regulatory regions. In addition, these molecules (named epi-miRNAs) were recently found to regulate epigenetic enzymes, such as DNA methyltransferases and histone deacetylases. Thus, it is possible that epi-miRNAs could indirectly affect the expression of cancer-related genes (Fabbri & Callin, 2010).

In summary, epigenetics is one of the most promising fields in biomedical research. Novel strategies for risk assessment, early detection and new therapeutic targets may be revealed by epigenetic studies (Boumber & Issa, 2011). This chapter will summarize the common epigenetic aberrations that are detected in bladder cancer, their translational implications and possible epigenetic therapies.

2. Translational implications of epigenetic changes in bladder cancer

Bladder cancer is the fifth most commonly diagnosed non-cutaneous solid tumor and the second most common in the urological tract. Although many tumors that originate in this organ are superficial, with low risks of metastasis, bladder cancer has a high recurrence risk; the 4-year recurrence rate for patients with superficial tumors is 50%. Currently, the diagnosis of bladder cancer is based on histological, pathological and morphological parameters and provides only a generalized outcome for patients (Tanaka & Sonpadvde, 2011). The gold standard for detecting bladder cancer is cystoscopic examination, but this analysis is costly, causes discomfort to the patient (invasive method) and has variable sensitivity, providing only a generalized outcome to patients. In addition, the sensitivity of the cytological analysis is questionable, especially in cases of low-grade carcinoma (Kim & Kim, 2009). With the advent of targeted therapy, molecular biomarkers are becoming increasingly important in both clinical research and practice. These markers are being identified with the purpose of reducing the need for invasive follow-up examinations and also to anticipate the prognosis of individual patients. Furthermore, the early diagnosis of bladder cancer by non-invasive methods could allow for more effective treatment and optimize the success of surgical therapy.

The DNA methylation of CpG islands that are mapped to promoter regions of specific genes, such as tumor suppressor genes, has been extensively reported in many cancer types. In bladder cancer, this epigenetic event has been related to tumor development, staging, recurrence, progression and clinical outcome. More specifically, DNA methylation has been strongly associated with higher stages, high rates of tumor progression and high mortality in patients with this cancer. As was demonstrated by Wolff et al. (2010), the analysis of epigenetic backgrounds can allow for the differentiation between noninvasive and invasive tumors by the identification of the different epigenetic characteristics that are present, such as the extensive DNA hypomethylation that is observed in noninvasive tumors compared to the high rates of DNA hypermethylation in invasive urothelial cancer. This may explain why ~15% of tumors will progress to invasive disease and have poor prognosis, while others will remain with low rates of generate metastasis.

Currently, some histone modifications and the aberrant expression of miRNAs have been linked to tumorigenesis and have also been identified to be reliable and strong biomarkers for bladder cancer. MicroRNAs are specifically interesting because they are very stable in body fluids due to their small sizes and thus are resistant to degradation by nucleases, which are present in large quantities in urine (Tilki et al., 2011).

2.1 Candidate epigenetic biomarkers in the diagnosis of bladder cancer

Because DNA methylation is chemically and biologically stable and can be detected early in the carcinogenesis process, this epigenetic change has been considered to be a valuable potential diagnostic marker that is feasible to assess in clinical routine analysis through the investigation of exfoliated cells in the urine or blood of patients with bladder cancer and appears to be more sensitive than conventional cytology. A number of genes have been identified as being hypermethylated in the urine or tissue samples of cancer patients compared to healthy tissues, indicating that the down-regulation of these genes has some clinical relevance to the origin and development of the disease (Table 1).

One example is the *RUNX3* (runt-related transcription factor 3) gene, which has been mapped to 1p36 and is thought to be a tumor suppressor gene that is frequently deleted or transcriptionally silenced in patients with cancer. In a study that analyzed 124 tumor tissue samples, 73% were found to have a methylation-positive pattern compared to the methylation-free pattern that was exhibited by the normal bladder mucosa. Moreover, the methylation of this gene was found to confer a significant increase (100-fold) in the risk of tumor development (Kim et al., 2005), suggesting that it may have potential as a potent bladder cancer detection marker.

Our group also contributed to the literature surrounding epigenetic markers in bladder cancer. We discovered high rates of DNA methylation in exfoliated urinary cells, in which the *RARB* gene had a sensitivity of 95% and specificity of 71% for detecting the presence of cancer (Negraes et al., 2008). These results are concordant with the increased methylation frequencies that have been previously described (Chan et al., 2002; Hoque et al., 2006) and suggest that this gene could be considered as a diagnostic biomarker. It encodes a member of the thyroid-steroid hormone receptor superfamily of nuclear transcriptional regulators that binds retinoic acid (the biologically active form of vitamin A) and also mediates cellular signaling during embryonic morphogenesis and cell growth and differentiation. It is thought that this protein limits the growth of many cell types by regulating gene expression (Soprano et al., 2004).

In the study conducted by Renard et al. (2010), it was demonstrated that 2 genes (*TWIST1* and *NID2*) were frequently methylated in urine samples collected from bladder cancer patients, including those with early-stage and low-grade diseases, with a specificity of 93% and sensitivity of 90%, which was an improvement from the cytological method of detection (48%).

Besides the identification of DNA hypermethylation at a single *locus*, some authors have demonstrated that several genes may be analyzed together to generate a profile of hypermethylated genes. These profiles may be able to allow for a more sensitive and reliable marker for the detection of bladder cancer (Table 1). Based on this, Chan et al. (2002) discovered that the sensitivity of the methylation analysis (90.9%) of four genes (*DAPK1*, *RARB*, *CDH1* and *CDKN2A*) was higher than that of urine cytology (45.5%) for cancer detection and was more striking in low-grade cases (100% versus 11.1%).

Similarly, Urakami et al. (2006) found that the identification of the increased methylation of six Wnt-antagonist genes (*SFRP1*, *SFRP2*, *SFRP4*, *SFRP5*, *WIF1* and *DKK3*) could predict bladder tumors with a sensitivity of 77.2% and specificity of 66.7%. These genes are known to inhibit Wnt signaling by binding to specific molecules that act in this pathway. The DNA methylation and consequent functional loss of these genes may result in the activation of the Wnt signaling pathway and promote the dysregulation of cell proliferation and differentiation. The authors also discovered that two of these genes (*SFRP2* and *DKK3*) were able to act as independent predictors of bladder tumors ($P < 0.05$ and $P < 0.01$, respectively).

Friedrich et al. (2004) also suggested that the presence of a combination of DNA methylation at the 5′ regions of three apoptosis-associated genes (*DAPK1, BCL2* and *TERT*) in urine sediment could be diagnostic of bladder cancer with a sensitivity of 78%, suggesting that this combined methylation analysis was a highly sensitive method for the noninvasive detection of bladder cancer.

In addition, Hoque et al. (2006) proposed a two-stage predictor for the classification of bladder cancer that was based on an investigation of a panel composed of nine genes (*APC, ARF, CDH1, GSTP1, MGMT, CDKN2A, RARB, RASSF1A* and *TIMP3*) in urine sediment. In the first stage, patients who presented with DNA methylation in the promoters of at least one of four specific genes (*CDKN2A, ARF, MGMT* and *GSTP1*) were classified as having cancer (100% specificity). Moreover, patients with no methylation in these genes were subjected to a second stage of investigation with a logistic prediction of risk scores based on the promoter methylation of the five remaining genes (sensitivity of 82% and specificity of 96%).

Three of these genes had previously been investigated by Dulaimi et al. (2004), who demonstrated the feasibility of obtaining reproducible highly sensitive (87%) and 100% positive identifications of hypermethylation in a panel composed of the *APC, RASSF1A* and *CDKN2A* tumor suppressor genes in urine in cases of early-stage disease. In addition to *RASSF1A* (a tumor suppressor gene that is frequently inactivated in several cancer types), the other two genes chosen were involved in the $p53/p14^{ARF}$ tumor suppressor gene pathway (*CDKN2A* gene) (Sherr & McCormick, 2002) and the Wnt signaling pathway (*APC* gene) (Taipale & Beachy, 2001). The evaluation of this panel yielded superior results compared to those of cytology in the detection of bladder cancer. Yates et al. (2006) also investigated the *APC, RASSF1A* and *CDH1* genes in urine. This panel generated a lower sensitivity (69%) and specificity (60%) than the former; however, the diagnostic accuracy was 86%.

Many of the genes that have been chosen to be investigated in combined analyses to generate panels have frequently been suggested to be individually methylated in bladder cancer, such as *RASSF1A*. The DNA methylation of this gene had previously been reported to be able to detect bladder cancer in urine samples with 100% sensitivity by Chan et al. 2003). The authors advocated that the detection of gene methylation using multiple markers could increase both the sensitivity and specificity of cancer detection, and the addition of *RASSF1A* to this panel could improve the diagnostic accuracy even further.

Yu et al. (2007) discovered that the methylation of a panel composed by 11 genes (*SALL3, CFTR, ABCC6, HPSE, RASSF1A, MT1A, ALX4, CDH13, RPRM, APBA1* and *BRCA1*) in urine sediments showed positive correlations with diagnosis in 121 out of 132 bladder cancer cases with a sensitivity of 91.7% and accuracy of 87%. Remarkably, this approach was able to detect more than 75% of tumors at stage 0a and 88% of stage I tumors, indicating the value of this panel in the early diagnosis of bladder cancer.

Likewise, a three-gene (*GDF15, TMEFF2* and *VIM*) panel was able to detect bladder cancer in urine samples with a sensitivity of 94% and specificity of 100% (Costa et al., 2010), exceeding the detection rates that are normally obtained using conventional cytopathology and cytology. This panel of genes was selected based on stringent criteria after a screening test that employed a genome-wide approach and was distinctive because it was able to detect bladder cancer by noninvasive methods even when patients with kidney or prostate cancer were used as controls. These three genes are biologically relevant to carcinogenesis because *TMEFF2* (mapped at 2q32.3) and *VIM* (mapped at 10p13) were previously found to be silenced by promoter methylation in esophageal, colorectal (Shirahata et al., 2009; Tsunoda et al., 2009) and bladder cancer (Hellwinkel et al., 2008). *GDF15* (mapped to 19p13.11) is a member of the transforming growth factor (TGF)-β superfamily and may act as a tumor suppressor gene in early-stage cancers (Eling et al., 2006).

Another biomarker of interest for the detection of urothelial cancer, according to Ellinger et al. (2008), is cell-free serum DNA methylation. The authors detected that the diagnostic accuracy of this marker increased when hypermethylation at multiple gene sites was assessed simultaneously, particularly at the *GSTP1, RARRES1* or *APC* genes (80% sensitivity and 93% specificity).

The list of aberrant epigenetically regulated genes continues to grow. Is important to note that the same genes have been investigated by different groups, and the methylation rates found may vary from one report to another. Results may reflect the distinct methodologies employed, the numbers and types of samples (urine, surgical tissue and/or serum) as well as disease classifications. Nevertheless, the reports above highlight the high potential of DNA methylation markers for the effective early detection of bladder cancer using noninvasive urine tests.

The measurement of global cytosine methylation rates (%5-mC) concomitantly with the DNA methylation of specific genes could be a useful biomarker to assess a patient's susceptibility to bladder cancer. In a large case-control study conducted by Moore et al. 2008), the DNA hypomethylation of leukocytes was strongly associated with an increased bladder cancer risk, and this association was independent of smoking and other assessed risk factors.

Recently, evidence has emerged that circulating miRNAs are present in human body fluids (as urine) in concentrations that are subject to variation during cancer pathogenesis or development (Iguchi et al., 2010), as was reported by Dudziec et al. (2011). The authors discovered that the combined low expression levels of miR-152, -328 and -1224-3p allowed for accurate diagnosis with 81% sensitivity and 75% specificity. These miRNAs were found to be epigenetically regulated by DNA methylation at CpG islands and the shores (regions of less dense CpG dinucleotides) that surrounded them following a genome-wide screening. In addition, Hanke et al. (2010) found that the ratio of miR-126:miR-152 enabled the detection of bladder cancer from urine samples with a specificity of 82% and a sensitivity of 72%; thus, they may be used as a tumor markers for this disease.

In addition, Yamada et al. (2011) identified one microRNA (miR-96) that may be a useful diagnostic marker with high sensitivity and specificity (71.0% and 89.2%, respectively) when assessed in combination with urinary cytology (80% diagnostic accuracy). This molecule, which has been mapped to 7q32, is a putative onco-miRNA that has been demonstrated to be able to down-regulate tumor suppressor genes. It was found to be up-regulated in a previous study conducted by the same group (Ichimi et al., 2009), in which the microRNA expression signatures that are specific to bladder cancer were determined, and a subset of 7 microRNAs (miR-145, miR-30a-3p, miR-133a, miR-133b, miR-195, miR-125b and miR-199a*) that are significantly down-regulated in bladder cancer were validated. These microRNAs were sufficiently sensitive (>70%) and specific (>75%) to distinguish bladder cancer from normal epithelium.

As mentioned above, not only the DNA methylation but also the expression profile of the miRNA molecules have been closely associated with the diagnosis of bladder cancer.

Epigenetic biomarker	Samples	Sensitivity/ specificity/ OR	Supporting literature
DNA methylation			
RASSF1A	Urine	Sensitivity: 100%	Chan et al., 2003
RUNX3	Tissue	OR 107.55 (95% CI, 6.33-1827.39)	Kim et al., 2005
RARB	Bladder washing (exfoliated cells)	OR/Sensitivity/specificity: 48.89/95%/71%	Negraes et al., 2008
TWIST1 and NID2	Urine	Sensitivity/specificity: 90%/93%	Renard et a., 2010
DAPK1, RARB, CDH1 and CDKN2A	Urine	Sensitivity/specificity: 90.9%/76.4%	Chan et al., 2002
APC, RASSF1A and CDKN2A	Urine	Sensitivity/specificity: 87%/100%	Dulaimi et al., 2004
DAPK1, BCL2 and TERT	Urine	Sensitivity: 78%	Friedrich et al., 2004
APC, ARF, CDH1, GSTP1, MGMT, CDKN2A, RARB, RASSF1A and TIMP3	Urine	1st stage sensitivity: 100% 2nd stage Sensitivity/specificity: 82%/96%	Hoque et al., 2006
SFRP1, SFRP2, SFRP4, SFRP5, WIF1, DKK3	Tissue	Sensitivity/specificity: 77.2%/66.7%	Urakami et al., 2006
APC, RASSF1A and	Urine	Sensitivity/specificity:	Yates et al., 2006

Epigenetic biomarker	Samples	Sensitivity/ specificity/ OR	Supporting literature
CDH1		69%/60%	
SALL3, CFTR, ABCC6, HPSE, RASSF1A, MT1A, ALX4, CDH13, RPRM, APBA1 and BRCA1	Urine	Sensitivity/especificity: 91.7%/87%	Yu et al., 2007
GSTP1, RARRES1, APC	Cell-free serum DNA	Sensitivity/specificity: 80%/93%	Ellinger et al., 2008
GDF15, TMEFF2 and VIM	Urine	Sensitivity/specificity: 94%/100%	Costa et al., 2010
%5-mC of leukocytes	Blood cells	OR 1.38 (95% CI:1.05–1.08, p=0.02)	Moore et al., 2008
miRNAs			
miR-145, miR-30a-3p, miR-133a, miR-133b, miR-195, miR-125b and miR-199a*	Tissue	Sensitivity/specificity: >70%/>75%	Ichimi et al., 2009
RNA ratio of miR-126:miR-152	Urine	Sensitivity/specificity: 72%/82%	Hanke et al., 2010
miR-152, -328 and -1224	Urine	Sensitivity/specificity: 81%/75%	Dudziec et al., 2011
miR-96	Urine	Sensitivity/specificity: 71%/89.2%	Yamada et al., 2011

Table 1. Epigenetic diagnostic markers in bladder cancer. The genes were described as official symbols according recommendations of Guidelines for Human Gene Nomenclature. More information about specific genes can be achieved at http://www.genenames.org/guidelines.html.

2.2 Candidate epigenetic biomarkers in the prognosis of bladder cancer

The knowledge of prognostic factors is of great importance for the determination of therapeutic strategies and to enable the application of different modalities of therapy in cancer treatment. In cases of bladder cancer, patients are monitored for recurrence or progression by periodic cystoscopy and urine cytological analysis, the frequencies of which vary depending on the risk factors that are associated with the disease. Thus, the discovery of more sensitive and non-invasive tumor markers that can help to predict tumor recurrence, progression and metastasis are required, and epigenetic alterations may be promising new potential prognostic markers for bladder cancer.

Bladder tumors may be superficial, with low risks of metastasis, but may have high recurrence risks (McConkey et al., 2010). Several genes that are related to the progression and prognosis of bladder cancer have been identified in bladder washes, urine and tumor tissues using various molecular and epigenetic approaches (Mitra et al., 2006) and are considered to be potential markers (Table 2).

Maruyama et al. (2001) determined the methylation statuses of 10 genes in 98 fresh bladder tumor tissues and found that multiple genes are methylated during the process of bladder cancer development. Their results also indicated that the frequent methylation of four genes (*CDH1*, *CDH13*, *RASSF1A* and *APC*) together with high MIs (median methylation index) were correlated with poor prognosis (tumors showed high grade, nonpapillary growth patterns, muscle invasions, advanced tumor stages and aneuploidies). In addition, the methylation of *CDH1*, *FHIT* and high MIs were associated with reduced patient survival rates.

In a study performed by Catto et al. (2005) that employed a large cohort of urothelial carcinomas, CpG hypermethylation at *DAPK* was associated with higher progression rates (log-rank P = .014) in all of the transitional-cell carcinoma (TCC) samples that were investigated compared to unmethylated samples at this *locus*.

In another study, Christoph et al. (2006) selected related genes as targets of p53 in the apoptotic cycle to perform a quantitative analysis of 110 tumor samples. The authors found that *APAF1* methylation levels were correlated with tumor stages and grades. In addition, the methylation levels of the *APAF1* and *IGFBP3* genes enabled tumors with higher recurrence risks to be distinguished from low-risk tumors in non-muscle-invasive and muscle-invasive tumors. The epigenetic inactivation of pro-apoptotic genes may be important events that are related to the progression and increased aggressiveness of tumors that are hypermethylated in these *loci*.

In addition, the hypermethylation of the promoter region of the *TIMP3* gene detected in urine sediments was found to be associated with an increased risk of death (Hoque et al., 2008). Other genes also have been found to undergo aberrant promoter methylation and were associated with poor prognosis in bladder cancer, including the hypermethylation of the *RUNX3* promoter, which was correlated with the development of invasive tumors, tumor progression and cancer specific-survival in patients with TCC (Kim et al., 2008). The methylation of this gene was also shown to be related to an increased risk of developing bladder cancer (Kim et al., 2005), suggesting that this gene not only suppresses the aggressiveness of tumors but also inhibits the tumor development.

Beyond to the tumor size and grade parameters, response to treatment is also an important prognostic factor because multidrug resistance to chemotherapy is a major obstacle in the treatment of cancer patients. Tada et al. (2000) showed that the overexpression of the *ABCB1* gene may be a prognostic factor indicating recurrence in bladder cancer, and the hypomethylation of the promoter of this gene may be necessary for the development of increased *ABCB1* mRNA levels and multidrug resistance.

Global DNA hypomethylation is also a common phenomenon that has been reported in bladder cancer (Seifert et al., 2007). The loss of DNA methylation in repetitive sequences may account for a majority of the global hypomethylation that characterizes a large percentage of human cancers. Neuhausen et al. (2006) found that the hypomethylation of LINE-1 retrotransposons was present in 90% of the urothelial carcinoma specimens that were studied, and the absence of this epigenetic change was indicative of a better clinical prognosis. In a high-throughput DNA methylation analysis, a distinct hypomethylation pattern was found in non-invasive (Ta-T1) urothelial tumors compared to both normal urothelium and invasive tumors (Wolff et al., 2010). These researchers found a substantial number of probes to be hypomethylated in non-invasive tumors only, suggesting that lower levels of DNA methylation may be related to a less malignant phenotype.

A particularly interesting example of epigenetic regulation is genomic imprinting, in which one copy of a gene is silenced in a manner determined by its parental origin. Thus, imprinted genes show parental-specific monoallelic expression. The loss of allele-specific expression pattern is termed as loss of imprinting (LOI), an event described in several types of pediatric and adult cancers (Monk, 2010). LOI has already been identified as an

Clinical – histolopathological parameters	Epigenetic biomarker	Supporting literature
Grade	**DNA methylation** *CDKN2A, BCL2, TERT, EDNRB, CDH1, RASSF1A, APC, CDH13*	Maruyama et al., 2001; Domínguez et al., 2002; Friedrich et al., 2004
Stage	**DNA methylation** *TIMP3, CDKN2A, RASSF1A, BCL2, OPCML, CDH1, APC, CDH13* **Histone modification** H4K20me1	Maruyama et al., 2001; Domínguez et al., 2002; Friedrich et al., 2004; Hoque et al., 2008; Schneider et al. 2011; Duarte-Pereira et al., 2011
Recurrence	**DNA methylation** *DAPK1, H19, TIMP3*	Ariel *et al.*, 2000; Tada et al., 2002; Friedrich et al., 2005
Survival	**DNA methylation** *TIMP3, OPCML, RUNX3, FHIT, CDH1* **Histone modification** H4K20me3	Maruyama et al., 2001; Kim et al., 2008; Hoque et al., 2008; Schneider et al. 2011; Duarte-Pereira et al., 2011
Metastasis	**DNA methylation** *TIMP3* **miRNA expression** miR-452, miR-452*	Hoque et al., 2008; Veerla et al., 2009
Muscle invasion	**DNA methylation** *CDKN2A, CDH1, RASSF1A, APC, CDH13* **miRNA expression** miR-222, miR-125b	Maruyama et al., 2001; Domínguez et al., 2002; Veerla et al., 2009
Tumor progression	**DNA methylation** *RASSF1A, CDH1, TNFRSF25, EDNRB, APC, DAPK1, H19* **Histone modification** H3K4me1, H4K20me1, H4K20me2, H4K20me3 **miRNA expression** Set of miR-21, miR-510, miR-492, miR-20a, miR-198 and set of miR-455-5p, miR-143, miR-145, miR-125b, miR-503	Catto et al., 2005; Yates et al., 2007; Dyrskjøt et al., 2009; Schneider et al. 2011

Table 2. Epigenetic prognostic markers in bladder cancer. The genes were described as official symbols according recommendations of Guidelines for Human Gene Nomenclature. More information about specific genes can be achieved at http://www.genenames.org/guidelines.html.

epimarker of cancer development. The *IGF2* and *H19* imprinted genes have been well documented in the literature. Some studies showed that the *H19* gene is involved in the development of bladder cancer (Ariel et al., 1995; Elkin et al., 1995) and is associated with high recurrence risks for this tumor type (Ariel et al., 2000). Furthermore, insulin-like growth factor-II (IGF-II) loss of imprinting (LOI) in a series of paired tumoral and normal adjacent bladder tissues and E-cadherin (*CDH1*) immunolocalization suggested a possible mechanism underlying E-cadherin relocalization to the cytoplasm, that is, the presence of aberrant levels of IGF-II due in some cases to *IGF2* LOI (Gallagher et al., 2008). Furthermore, the finding of LOI in the tumoral adjacent normal samples holds promise of *IGF2* LOI as a predictor of tumor development.

Others epigenetic mechanisms in cancer patients remain less comprehensively understood. One of these epigenetic changes involves the histone modifications, which include changes in their levels and distribution at gene promoters, gene coding regions, repetitive DNA sequences and other genomic elements (Kurdistani, 2011). In a recent study, Schneider et al. (2011) found that global levels of H3K4me1, H4K20me1, H4K20me2 and H4K20me3 were decreased compared to normal urothelium. The distribution of these histone modifications were associated with the risk of metastasis in muscle-invasive compared to non-muscle-invasive bladder cancers. The authors also showed that H4K20me1 levels were increased in patients with non-muscle-invasive bladder cancer with advanced pT stages and less differentiated bladder cancer, and H4K20me3 levels were significantly correlated with mortality after radical cystectomy in patients with muscle-invasive cancer.

Recently, several groups have questioned whether the miRNA expression profiles or even single miRNAs could act as useful biomarkers not only for cancer diagnosis but also for prognosis and treatment optimization (Lu et al., 2005; Calin & Croce, 2006). Dyrskjøt et al. (2009) identified the aberrant expression of several miRNAs in 106 samples from patients with different stages of bladder cancer and associated their profiles with disease progression. Among the miRNAs that were differentially expressed in normal bladder tissue compared to that of bladder cancer, two subsets [(miR-21, miR-510, miR-492, miR-20a, miR-198) and (miR-455-5p, miR-143, miR-145, miR-125b, miR-503)] were up- and down-regulated by two-fold, respectively. In another large-scale study that evaluated miRNA expression, high expression levels of miR-222 and miR-125b were observed in muscle-invasive tumors, and miR-452 and miR-452* were shown to be over-expressed in node-positive tumors (Veerla et al., 2009).

Moreover, aberrant DNA methylation has been implicated in the deregulation of several miRNAs in different types of cancer (Lujambio et al., 2007). Wiklund et al. (2011) studied this relationship and found that the miR-200 family and miR-205 are concurrently silenced and that DNA hypermethylation would be associated with the silencing of these microRNAs in invasive bladder tumors. They also found that the loss of miR-200c expression was associated with disease progression of muscle-invasive cancers and with poor prognosis.

3. The promise of epigenetic therapy

The knowledge of epigenetic alterations that are associated with human cancers and their potential reversibility has prompted the development of drugs that target epigenetic enzymes. Either natural or synthetic modulators can be utilized to restore normal epigenetic and gene expression patterns; for example, by restoring the expression of the frequently silenced *RUNX3* gene, which is considered to be good target for this new therapeutic modality since the loss of its function in cancer cells due to genetic mutations is a rare event (Kim et al., 2005). The epigenetic therapy can be used alone or in combination with other therapeutic modalities, such as chemotherapy, immunotherapy or radiotherapy. This approach will eventually lead to targeted therapies that are suited for specific molecular defects, thereby significantly decreasing the morbidity associated with bladder cancer in addition to other cancers (Balmain, 2002; Kim & Kim, 2009; Mund & Lyko, 2010). Two principal classes of epigenetic drugs have been demonstrated to be clinically relevant: DNA methyltransferase (DNMT) inhibitors and histone deacetylase (HDAC) inhibitors (Esteller, 2005) (Table 3). Novel epigenetic compounds that are of potential interest as clinical therapeutic drugs include the histone acetyltransferase inhibitors, such as anacardic acid, curcumin and peptide CoA conjugates. In addition, histone methyltransferase inhibitors and HDACis that are specific for SIRT1 (class III HDAC), such as nicotinamide and splitomycin, are now under intense analysis (Ballestar & Esteller, 2008; Greiner et al., 2005).

3.1 DNMTs inhibitors

Genes that are silenced by DNA hypermethylation may be reactivated by small molecules that are called DNMT inhibitors. These agents may be structural analogues of the nucleoside deoxycytidine or non-nucleoside analogues. The analogues, after being phosphorylated by kinases that convert the nucleosides into nucleotides, can be incorporated into DNA and subsequently inhibit DNMT activity by forming a covalent bond with the cysteine residue in the active DNMT site. However, it has also been shown that such incorporation may lead to instabilities in DNA structure and even DNA damage (Bouchard & Momparler, 1983; Goffin & Eisenhauer, 2002).

Two prominent examples are the cytosine analogs 5-azacytidine (azacytidine, Vidaza) and 2′-deoxy-5-azacytidine (decitabine, Dacogen), which are potent inhibitors of DNMTs (Table 3) and have been approved by the FDA (Food and Drug Administration) for the treatment of myelodysplastic syndrome, a pre-leukemic bone marrow disorder (Lübbert, 2000). Various additional molecules has been found to possess better stability and less toxicity and are currently being investigated as DNMT inhibitors in preclinical experiments, such as dihydro-5-azacytidine, arabinofuranosyl-5-azacytosine (fazarabine) and zebularine (Cheng et al., 2003).

Azacytidine and decitabine have been widely used in cell culture systems to reverse DNA hypermethylation and restore silenced gene expression. However, results from *in vivo* studies are not satisfactory, especially with solid tumors in which limited efficacy has been encountered. In general, both agents are unstable in aqueous solutions, have short half-lives and need to be freshly prepared before administration. In addition, both drugs have relatively poor bioavailabilities and high cytotoxic effects with potential risks, such as myelotoxicity, mutagenesis, and tumorigenesis, which have limited their clinical applications (Jackson-Grusby et al., 2007).

Despite this discouraging data, the orally administered zebularine shows some promise. It was shown to suppress the growth of TCC in bladder xenografts in nude mice and was less toxic than other nucleoside analogues. In addition, when zebularine was given at a lower dose after an initial dose of decitabine, a profound demethylation of the *CDKN2A* gene promoter was observed. These results provide a rationale for the strategy of combining an initial administration of a parenteral DNMT inhibitor with a subsequent low dose of oral zebularine (Cheng et al., 2004; Zhang et al., 2006). Another group of compounds are called non-nucleoside analogues. These small molecules inhibit DNA methylation by binding directly to the catalytic site of the DNMT enzyme without being incorporated into the DNA. The local anesthetic procaine and its derivative procainamide, which is an approved antiarrhythmic drug, have exhibited demethylating activities. For example, Lin et al. (2001) reported that procainamide was able to restore GSTP1 gene expression by reversing the hypermethylation of the promoter CpG islands of androgen-sensitive human prostate adenocarcinoma (LNCaP) cells in vitro and in vivo. Because these agents do not incorporate into DNA, it is expected that they may have less genotoxicity than nucleoside DNMT inhibitors. In addition, (-)-epigallocatechin-3-gallate (EGCG), the main polyphenol compound in green tea, also acts as DNMT inhibitor . Cancer cells treated with micromolar concentrations of EGCG showed reduced DNA methylation and the increased transcription of tumor suppressor genes. However, it is still unknown whether EGCG has a direct inhibitory effect on DNMTs (Fang et al., 2003; Villar-Garea et al., 2003).

3.2 HDAC inhibitors

A variety of structurally distinct groups of compounds have been identified as histone deacetylase inhibitors (HDACi) (Table 3). These compounds inhibit histone deacetylase activity by binding to the catalytic site of the enzyme and chelating zinc ions because they share similar structures with the substrates (Finnin et al., 1999). Similar to their effects on gene expression and differentiation, HDACi have also been shown to be efficient inducers of apoptosis in several cellular systems. The precise mechanism of this effect is under investigation, and it has been suggested that they may affect cellular oxidative stress and DNA damage induction. They have shown impressive activities in preclinical studies as well as selectivity for neoplastic cells. Many HDACi are being tested in clinical trials for various malignancies (Bolden et al., 2006; Xu et al., 2007).

The class of the HDAC inhibitors is divided into four groups: hydroxamic acids, cyclic tetrapeptides, short-chain fatty acids and benzamides. The hydroxamate compounds are more potent and have higher inhibitory effects. Trichostatin A from *Streptomyces hygroscopicus* is active at nanomolar concentrations, while the synthetic compounds, such as suberoylanilide hydroxamic acid (SAHA), can function in low micromolar or nanomolar ranges. Cyclic tetrapeptides are very potent compounds and can inhibit histone deacetylase at nanomolar concentrations. Short-chain fatty acid compounds usually require millimolar concentrations to inhibit histone deacetylase activities in vivo; therefore, their clinical applicability could be limited. The fourth class is the benzamides, such as MS-275 and CI-994, which are effective at micromolar concentrations (Rosato et al., 2003; Zhang et al., 2006).

The clinical potentials of histone deacetylase inhibitors have been suggested by several promising in vivo studies. For example, SAHA was FDA approved in Oct. 2006 for the treatment of cutaneous T cell lymphoma (CTCL), and it is under a phase I clinical trial for use in patients with TCC (Mann et al., 2007). Preliminary reports have indicated that 2 out of 6 patients with metastatic TCC disease have had objective tumor regression and tumor-related symptom relief (Kelly et al., 2003). The induction of CDKN1A messenger RNA and

Group	Drug	Clinical status
DNMT inhibitor		
Nucleoside analogues	5-Azacyticine	Approved 2004 for MDS
	2′-Deoxy-5-azacytidine	Approved 2006 for MDS
	Zebularine	Preclinical
Non-nucleoside analogues	Hydralazine	Phase I > II for cervical Ca
	MG98	Phase I > II for advanced metastatic tumors
	Procaine	Preclinical
	RNAi	Preclinical
	Epigallocatichin-3-gallate	Preclinical
	Psammaplin A	Preclinical
HDAC inhibitor		
Hydroxamic acids	Suberoylanilide hydroxamic acid (SAHA)	Approved 2006 for CTCL
	Panobinostat	Phase I > II > III for breast Ca, gliomas, prostate Ca, NSCLC, CTCL, leukemia
	Belinostat	Phase I > II for ovarian Ca, CTCL, lymphoma, multiple myeloma, leukemia
	Trichostatin A	Preclinical
Cyclic tetrapeptides	Depsipeptide, Romidepsin	Approved 2009 for CTCL
Short-chain fatty acids	Valproic acid	Phase I > II > III for melanoma, myelodysplastic syndrome, leukemia, chronic lymphocytic leukemia, cervical Ca, breast Ca
	AN-9	Phase I > II for malignant melanoma, leukemia, lymphoma, NSCLC
Benzamides	Entinostat	Phase I > II for breast Ca, acute lymphoblastic leukemia, Hodgkin's lymphoma, MDS, renal Ca, colorectal Ca, lung Ca
	Mocetinostat	Phase I > II for breast Ca, NSCLC, prostate Ca, stomach Ca, non-Hodgkin's lymphoma, Hodgkin's lymphoma, AML, CLL, lymphoma
	N-Acetyldinaline	Phase I > II > III for multiple myeloma, lung Ca, pancreatic Ca

Table 3. List of the main DNMT and HDAC inhibitors and their current clinical trial status. MDS: myelodysplastic syndrome, CTCL: cutaneous T cell lymphoma, NSCLC: non small cell lung cancer, AML: acute myeloid leukemia, CLL: Chronic lymphocytic leukemia, Ca: cancer. Clinical status source: clinicaltrials.gov.

protein levels in T24 cells following SAHA exposure mediated by increased acetyl H3 and H4 levels in the respective promoter region may contribute to its tumor inhibitory effect

(Richon et al., 2000). Other researchers have reported similar inhibitory effects on bladder tumor growth using trichostatin A and pyroxamide on T24 cells. Additionally, trichostatin A is able to suppress 70% of tumor growth with no detectable toxicity in EJ and UM-UC-3 xenograft models (Canes et al., 2005).

3.3 Combination therapy

The emerging concept of gene silencing involves the interaction of multiple factors that may act in a sequential manner. It is also known that a single agent may not be able to eradicate a tumor mass that is derived from a very heterogeneous population of cells. Moreover, the adverse toxic effects that are caused by single-agent treatments, especially at high doses, call for a rationalized therapeutic approach with low-dosage drug combinations. Accumulating evidence has shown that the combination of histone deacetylase inhibitors and DNMT inhibitors is very effective (and synergistic) in inducing apoptosis, differentiation and/or cell growth arrest in various human cancer cell lines (Gottlicher et al., 2001; Mei et al., 2004; Stirzaker et al., 2004).

In urologic cancers, Cameron et al. (1999) showed that the combination of decitabine and trichostatin A stimulated a synergistic reactivation of several tumor suppressor genes. Dunn et al. (2005) reported that the combination of DNMT inhibitors and histone deacetylase inhibitors was able to reactivate the sensitivities of LNCaP cells to interferon treatment by the re-expression of JAK1 kinase, which is a key mediator of both interferon-gamma and interferon-alpha/beta receptor-elicited effects. Another strategy is to combine either histone deacetylase inhibitors or DNMT inhibitors with conventional therapies, as was demonstrated by Zhang et al. (2007), who indicated that the combination of FK228 (a HDAC inhibitor) and docetaxel (chemotherapeutic drug) caused a synergistic growth inhibition in androgen-independent prostate cancer cell lines. Moreover, single treatments with SAHA or MS-275 show enhanced radiation-induced cytotoxicity in DU-145 cells both *in vitro* and *in vivo* (Chinnaiyan et al., 2005).

4. Future

There is a great deal of evidence that demonstrates the connections between epigenetic modification enzymes and cancer. Epigenetic alterations contribute to tumorigenesis by the activation of oncogenes or inactivation of tumor suppressor genes. The identification of molecules that can modulate epigenetic enzymes could lead to the prevention of oncogene transcription and activation of tumor repressors, and thus it is an important topic to research (Zheng, 2008).

A major impediment to the use of such drugs is that they are nonspecific and may reactivate genes non-discriminately. However, this does not seem to be a problem in the present case because DNA methylation inhibitors only act on dividing cells and leave normal, non-dividing cells unaffected. Also, it seems that the drugs preferentially activate genes that have become abnormally silenced in cancer. Further studies are required to establish an unambiguous proof of concept for epigenetic cancer therapies (Jones & Baylin, 2007; Liang et al., 2002; Mund & Lyko, 2010).

For future clinical applications, researchers should focus on several aspects, including the biomarkers that predict drug responses. Researchers should also focus on the screening of new, more effective and less toxic agents. The psammaplin, for example, a family of bromotyrosine derivatives that have been extracted from the marine sponge *Pseudoceratina purpurea*, appear to be a novel class of compounds with the ability to inhibit both DNMT and histone deacetylase activities (Pina et al., 2003).

In addition, exploring the silencing of specific genes by RNA interference for key epigenetic regulatory complexes could enhance therapeutic indices. For example, DNMT-specific siRNA (single-interfering RNA) is able to elicit the demethylation of several epigenetically silenced genes. Additionally, the treatment of cultured cells *in vivo* with demethylating agents, either alone or in combination with HDACi, has been shown to re-activate the expression of tumor-suppressor miRNAs, such as miR-124a and miR-127, causing the corresponding repression of their oncogenic targets. Although the successful delivery of siRNAs to solid tumors has yet to be achieved, designing small-molecule siRNAs to mimic tumor-suppressor miRNAs could be a potential method to selectively repress the expression of oncogenes (Leu et al., 2003; Saito et al., 2006).

In the next decade, with the availability of gene profiling databases of epigenetic modifiers, it is expected that epigenetic therapy will be translated from the bench to the clinical arena and become a real alternative to conventional cancer treatments (Rodríguez-Paredes & Esteller, 2011; Zhang et al., 2006).

In summary, the field of epigenetic biomarker studies is still new but shows promise in the clinical management of cancer. Valuable progress has been made on this end, and the combination of existing and newly discovered biomarkers will likely allow for more accurate diagnosis. Thus, patients will be able to benefit from this new era of personalized medicine, in which biomarkers will allow for direct treatments with more effective therapeutic agents.

5. References

Ariel, I.; Sughayer, M.; Fellig, Y.; Pizov, G.; Ayesh, S.; Podeh, D.; Libdeh, B.A.; Levy, C.; Birman, T.; Tykocinski, M.L.; de Groot, N. & Hochberg, A. (2000). The imprinted H19 gene is a marker of early recurrence in human bladder carcinoma. *Molecular Pathology*, Vol.53, No.6, pp. 320-323.

Ariel, I.; Lustig, O.; Schneider, T.; Pizov, G.; Sappir, M.; De-Groot, N. & Hochberg, A. (1995). The imprinted H19 gene as a tumor marker in bladder carcinoma. *Urology*, Vol.45, No.2, pp. 335-338.

Ballestar, E. (2011). An introduction to epigenetics. *Advances in Experimental Medicine and Biology*, Vol.711, pp. 1-11.

Ballestar, E. & Esteller, M. (2008). Epigenetic gene regulation in cancer. *Advances in Genetics*, Vol.61, pp.247-67.

Balmain, A. (2002). Cancer: new-age tumour suppressors. *Nature*, Vol.417, No.6886, pp.235-7.

Bolden, J.E.; Peart, M.J. & Johnstone, R.W. (2006). Anticancer activities of histone deacetylase inhibitors. *Nature Reviews Drug Discovery*, Vol.5, No.9, pp.5 769–784.

Bouchard, J. & Momparler, R.L. (1983). Incorporation of 5-Aza-2'-deoxycytidine-5'-triphosphate into DNA. Interactions with mammalian DNA polymerase alpha and DNA methylase. *Molecular Pharmacology*. Vol.24, No.1, pp.109–14.

Boumber, Y. & Issa, J.P. (2011) Epigenetics in cancer: what's the future? *Oncology (Williston Park)*, Vol.25, No.3, pp. 220-6.

Calin, G.A. & Croce, C.M. (2006). MicroRNA signatures in human cancers. *Nature Review Cancer*, Vol.6, No.11, pp. 857-866.

Cameron, E.E.; Bachman, K.E.; Myöhänen, S.; Herman, J.G. & Baylin, S.B. (1999). Synergy of demethylation and histone deacetylase inhibition in the re-expression of genes silenced in cancer. *Nature Genetics*, Vol.21, No.1, pp.103-7.

Canes, D.; Chiang, G.J.; Billmeyer, B.R.; Austin, C.A.; Kosakowski, M.; Rieger-Christ, K.M.; Libertino, J.A. & Summerhayes, I.C. (2005). Histone deacetylase inhibitors upregulate plakoglobin expression in bladder carcinoma cells and display antineoplastic activity in vitro and in vivo. *International Journal of Cancer*, Vol.113, No.5, pp.841-8.

Catto, J.W.; Azzouzi, A.R.; Rehman, I.; Feeley, K.M.; Cross, S.S.; Amira, N.; Fromont, G.; Sibony, M.; Cussenot, O.; Meuth, M. & Hamdy, F.C. (2005). Promoter hypermethylation is associated with tumor location, stage, and subsequent progression in transitional cell carcinoma. *Journal of Clinical Oncology*, Vol.23, No.13, pp. 2903-2910

Chan, M.W.; Chan, L.W.; Tang, N.L.; Tong, J.H.; Lo, K.W.; Lee, T.L.; Cheung, H.Y.; Wong, W.S.; Chan, P.S.; Lai, F.M. and To, K.F. (2002). Hypermethylation of multiple genes in tumor tissues and voided urine in urinary bladder cancer patients. *Clinical Cancer Research*, Vol.8, No.2, pp.464-470.

Chan, M.W.; Chan, L.W.; Tang, N.L.; Lo, K.W.; Tong, J.H.; Chan, A.W.; Cheung, H.Y.; Wong, W.S.; Chan, P.S.; Lai, F.M. & To, K.F. (2003). Frequent hypermethylation of promoter region of RASSF1A in tumor tissues and voided urine of urinary bladder cancer patients. *International Journal of Cancer*, Vol.104, No.5, pp.611-6.

Cheng, J.C.; Matsen, C.B.; Gonzales, F.A.; Ye, W.; Greer, S.; Marquez, V.E.; Jones, P.A. & Selker, E.U. (2003). Inhibition of DNA methylation and reactivation of silenced genes by zebularine. *Journal of the National Cancer Institute*, Vol.95, No.5, pp.399-409.

Cheng, J.C.; Weisenberger, D.J.; Gonzales, F.A.; Liang, G.; Xu, G.L., Hu, Y.G., Marquez, V.E. & Jones, P.A. (2004). Continuous zebularine treatment effectively sustains demethylation in human bladder cancer cells. *Molecular and Cellular Biology*, Vol.24, No.3, pp.1270-8.

Chinnaiyan, P.; Vallabhaneni, G.; Armstrong, E.; Huang, S.M. & Harari, P.M. (2005). Modulation of radiation response by histone deacetylase inhibition. *International Journal of Radiation Oncology, Biology, Physics*, Vol.62, No.1, pp.223-9.

Christoph, F.; Weikert, S.; Kempkensteffen, C.; Krause, H.; Schostak, M.; Miller, K. & Schrader, M. (2006). Regularly methylated novel pro-apoptotic genes associated with recurrence in transitional cell carcinoma of the bladder. *International Journal of Cancer*, Vol.119, No.6, pp. 1396-1402.

Costa, V.L.; Henrique, R.; Danielsen, S.A.; Duarte-Pereira, S.; Eknaes, M.; Skotheim, R.I.; Rodrigues, A.; Magalhães, J.S.; Oliveira, J.; Lothe, R.A.; Teixeira, M.R.; Jerónimo, C. & Lind, G.E. (2010) Three epigenetic biomarkers, GDF15, TMEFF2, and VIM, accurately predict bladder cancer from DNA-based analyses of urine samples. *Clinical Cancer Research*, Vol.16, No.23, pp.5842-51.

Domínguez, G.; Carballido, J.; Silva, J.; Silva, J.M.; García, J.M.; Menéndez, J.; Provencio, M.; España, P. & Bonilla, F. (2002). p14ARF promoter hypermethylation in plasma DNA as an indicator of disease recurrence in bladder cancer patients. *Clinical Cancer Research*, Vol.8, No.4, pp. 980-985.

Duarte-Pereira, S.; Paiva, F.; Costa, V.L.; Ramalho-Carvalho, J.; Savva-Bordalo, J.; Rodrigues, A.; Ribeiro, F.R.; Silva, V.M.; Oliveira, J.; Henrique, R. & Jerónimo, C. (2011). Prognostic value of opioid binding protein/cell adhesion molecule-like promoter methylation in bladder carcinoma. *European Journal of Cancer*, Vol.47, No.7, pp. 1106-1114.

Dudziec, E.; Miah, S.; Choudhry, H.M.; Owen, H.C.; Blizard, S.; Glover, M.; Hamdy, F.C. & Catto, J.W. (2011). Hypermethylation of CpG islands and shores around specific microRNAs and mirtrons is associated with the phenotype and presence of bladder cancer. *Clinical Cancer Research*, Vol.17, No.6, pp.1287-96.

Dulaimi, E.; Uzzo, R.G.; Greenberg, R.E.; Al-Saleem, T.; Cairns, P. (2004). Detection of bladder cancer in urine by a tumor suppressor gene hypermethylation panel. *Clinical Cancer Research*, Vol.10, No.6, pp.1887-1893

Dunn, G.P.; Sheehan, K.C.; Old, L.J. & Schreiber, R.D. (2005). IFN unresponsiveness in LNCaP cells due to the lack of JAK1 gene expression. *Cancer Research*, Vol.65, No.8, pp.3447–53.

Dyrskjøt, L.; Ostenfeld, M.S.; Bramsen, J.B.; Silahtaroglu, A.N.; Lamy, P.; Ramanathan, R.; Fristrup, N.; Jensen, J.L.; Andersen, C.L.; Zieger, K.; Kauppinen, S.; Ulhøi, B.P.; Kjems, J.; Borre, M. & Orntoft, T.F. (2009). Genomic profiling of microRNAs in bladder cancer: miR-129 is associated with poor outcome and promotes cell death in vitro. *Cancer Research*, Vol.69, No.11, pp.4851-4860.

Eling, T.E.; Baek, S.J.; Shim, M. & Lee, C.H. (2006). NSAID activated gene (NAG-1), a modulator of tumorigenesis. *Journal of Biochemistry and Molecular Biology*, Vol.39, No.6, pp.649-55.

Elkin, M.; Shevelev, A.; Schulze, E.; Tykocinsky, M.; Cooper, M.; Ariel, I.; Pode, D.; Kopf, E.; de Groot, N. & Hochberg, A. (1995). The expression of the imprinted H19 and IGF-2 genes in human bladder carcinoma. *FEBS Letters*, Vol.374, No.1, pp. 57-61.

Ellinger, J.; El Kassem, N.; Heukamp, L.C.; Matthews, S.; Cubukluoz, F.; Kahl, P.; Perabo, F.G.; Müller, S.C.; von Ruecker, A. & Bastian, P.J. (2008). Hypermethylation of cell-free serum DNA indicates worse outcome in patients with bladder cancer. *The Journal of Urology*, Vol.179, No.1, pp.346-52.

Esteller, M. (2005). DNA methylation and cancer therapy: New developments and expectations. *Current Opinion in Oncology*, Vol.17, No.1, pp.55–60.

Fabbri, M. & Calin, G.A. (2010). Epigenetics and miRNAs in human cancer. *Advances in Genetics*. Vol.70, pp.87-99.

Fang, M.Z.; Wang, Y.; Ai, N.; Hou, Z.; Sun, Y.; Lu, H.; Welsh, W. & Yang, C.S. (2003). Tea polyphenol (-)-epigallocatechin-3-gallate inhibits DNA methyltransferase and reactivates methylation-silenced genes in cancer cell lines. *Cancer Research*, Vol.63, No.22, pp.7563–70.

Fernandez, A.F.; Assenov, Y.; Martin-Subero, J.I.; Balint, B.; Siebert, R.; Taniguchi, H.; Yamamoto, H.; Hidalgo, M.; Tan, A.C.; Galm, O.; Ferrer, I.; Sanchez-Cespedes, M.; Villanueva, A.; Carmona, J.; Sanchez-Mut, J.V.; Berdasco, M.; Moreno, V.; Capella, G.; Monk, D.; Ballestar, E.; Ropero, S.; Martinez, R.; Sanchez-Carbayo, M.; Prosper, F.; Agirre, X.; Fraga, M.F.; Graña, O.; Perez-Jurado, L.; Mora, J.; Puig, S.; Prat, J.; Badimon, L.; Puca, A.A.; Meltzer, S.J.; Lengauer, T.; Bridgewater, J.; Bock, C. & Esteller, M. (2011). A DNA methylation fingerprint of 1628 human samples. *Genome Research*, Epub ahead of print.

Finnin, M.S.; Donigian, J.R.; Cohen, A.; Richon, V.M.; Rifkind, R.A.; Marks, P.A.; Breslow, R. & Pavletich, N.P. (1999). Structures of a histone deacetylase homologue bound to the TSA and SAHA inhibitors. *Nature*, Vol.401, No.6749, pp.88–93.

Friedrich, M.G.; Weisenberger, D.J.; Cheng, J.C.; Chandrasoma, S.; Siegmund, K.D.; Gonzalgo, M.L.; Toma, M.I.; Huland, H.; Yoo, C.; Tsai, Y.C.; Nichols, P.W.; Bochner, B.H.; Jones, P.A. & Liang, G. (2004). Detection of methylated apoptosis-associated genes in urine sediments of bladder cancer patients. *Clinical Cancer Research*, Vol.10, No.22, pp.7457-65.

Friedrich, M.G.; Chandrasoma, S.; Siegmund, K.D.; Weisenberger, D.J.; Cheng, J.C.; Toma, M.I.; Huland, H.; Jones, P.A. & Liang, G. (2005). Prognostic relevance of methylation markers in patients with non-muscle invasive bladder carcinoma. *European Journal of Cancer*, Vol.41, No.17, pp. 2769-2778.

Gallagher, E.M.; O'Shea, D.M.; Fitzpatrick, P.; Harrison, M.; Gilmartin, B.; Watson, J.A.; Clarke, T.; Leonard, M.O.; McGoldrick, A.; Meehan, M.; Watson, C.; Furlong, F.; O'Kelly, P.; Fitzpatrick, J.M.; Dervan, P.A.; O'Grady, A.; Kay, E.W. & McCann, A. (2008). Recurrence of urothelial carcinoma of the bladder: a role for insulin-like growth factor-II loss of imprinting and cytoplasmic E-cadherin immunolocalization. *Clinical Cancer Research*, Vol.14, No.21, pp.6829-6838.

Goffin, J. & Eisenhauer, E. (2002). DNA methyltransferase inhibitors-state of the art. *Annals of Oncology*, Vol.13, No.11, pp.1699 –716.

Gottlicher, M.; Minucci, S.; Zhu, P.; Krämer, O.H.; Schimpf, A.; Giavara, S.; Sleeman, J.P.; Lo Coco, F.; Nervi, C.; Pelicci, P.G. & Heinzel, T. (2001). Valproic acid defines a novel class of HDAC inhibitors inducing differentiation of transformed cells. *The EMBO Jornal*, Vol.20, No.24, pp.6969 –78.

Greiner, D.; Bonaldi, T.; Eskeland, R.; Roemer, E. & Imhof, A. (2005). Identification of a specific inhibitor of the histone methyltransferase SU (VAR) 3–9. *Nature Chemichal Biology*, Vol.1, No.3, pp.143–45.

Hanke, M.; Hoefig, K.; Merz, H.; Feller, A.C.; Kausch, I.; Jocham, D.; Warnecke, J.M. & Sczakiel, G. (2010) A robust methodology to study urine microRNA as tumor marker: microRNA-126 and microRNA-182 are related to urinary bladder cancer. *Urologic Oncology*, Vol.28, No.6, pp.655-61.

Hellwinkel, O.J.; Kedia, M.; Isbarn, H.; Budäus, L. & Friedrich, M.G. (2008) Methylation of the TPEF- and PAX6-promoters is increased in early bladder cancer and in normal mucosa adjacent to pTa tumours. *BJU International*, Vol.101, No.6, pp.753-7.

Hoque, M.O.; Begum, S.; Topaloglu, O.; Chatterjee, A.; Rosenbaum, E.; Van Criekinge, W.; Westra, W.H.; Schoenberg, M.; Zahurak, M.; Goodman, S.N. & Sidransky, D. (2006).

Quantitation of promoter methylation of multiple genes in urine DNA and bladder cancer detection. *Journal of the National Cancer Institute*, Vol.98, No.14, pp.996-1004.

Hoque, M.O.; Begum, S.; Brait, M.; Jeronimo, C.; Zahurak, M.; Ostrow, K.L.; Rosenbaum, E.; Trock, B.; Westra, W.H.; Schoenberg, M.; Goodman, S.N. & Sidransky, D. (2008). Tissue inhibitor of metalloproteinases-3 promoter methylation is an independent prognostic factor for bladder cancer. *Journal of Urology*, Vol.179, No.2, pp.743-747.

Ichimi, T.; Enokida, H.; Okuno, Y.; Kunimoto, R.; Chiyomaru, T.; Kawamoto, K.; Kawahara, K.; Toki, K.; Kawakami, K.; Nishiyama, K.; Tsujimoto, G.; Nakagawa, M. & Seki, N. (2009). Identification of novel microRNA targets based on microRNA signatures in bladder cancer. *International Journal of Cancer*, Vol.125, No.2, pp.345-52.

Iguchi, H.; Kosaka, N. & Ochiya, T. (2010). Versatile applications of microRNA in anti-cancer drug discovery: from therapeutics to biomarkers. *Current Drug Discovery Technologies*, Vol.7, No.2, pp.95-105.

Jackson-Grusby, L.; Laird, P.W.; Magge, S.N.; Moeller, B.J. & Jaenisch, R. (1997). Mutagenicity of 5-aza-2'-deoxycytidine is mediated by the mammalian DNA methyltransferase. *Proceedings of the National Academy of Sciences of the United States of America*, Vol.94, No.9, pp.4681-5.

Jones, P.A. & Baylin, S.B. (2007). The epigenomics of cancer. *Cell*, Vol.128, No.4, pp.683-92.

Kelly, W.K.; Richon, V.M.; O'Connor, O.; Curley, T.; MacGregor-Curtelli, B.; Tong, W.; Klang, M.; Schwartz, L.; Richardson, S.; Rosa, E.; Drobnjak, M.; Cordon-Cordo, C.; Chiao, J.H.; Rifkind, R.; Marks, P.A. & Scher, H. (2003). Phase I clinical trial of histone deacetylase inhibitor: Suberoylanilide hydroxamic acid administered intravenously. *Clinical Cancer Research*, Vol.9, No.10 Pt 1, pp.3578-88.

Kim, W.J. & Kim, Y.J. Epigenetic biomarkers in urothelial bladder cancer. (2009). *Expert Review of Molecular Diagnostics*. Vol.9, No.3, pp.259-69.

Kim, Y.K. & Kim, W.J. (2009). Epigenetic markers as promising prognosticators for bladder cancer. *International Journal of Urology*, Vol.16, No.1, pp.17-22.

Kim, E.J.; Kim, Y.J.; Jeong, P.; Ha, Y.S.; Bae, S.C. & Kim, W.J. (2008). Methylation of the RUNX3 promoter as a potential prognostic marker for bladder tumor. *Journal of Urology*, Vol.180, No.3, pp. 1141-1145.

Kim, W.J.; Kim, E.J.; Jeong, P.; Quan, C.; Kim, J.; Li, Q.L.; Yang, J.O.; Ito, Y. & Bae, S.C. (2005). RUNX3 inactivation by point mutations and aberrant DNA methylation in bladder tumors. *Cancer Research*, Vol.65, No.20, pp.9347-54.

Kouzarides T. (2007). Chromatin modifications and their functions. *Cell*, Vol.128, No.4, pp. 693-705.

Kurdistani, S.K. (2011). Histone modifications in cancer biology and prognosis. *Progress in Drug Research*, Vol.67, pp.91-106.

Leu, Y.W.; Rahmatpanah, F.; Shi, H.; Wei, S.H.; Liu, J.C.; Yan, P.S. & Huang, T.H. (2003). Double RNA interference of DNMT3b and DNMT1 enhances DNA demethylation and gene reactivation. *Cancer Research*, Vol.63, No.19, pp.6110 –5.

Liang, G.; Gonzales, F.A.; Jones, P.A.; Orntoft, T.F. & Thykjaer, T. (2002). Analysis of gene induction in human fibroblasts and bladder cancer cells exposed to the methylation inhibitor 5-aza-20-deoxycytidine. *Cancer Research,* Vol.62, No.4, pp.961–966.

Lin, X.; Asgari, K.; Putzi, M.J.; Gage, W.R.; Yu, X.; Cornblatt, B.S.; Kumar, A.; Piantadosi, S.; DeWeese, T.L.; De Marzo, A.M. & Nelson, W.G. (2001). Reversal of GSTP1 CpG island hypermethylation and reactivation of pi-class glutathione S-transferase (GSTP1) expression in human prostate cancer cells by treatment with procainamide. *Cancer Research,* Vol.61, No.24, pp.8611– 6.

Lu, J.; Getz, G.; Miska, E.A.; Alvarez-Saavedra, E.; Lamb, J.; Peck, D.; Sweet-Cordero, A.; Ebert, B.L.; Mak, R.H.; Ferrando, A.A.; Downing, J.R.; Jacks, T.; Horvitz, H.R. & Golub, T.R. (2005). MicroRNA expression profiles classify human cancers. *Nature,* Vol.435, No.7043, pp. 834-8.

Lübbert, M. (2000). DNA methylation inhibitors in the treatment of leukemias, myelodysplastic syndromes and hemoglobinopathies: Clinical results and possible mechanisms of action. *Current Topics in Microbiology and Immunology,* Vol.249, pp.135– 64.

Lujambio, A.; Ropero, S.; Ballestar, E.; Fraga, M.F.; Cerrato, C.; Setien, F.; Casado, S.; Suarez-Gauthier, A.; Sanchez-Cespedes, M.; Git, A.; Spiteri, I.; Das, P.P.; Calds, C.; Miska, E. & Esteller, M. (2007). Genetic unmasking of an epigenetically silenced microRNA in Human cancer cells. *Cancer Resesrch,* Vol.67, No.4, pp.1424-1429.

Maruyama, R.; Toyooka, S.; Toyooka, K.O.; Harada, K.; Virmani, A.K.; Zöchbauer-Müller, S.; Farinas, A.J.; Vakar-Lopez, F.; Minna, J.D.; Sagalowsky, A.; Czerniak, B. & Gazdar, A.F. (2001). Aberrant promoter methylation profile of bladder cancer and its relationship to clinicopathological features. *Cancer Research,* Vol.61, No.24, pp. 8659-8663.

Mann, B.S.; Johnson, J.R.; Cohen, M.H.; Justice, R. & Pazdur, R. (2007). FDA approval summary: vorinostat for treatment of advanced primary cutaneous T-cell lymphoma. *Oncologist.* Vol.12, No.10, pp.1247-1252.

McConkey, D.J.; Lee, S.; Choi, W.; Tran, M.; Majewski, T.; Lee, S.; Siefker-Radtke, A.; Dinney, C. & Czerniak, B. (2010). Molecular genetics of bladder cancer: Emerging mechanisms of tumor initiation and progression. *Urologic Oncology,* Vol.28, No.4, pp. 429-440.

Mei, S.; Ho, A.D. & Mahlknecht, U. (2004). Role of histone deacetylase inhibitors in the treatment of cancer. *International Journal of Oncology,* Vol.25, No.6, pp.1509 –19.

Mitra, A.P.; Datar, R.H & Cote, R.J. (2006). Molecular pathways in invasive bladder cancer: new insights into mechanisms, progression, and target identification. *Journal of Clinical Oncology,* Vol.24, No.35, pp.5552-5564.

Monk D. (2010). Deciphering the cancer imprintome. *Briefings in Functional Genomics and Proteomics,* Vol.9, No.4, pp.329-339.

Moore, L.E.; Pfeiffer, R.M.; Poscablo, C.; Real, F.X.; Kogevinas, M.; Silverman, D.; García-Closas, R.; Chanock, S.; Tardón, A.; Serra, C.; Carrato, A.; Dosemeci, M.; García-Closas, M.; Esteller, M.; Fraga, M.; Rothman, N. & Malats, N. (2008). Genomic DNA hypomethylation as a biomarker for bladder cancer susceptibility in the Spanish

Bladder Cancer Study: a case-control study. *The Lancet Oncology,* Vol.9, No.4, pp.359-66.

Mund, C. & Lyko, F. (2010). Epigenetic cancer therapy: Proof of concept and remaining challenges. *Bioessays,* Vol.32, No.11, pp.949-57.

Negraes, P.D.; Favaro, F.P.; Camargo, J.L.; Oliveira, M.L.; Goldberg, J.; Rainho, C.A.; Salvadori, D.M. (2008). DNA methylation patterns in bladder cancer and washing cell sediments: a perspective for tumor recurrence detection. *BMC Cancer.* Vol.8, pp.238-250.

Neuhausen, A.; Florl, A.R.; Grimm, M.O. & Schulz, W.A. (2006). DNA methylation alterations in urothelial carcinoma. *Cancer Biology and Therapy,* Vol.5, No.8, pp. 993-1001.

Pina, I.C.; Gautschi, J.T.; Wang, G.Y.; Sanders, M.L.; Schmitz, F.J.; France, D.; Cornell-Kennon, S.; Sambucetti, L.C.; Remiszewski, S.W.; Perez, L.B.; Bair, K.W. & Crews, P. (2003). Psammaplins from the sponge Pseudoceratina purpurea: Inhibition of both histone deacetylase and DNA methyltransferase. *The Journal of Organic Chemistry,* Vol.68, No.10, pp.3866 –73.

Portela, A. & Esteller, M. (2010). Epigenetic modifications and human disease. *Nature Biotechnology,* Vol.28, No.10, pp. 1057-68.

Renard, I.; Joniau, S.; van Cleynenbreugel, B.; Collette, C.; Naômé, C.; Vlassenbroeck, I.; Nicolas, H.; de Leval, J.; Straub, J.; Van Criekinge, W.; Hamida, W.; Hellel, M.; Thomas, A.; de Leval, L.; Bierau, K. & Waltregny, D. (2010). Identification and validation of the methylated TWIST1 and NID2 genes through real-time methylation-specific polymerase chain reaction assays for the noninvasive detection of primary bladder cancer in urine samples. *European Urology,* Vol.58, No.1, pp.96-104.

Richon, V.M.; Sandhoff, T.W.; Rifkind, R.A. & Marks, P.A. (2000). Histone deacetylase inhibitor selectively induces p21WAF1 expression and gene-associated histone acetylation. *Proceedings of the National Academy of Sciences of the United States of America,* Vol.97, No.18, pp.10014–9.

Rodríguez-Paredes, M. & Esteller, M. (2011). Cancer epigenetics reaches mainstream oncology. *Nature Medicine.* Vol.17, No.3, pp.330-339.

Rosato, R.R.; Almenara, J.A. & Grant, S. (2003). The histone deacetylase inhibitor MS-275 promotes differentiation or apoptosis in human leukemia cells through a process regulated by generation of reactive oxygen species and induction of p21CIP1/WAF1. *Cancer Research,* Vol.63, No.13, pp.3637–45.

Saito, Y.; Liang, G.; Egger, G.; Friedman, J.M.; Chuang, J.C.; Coetzee, G.A. & Jones, P.A. (2006). Specific activation of microRNA-127 with downregulation of the proto-oncogene BCL6 by chromatin-modifying drugs in human cancer cells. *Cancer Cell,* Vol. 9, No.6, pp. 435–43.

Sawan, C.; Vaissière, T.; Murr, R. & Herceg, Z. (2008). Epigenetic drivers and genetic passengers on the road to cancer. *Mutation Research,* Vol.642, No.1-2, pp. 1-13.

Schneider, A.C.; Heukamp, L.C.; Rogenhofer, S.; Fechner, G.; Bastian, P.J.; von Ruecker, A.; Müller, S.C. & Ellinger, J. (2011). Global histone H4K20 trimethylation predicts cancer-specific survival in patients with muscle-invasive bladder cancer. *British Journal of Urology International*, doi:10.1111/j.1464-410X.2011.10203.x.

Seifert, H.H.; Schmiemann, V.; Mueller, M.; Kazimirek, M.; Onofre, F.; Neuhausen, A.; Florl, A.R.; Ackermann, R.; Boecking, A.; Schulz, W.A. & Grote, H.J. (2007). In situ detection of global DNA hypomethylation in exfoliative urine cytology of patients with suspected bladder cancer. *Experimental and Molecular Pathology*, Vol.82, No.3, pp. 292-297.

Sherr, C.J. & McCormick, F. (2002). The RB and p53 pathways in cancer. *Cancer Cell*, Vol.2, No.2, pp.103–12.

Shirahata, A.; Sakata, M.; Sakuraba, K.; Goto, T.; Mizukami, H.; Saito, M.; Ishibashi, K.; Kigawa, G.; Nemoto, H.; Sanada, Y. & Hibi, K. (2009). Vimentin methylation as a marker for advanced colorectal carcinoma. *Anticancer Research*, Vol.29, No.1, pp.279-81.

Soprano, D.R.; Qin, P. & Soprano, K.J. Retinoic acid receptors and cancers. (2004). *Annual Review of Nutrition*, Vol.24, pp.201-21.

Stirzaker, C.; Song, J.Z.; Davidson, B. & Clark, S.J. (2004). Transcriptional gene silencing promotes DNA hypermethylation through a sequential change in chromatin modifications in cancer cells. *Cancer Research*, Vol.64, No.11, pp.3871-7.

Tada, Y.; Wada, M.; Kuroiwa, K.; Kinugawa, N.; Harada, T.; Nagayama, J.; Nakagawa, M.; Naito, S. & Kuwano, M. (2000). MDR1 gene overexpression and altered degree of methylation at the promoter region in bladder cancer during chemotherapeutic treatment. *Clinical Cancer Research*, Vol.6, No.12, pp. 4618-4627.

Tada, Y.; Wada, M.; Taguchi, K.; Mochida, Y.; Kinugawa, N.; Tsuneyoshi, M.; Naito, S. & Kuwano, M. (2002). The association of death-associated protein kinase hypermethylation with early recurrence in superficial bladder cancers. *Cancer Research*, Vol.62, No.14, pp. 4048-4053.

Taipale, J. & Beachy, P.A. (2001). The Hedgehog and Wnt signalling pathways in cancer. *Nature*, Vol.411, No.6835, pp.349–54.

Tanaka, M.F. & Sonpavde, G. (2011). Diagnosis and management of urothelial carcinoma of then bladder. *Postgraduate Medicine*, Vol.123, No.3, pp. 43-55.

Tilki, D.; Burger, M.; Dalbagni, G.; Grossman, H.B.; Hakenberg, O.W.; Palou, J.; Reich, O.; Rouprêt, M.; Shariat, S.F. & Zlotta, A.R. (2011). Urine Markers for Detection and Surveillance of Non-Muscle-Invasive Bladder Cancer. *European Urology*, doi:10.1016/j.eururo.2011.05.053.

Tsunoda, S.; Smith, E.; De Young, N.J.; Wang, X.; Tian, Z.Q.; Liu, J.F.; Jamieson, G.G. & Drew, P.A. (2009). Methylation of CLDN6, FBN2, RBP1, RBP4, TFPI2, and TMEFF2 in esophageal squamous cell carcinoma. *Oncology Reports*, Vol.21, No.4, pp.1067-73.

Urakami, S.; Shiina, H.; Enokida, H.; Kawakami, T.; Kawamoto, K.; Hirata, H.; Tanaka, Y.; Kikuno, N.; Nakagawa, M.; Igawa, M. & Dahiya, R. (2006). Combination analysis of hypermethylated Wnt-antagonist family genes as a novel epigenetic biomarker panel for bladder cancer detection. *Clinical Cancer Research*, Vol. 12, No.7 Pt 1, pp.2109-16.

'aleri, N.; Vannini, I.; Fanini, F.; Calore, F.; Adair, B. & Fabbri, M. (2009). Epigenetics, miRNAs, and human cancer: a new chapter in human gene regulation. *Mammalian genome: official journal of the International Mammalian Genome Society*, Vol.20, No.9-10, pp. 573-80.

'eerla, S.; Lindgren, D.; Kvist, A.; Frigyesi, A.; Staaf, J.; Persson, H.; Liedberg, F.; Chebil, G.; Gudjonsson, S.; Borg, A.; Månsson, W.; Rovira, C. & Höglund, M. (2009). MiRNA expression in urothelial carcinomas: important roles of miR-10a, miR-222, miR-125b, miR-7 and miR-452 for tumor stage and metastasis, and frequent homozygous losses of miR-31. *International Journal of Cancer*, Vol.124, No.9, pp. 2236-2242.

'illar-Garea, A.; Fraga, M.F.; Espada, J. & Esteller, M. (2003). Procaine is a DNAdemethylating agent with growth-inhibitory effects in human cancer cells. *Cancer Research*, Vol.63, No.16, pp.4984 –9.

Viklund, E.D.; Bramsen, J.B.; Hulf, T.; Dyrskjøt, L.; Ramanathan, R.; Hansen, T.B.; Villadsen, S.B.; Gao, S.; Ostenfeld, M.S.; Borre, M.; Peter, M.E.; Ørntoft, T.F.; Kjems, J. & Clark, S.J. (2011). Coordinated epigenetic repression of the miR-200 family and miR-205 in invasive bladder cancer. *International Journal of Cancer*, Vol.128, No.6, pp. 1327-1334.

Volff, E.M.; Chihara, Y.; Pan, F.; Weisenberger, D.J.; Siegmund, K.D.; Sugano, K.; Kawashima, K.; Laird, P.W.; Jones, P.A. & Liang, G. (2010). Unique DNA methylation patterns distinguish noninvasive and invasive urothelial cancers and establish an epigenetic field defect in premalignant tissue. Cancer Research, Vol.70, No.20, pp.8169-78.

Xu, W.S.; Parmigiani, R.B. & Marks, P.A. (2007). Histone deacetylase inhibitors: molecular mechanisms of action, *Oncogene*, Vol.26, No.37, pp.5541–5552.

Yamada, Y.; Enokida, H.; Kojima, S.; Kawakami, K.; Chiyomaru, T.; Tatarano, S.; Yoshino, H.; Kawahara, K.; Nishiyama, K.; Seki, N. & Nakagawa, M. (2011). MiR-96 and miR-183 detection inurine serve as potential tumor markers of urothelial carcinoma: correlation with stage and grade, and comparison with urinary cytology. *Cancer Science*, Vol.102, No.3, pp.522-9.

Yates, D.R.; Rehman, I.; Meuth, M.; Cross, S.S.; Hamdy, F.C. & Catto, J.W. (2006) Methylational urinalysis: a prospective study of bladder cancer patients and age stratified benign controls. *Oncogene*, Vol.25, No.13, pp.1984-8.

Yates, D.R.; Rehman, I.; Abbod, M.F.; Meuth, M.; Cross, S.S.; Linkens, D.A.; Hamdy, F.C. & Catto, J.W. (2007). Promoter hypermethylation identifies progression risk in bladder cancer. *Clinical Cancer Research*, Vol.13, No.7, pp. 2046-53.

Yu, J.; Zhu, T.; Wang, Z.; Zhang, H.; Qian, Z.; Xu, H.; Gao, B.; Wang, W.; Gu, L.; Meng, J.; Wang, J.; Feng, X.; Li, Y.; Yao, X. & Zhu, J. (2007). A novel set of DNA methylation markers in urine sediments for sensitive/specific detection of bladder cancer. *Clinical Cancer Research*, Vol.13, No.24, pp.7296-304.

Zhang, Z.; Karam, J.; Frenkel, E.; Sagalowsky, A. & Hsieh, J.T. (2006). The application of epigenetic modifiers on the treatment of prostate and bladder cancer. *Urologic Oncology*, Vol.24, No.2, pp.152-60.

Zhang, Z.; Stanfield, J.; Frenkel, E.; Kabbani, W. & Hsieh, J.T. (2007). Enhanced therapeutic effect on androgen-independent prostate cancer by depsipeptide (FK228), a histone deacetylase inhibitor, in combination with docetaxel. Urology, Vol.70, No.2, pp.396-401.

Zheng, Y.G.; Wu, J.; Chen, Z. & Goodman, M. (2008). Chemical regulation of epigenetic modifications: opportunities for new cancer therapy. *Medicinal Research Reviews*, Vol.28, No.5, pp.645-87.

3

Biomarkers of Bladder Cancer in Urine: Evaluation of Diagnostic and Prognostic Significance of Current and Potential Markers

Daben Dawam
Medway NHS Foundation Trust
Medway Maritime Hospital
Associate Teaching Hospital, University of London,
United Kingdom

1. Introduction

The diagnosis of bladder cancer is generally made by cystoscopy and biopsy. Moreover, bladder cancer has a very high frequency of recurrence and therefore requires follow-up cystoscopy, along with urine cytology, as periodic surveillance to identify recurrence early. Cystoscopy is invasive and apt with complications like urine infection which sometimes lead to septicaemia with serious consequencies. Patient experience is most times not pleasant. Therefore, there needs to be a better way of surveillance for bladder cancer which is non-invasive and more acceptable to the patient experience. Consequently, urine biomarkers might be used to either supplement or supplant these tests.

Urinary bladder carcinoma, the fourth most common cancer in men and ninth most common in women results in significant morbidity and mortality.

Bladder cancer (urothelial carcinoma) typically presents as a tumour confined to the superficial mucosa of the bladder. The most common symptom of early bladder cancer is haematuria; however, urinary tract symptoms (i.e., urinary frequency, urgency and dysuria) may also occur. Most urologists follow the American Urological Association (AUA) guidelines for haematuria which recommend cystoscopic evaluation of all adults greater than 40 years old with microscopic haematuria and for those less than 40 years old with risk factors for developing bladder cancer. Confirmatory diagnosis of bladder cancer must by made by cystoscopic examination and biopsy which is considered to be the "gold standard."

At initial diagnosis, about 70 percent of patients have cancers confined to the epithelium or sub-epithelial connective tissue. Non-muscle invasive disease is usually treated with transurethral resection with or without intravesical therapy, depending on depth of invasion and tumour grade. However, there is a 75 percent incidence of recurrence in these patients with 10-15 percent progressing to muscle invasion over a five year period. Current follow-up protocols include flexible cystoscopy and urine cytology every three months for one to three years, every six months for an additional two to three years, and then annually, assuming no recurrence.

While urine cytology is a specific test (from 90 percent–100 percent), its sensitivity is lower, ranging from 50 percent–60 percent overall and is considered even lower for low-grade tumours. Therefore, there has been interest in identifying tumour markers in voided urine that would provide a more sensitive and objective test for tumour recurrence.

2. Background

Bladder cancer is very common, ranking second only to prostate cancer for cancers of the urinary tract. Approximately 54 000 new cases of bladder cancer are diagnosed and ~12 000 people die from this disease every year in the United States alone. Most patients are diagnosed with superficial tumours, which can be completely resected. However, two-thirds of these patients will experience recurrence within 5 years, and almost 90% will have a recurrence by 15 years. Early diagnosis leads to better clinical outcomes, underscoring the importance of finding new ways for screening the general population. Currently, potential bladder tumour markers can be used in various clinical scenarios, including (14):

- Serial testing for earlier detection of recurrence;
- Complementary testing to urine cytology to improve the detection rate;
- Providing a less expensive and more objective alternative to the urine cytology test; and
- Directing the cytoscopic evaluation of patient follow-up.

The gold standard for the detection of urothelial neoplasia is cytologic examination of urothelial cells from voided urine, urinary bladder washings, and urinary tract brushing specimens in combination with cystoscopic examination [12,13]. Because cystoscopy is an invasive procedure and urinary cytology suffers from low sensitivity and specificity, particularly for lower grade tumours, it is desirable to identify novel biomarkers for this cancer. Biochemical testing of urine is a non-invasive and less expensive procedure for diagnosing and monitoring this disease. Because none of the markers mentioned above has sufficient sensitivity and specificity, the quest for identifying additional bladder cancer biomarkers continues.

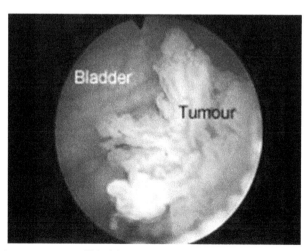

Fig. 1. Cystoscopic appearance of bladder tumour

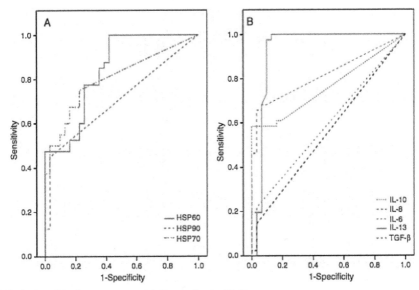

Fig. 2. Relationship between sensitivity and specificity

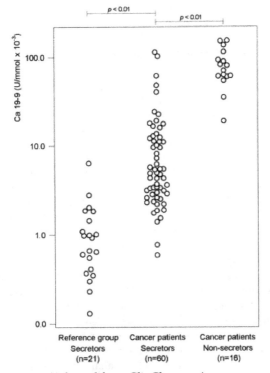

Fig. 3. Ca 19-9 levels in urine (Adapted from ClinChem.org)

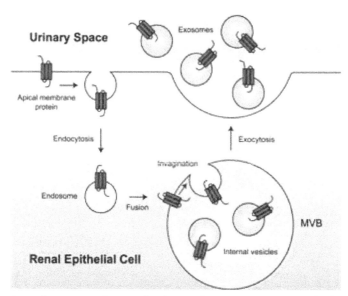

Fig. 4. Mechanism of cancer marker production and appearance in urine (Adapted from flipper.diff.org)

Kageyama et al. propose proteomic analysis of urine as a new way to identify bladder cancer biomarkers. Previously, Celis et al. utilised two-dimensional gel electrophoresis and developed a comprehensive database for bladder cancer profiles of both transitional and squamous cell carcinomas.

Biochemical testing of urine should be able to diagnose early bladder carcinoma because candidate informative molecules could be excreted into the urine during cancer development. Proteomic profiling of urine has been suggested as a diagnostic test for bladder carcinoma [11]. In addition, many other biochemical molecules or genetic markers have been discovered that could be used to diagnose bladder carcinoma with fair sensitivity and specificity. Such molecules (or methods) include, but are not limited to, the following (the approximate diagnostic sensitivities and specificities are in parentheses): BTA stat (68%; 66%); BTA-TRAK (71%; 62%); NMP22 (64%; 71%); telomerase (74%; 89%); HA-HAase (91%; 86%); Immunocyt (68%; 79%); F/FDP (68%; 86%); multicolor fluorescence in situ hybridization assays (84%; 90%); cytokeratins (76%; 84%); metalloproteinases (60%; 80%); and p53 mutation (32%; 100%). The most common noninvasive test, however, is voided urine cytology (VUC), which has a sensitivity of ~50% and a specificity of 97% [12]. This test has higher sensitivity for higher grade tumors.

Through their studies, Kageyama et al. were able to identify a potential tumour marker, calreticulin, which is found in the urine of patients with bladder carcinoma. The authors used a differential display method of bladder cancer vs healthy urothelial tissue and mass spectrometry to identify proteins that are increased in cancer tissue. In addition to calreticulin, an endoplasmic reticulum chaperone, they found nine other candidate proteins that could constitute new biomarkers for bladder carcinoma. The authors confirmed their data with quantitative Western blot analysis, immunoprecipitation, and immunohistochemistry. Their reported sensitivity and specificity were 73% and 86%, espectively, similar to the values reported for other biochemical bladder markers (see above). However, the diagnostic accuracy of their test was vulnerable to urinary tract infections.

The main question surrounding bladder cancer and urinary biomarkers is how these molecules can be used in clinical practice. Clearly, these tests are not useful for population screening because of their low sensitivity and specificity. In addition, none of the available tests is sufficiently accurate to replace cystoscopy in the investigation of a patient with a possible bladder tumour. VUC has relatively low sensitivity, especially for low-grade tumours, but it is currently the most specific test for bladder carcinoma. Consequently, when VUC is positive, it indicates a high-risk tumour that requires definitive treatment. VUC is currently used for monitoring of patients with known high-risk disease, and positive cytology with negative cystoscopy may indicate malignancy of the prostate or upper urinary tract.

Current guidelines suggest that low-risk patients should be surveyed once a year with cystoscopy and high-risk patients at 3-month intervals. Currently, cystoscopy is always combined with VUC. Because, as mentioned earlier, new urinary bladder tests such as BTA or NMP22 could detect lower-grade disease recurrence with higher sensitivity than VUC, it could be worthwhile to consider including one or more of these tests in the routine follow-up of patients with bladder carcinoma. However, large prospective studies will be necessary to test the clinical utility of these assays against cytology. Such trials could show the value of these new tests in reducing the frequency of cystoscopy and in contributing to the earlier and more sensitive detection of disease recurrence, leading to earlier therapeutic interventions and, fortunately, to improved clinical outcomes.

In conclusion, bladder cancer biomarkers have proliferated more than any other class of cancer markers over the last 10 years. We now have at hand a multitude of molecules that can be measured with automated, inexpensive, quantitative assays in urine. These markers may aid in the monitoring of patients with bladder carcinoma and have the potential to reduce the number of follow-up cystoscopy, thus reducing healthcare costs and patient discomfort and, at the same time, detecting relapsing disease more effectively than VUC. It is time to test these new possibilities with prospective clinical trials.

3. Evaluation of individual markers

Urine-based marker tests are being developed to fill some of the remaining needs. These newer tests are more accurate in detecting low-grade bladder cancer, so they are especially useful in monitoring for recurrence, may significantly improve and simplify workup, diagnosis, and follow-up, and hopefully allow for detection of disease at an earlier stage, thus improving the chances of curative therapy.

The urine marker assays discussed here have shown enhanced sensitivity in detecting bladder cancers. However, each still requires further validation and testing in clinical trials to determine how best to apply these tools for in individual patients. In recent years several of the newer tests are being used by urologists as another weapon in the arsenal. Although immunological markers are superior to standard urine cytology, at the present time urine bound tests are not specific enough to completely replace cystoscopy as a definite diagnostic tool.

In order to understand what these tests are about it's helpful to have an understanding of *Sensitivity vs. Specificity:*

A diagnostic test is one that predicts the presence of a disease. An ideal diagnostic test would always give the right answer, with a positive result in everyone with the disease and a negative result in everyone else - and would be quick, safe, simple, painless, reliable, and inexpensive, as well. Since no current diagnostic test is ideal, we need to evaluate each of them for their clinical usefulness. In practice, for any diagnostic test there is a trade-off between sensitivity and specificity. In cancer diagnosis, the need for this trade-off is rooted in the fact that cancer arises from our own tissues. It is not completely "foreign" to our systems like a virus or bacterium is.

It's important to remember that there are four possible results when a diagnostic test is run:

True positive - when the test is **positive** and the patient **does have** the disease

False positive - when the test is **positive** but the patient **does not have** the disease

True negative - when the test is **negative** and the patient **does not have** the disease

False negative - when the test is **negative** but the patient **does have** the disease

Here's another way of looking at this (often referred to as a "truth table"):

Test Result	The disease being tested for is present	The disease being tested for is not present
"Positive"	True positive	False positive
"Negative"	False negative	True negative

Calculating the disease sensitivity and specificity are ways of evaluating diagnostic tests, using the four possible results.

Sensitivity - is the ability of a test to correctly identify a positive specimen, and it tells you how good the test is at identifying the disease. Statistically, it's the proportion of patients with the disease who have a positive result, that is, the number of "true positives" out of all the situations where the disease is present.

For example, 100 patients with cancer are tested using a test that detects tumours. There are 80 positive results and 20 negative results. This means the test has a sensitivity of 80% - it correctly identified 80 of the 100 cancers - and it gave 20 false negative results.

Specificity - is the ability of a test to correctly identify a negative specimen, and it tells you how good the test is at identifying when the disease is absent. The statistical way of looking at this is the proportion of patients without the disease who have a negative test, that is, the number of "true negatives" out of all the situations where the disease is not present.

For example, 100 normal, healthy individuals are tested using a test that detects tumours. There are 80 positives and 20 negatives. This means the test has a specificity of 20% - it correctly identified 20 of the 100 negative specimens - and it gave 80 false positive results.

Both sensitivity and specificity are very important, and they can both be influenced by various factors, such as the characteristics of the population tested or the value used as a cut-off for the test (above which the test is positive and below which it is negative). A test with low sensitivity and many false negative results will fail to detect the tumour in a large portion of the patients being tested, while a test with low specificity with many false positive results may lead to unnecessary invasive or expensive procedures and cause undue alarm.

Many, but not all, patients report they would rather be "scared for nothing" than miss a tumour, and are therefore most interested in tests with high sensitivity.1

4. BTA stat test and the BTA TRAK assay

The original Bard BTA Test, which continues to be referred to in the literature from time to time, was a latex agglutination test detecting bladder tumour-associated antigen and is no longer distributed in the US. It is important to note that it has been replaced by two newer tests based on significantly improved technology with much better sensitivity and specificity.

Both of the new tests detect a human complement factor H-related protein (hCFHrp) which has been shown to be produced by several human bladder cancer cell lines, and by human bladder cancers, but not by other epithelial cell lines (Kinders, Clin Cancer Res 4:2511, 1998). It is thought that factor H acts to protect the tumor cell from the body's natural immune system (Corey, J Biol Chem 275:12917, 2000). Both the BTA stat and BTA TRAK tests can provide valuable but slightly different information for the bladder cancer patient and her doctor.

The BTA stat Test is a qualitative (positive or negative) test provided in a disposable format similar to a home pregnancy test. It uses five drops of urine and can be read in five minutes by the appearance of a coloured line in the patient window, while a coloured line appears in a "check" window to indicate the test is working properly. This test is cleared in the US for use by clinical laboratories, the physician or his staff right in the office, or even by the bladder cancer patient at home (with a physician's prescription). To date, it is the only tumour marker in the United States with this status. Besides being highly sensitive, fast, and easy to use, with a unique availability to be run by the physician and/or the patient, this test is significantly less costly than other diagnostic tests or cytology.

The BTA TRAK Assay is a quantitative immunoassay test and provides a numerical result of the hCFHrp level. Like the NMP22 test, urine must be sent to a reference laboratory where the test is performed by professional technologists. In addition to knowledge of the specific level, an advantage of the BTA TRAK test is the ability to monitor the rise or fall of hCFHrp.

Numerous clinical studies have been conducted with the new BTA tests. Most reports state findings in terms of "sensitivity" and "specificity." Briefly, sensitivity is the ability of the test to correctly identify a positive specimen, and specificity is the ability of the test to correctly identify a negative specimen.

4.1 BTA stat test studies

In the most recent study (June 2000) and the largest of its kind to date, Raitanen reported the overall sensitivity of BTA stat as 82%, and cytology as 30% . In another study, Pode reported 100% BTA stat sensitivity in tumors of stage T2 or higher, grade III, and all tumors greater than 2cm (Pode, J Urol 161:443, 1999). Specificity of the BTA stat Test has been reported as 72-95% (Sarosdy, Urology 50:349, 1997) and 98% in healthy individuals (Raitanen, Scand J Urol Nephrol 33:234, 1999).

4.2 BTA TRAK assay studies

In one study, the overall sensitivity of the BTA TRAK Assay was reported as 72% with a specificity of 75-97% (Ellis, Urology 50:882, 1997). Heicappell again reported an overall sensitivity of 72%, with 97% specificity in healthy individuals. He also reported that BTA

TRAK levels reflect tumour stage and grade, with levels in superficial bladder cancer at high risk of tumour progression significantly higher compared to low and intermediate grade superficial cancers (Heicappell, Eur Urol 35:81, 1999).

4.3 Comparison studies

In a study conducted at the Mayo Clinic, several urine tumour markers were evaluated, including urine cytology, BTA stat, NMP22, fibrin/fibrinogen degradation products (FDP), telomerase, chemiluminescent hemoglobin and hemoglobin dipstick. The telomerase test presented the highest combination of sensitivity and specificity for screening. However, other researchers have had difficulty reproducing the telomerase results of this study, possibly due to the technical difficulties of running the test. It's also important to note that telomerase is a "Research Use Only" test, and has not received FDA clearance for marketing in the US. In the same study, the BTA stat Test was shown to have the best overall sensitivity (74%), and the best sensitivity for T1-T3 and primary tumour detection (Ramakumar, J Urol 161:388, 1999).

Another comparison study (Giannopoulos, Urology 55:871, 2000) showed that the BTA stat Test was more sensitive than cytology in all stages and grades except G3, while NMP22 was more sensitive than cytology only in stage Ta and Grade 1 and 2. The BTA stat Test also had higher sensitivity than NMP22 in all stages and grades.

It is also important to note that in both of the BTA tests, and with NMP22 as well, results can be compromised if there is a urinary tract infection, inflammation, or kidney stones present, if there has been recent trauma to the bladder, or if the specimen is collected by catheter. The paper by Sharma, for example, shows the dramatic increase in specificity when these conditions are excluded from testing (Sharma, J Urol 162:53, 1999). As with any test, for the results to be most useful they should be interpreted in light of all the medical and clinical information available.

5. NMP22 'Bladder check'

In a study comparing cystoscopy, cytology, and Bladder Check; the NMP22/Bladderchek test had a considerably higher detection rate than cytology (67% vs. 20%). Cystoscopy detected 86% of bladder cancers.

More cost effective than cytology, the Bladder check test could also be a good adjunct to cystoscopy. The test costs in the range of $20 to $25, which Medicare reimburses for both bladder cancer monitoring and detection. It is a waived test under the Clinical Laboratory Improvement Amendments (CLIA).

While the test showed a high negative predictive value, it produced a false-positive result in 19 of the 194 patients without bladder cancer. Dr. Tomera advised that such patients need to be watched closely. Earlier data by Mark Soloway, MD, has shown that bladder cancer will be found in 70% of these individuals during the following 3 to 6 months (J Urol 1996; 156:363-7).

NMP22's core technology is based on the level of nuclear matrix proteins (NMPs) that are detected in body fluids. These levels are correlated to the presence of early-stage cancerous abnormalities, which have been validated in multiple clinical studies. The technology was discovered at the Massachusetts Institute of Technology and licensed to Matritech.

Biomarkers of Bladder Cancer in Urine: Evaluation of Diagnostic and Prognostic Significance of Current and Potential Markers

79

6. FISH

Florescence in situ hybridization (FISH) is an assay which uses a mixture of fluorescent labeled probes to assess urinary cells for chromosomal abnormalities associated with malignancy.

In a study at the Mayo clinic, researchers found that urine cytology detected cancerous cells in only 57 percent of the patients with bladder cancer while the FISH test picked up more than 95 percent of the high grade cancers, which are the most dangerous and important group of bladder cancers because they have a high probability of progressing to potentially incurable muscle-invasive bladder cancer. Cancers the test missed were low-grade tumours, which are less dangerous and have only a 3 to 5 percent chance of progressing to a higher stage tumour over five years. The FISH test also detected recurrence of the cancer three to six months earlier than by the cytology. This earlier detection capability should allow treatment to be initiated earlier and possibly give the patient a greater chance for survival, he said.

Fluorescence-in-situ-hybridization (FISH) for multiple centromeric probes has previously been shown to be a very sensitive test for diagnosing UC, however the test was limited by the requirement of multiple cytospins to evaluate 4 or more probe sets. Recently a new commercial test (VYSIS) for evaluating urinary cytology became available in which 4 probes are simultaneously evaluated on a per cell basis on a single cytospin. We performed a pilot study to test the efficacy of the new FISH test compared to standard urine cytology. This study showed that the multi-colour FISH probe test was more sensitive than cytology, easily performed and yielded a high number of cells with numerical chromosomal aberrations.

7. DiagnoCure's ImmunoCyt™ bladder cancer monitoring test

ImmunoCyt™ is a 510(k) cleared, by the FDA, qualitative direct immuno-cytofluorescence assay, intended for use in conjunction with cytology to increase the overall sensitivity for the detection of tumor cells exfoliated in the urine of patients previously diagnosed with bladder cancer.

ImmunoCyt™ contains a cocktail of three monoclonal antibodies labeled with fluorescent markers. The cocktail of antibodies have been shown to react with a mucin glycoprotein as well as to be specific to a glycoform of CEA. The test detects cellular markers specific for bladder cancer in exfoliated cells isolated from urine sample. This non-invasive test, when coupled with urine cytology proves to be more sensitive than urine cytology alone or other currently available tumour markers.

The current standard method for non-invasive detection of bladder cancer is urinary cytology, which consists of identifying the presence of cancer cells in urine. Urinary cytology has high specificity but poor sensitivity, typically no greater than 30% to 45%. This sensitivity varies according to the stage and grade of the tumor.

ImmunoCytT™is carried out in parallel with cytology to improve cytology's sensitivity at detecting tumour cells in the urine of patients, especially those with low stage, low grade tumors. The concomitant use of classical cytology and ImmunoCytTM can substantially improve the detection of bladder cancer. As shown in the ImmunoCytTM performance analysis (cumulative data from eleven publications and presentations from 3,203 cases), a sensitivity of 88% has been obtained when both cytology and ImmunoCyt™ were used together.

A multi-centre study in the United States, published in the Journal of Urology, concluded: ImmunoCyt™ enhances the sensitivity of cytology, which is a specific but not a sensitive method for detecting bladder cancer. The ability of this immuno-cytochemical test to detect low grade, superficial, small tumours makes it the most suitable available marker to test for monitoring strategies in patients with low risk bladder cancer. Performance of urine test in patients monitored for recurrence of bladder cancer: a multi-centre study in the United States.

8. FDP-Fibrin/Fibrinogen Degradation Products

FDP has shown high sensitivity even for low-grade and non-invasive tumours, and its diagnostic ability could be superior to NMP22 according to a recent study
The FDP test detects the presence of fibrin and fibrinogen degradation products in urine. It is a simple test that can be performed in the office, and results are available in about 10 minutes. Fibrin and fibrinogen degradation products are protein fragments generated by the action of the fibrinolytic system on fibrin and fibrinogen. Plasma proteins leak from blood vessels in tumours into the surrounding tissue. Clotting factors rapidly convert the fibrinogen in the plasma into an extravascular fibrin clot, which is degraded by plasmin and activated by urokinase. The FDP test can detect these degradation products and is positive in two thirds of patients with bladder cancer. The FDP assay is more accurate than urine cytology and has high specificity (negative in 96% of healthy subjects). The FDP test was found to be superior to the BTA test in at least one study*.
Telomerase is another substance currently being assessed for its potential usefulness in diagnosing transitional cell cancer (TCC) and in monitoring for recurrence. It will soon be made available to doctors and patients. Telomerase is a ribonucleoprotein enzyme responsible for production of telomeres, which are DNA sequences that occupy the ends of chromosomes and protect their integrity during DNA replication and may be involved in the immortalization of a cancer cell [3]

9. Comparison of screening methods in the detection of bladder cancer

In a study done in '99, researchers prospectively evaluated and compared the sensitivity and specificity of urine cytology, BTA stat, NMP22, fibrin/fibrinogen degradation products (FDP), telomerase, chemiluminescent hemoglobin and hemoglobin dipstick to detect bladder cancer ; within each tumour grade and stage telomerase had the strongest association with bladder cancer among all tests (69% overall concordance). Telomerase was positive in 91% of the patients (10 of 11) with carcinoma in situ. The combination of sensitivity and specificity (70 and 99%, respectively) was the highest for bladder cancer screening in these patients. Telomerase outperformed cytology, BTA stat, NMP22, FDP, chemiluminescent hemoglobin and hemoglobin dipstick in the prediction of bladder cancer. [4]
Telomerase - According to a study published in JAMA (2005; 294:2052-6) Italian researchers reported the assay showed 90% sensitivity and 88% specificity. Specificity increased to 94% for those aged 75 years or younger. The same predictive capacity of activity levels was observed for patients with low-grade tumours or with negative cytology results. In particular, sensitivity was 93%, 87%, and 89% for tumour grades 1, 2, and 3, respectively.

Although the test is proven to identify low-grade tumours, it is not recommended for use in routine screening programs because of the low incidence of bladder cancer and should be aimed at high-risk subgroups, noted the authors, from Morgagni-Pierantoni Hospital, Forli. Theoretically, urine telomerase appears more promising than do non-invasive tests for bladder cancer to date. The main advantages of the test, are that it is non-invasive, can be performed under local anaesthetic, and is significantly less expensive, at $20, than the approximately $100 for cystoscopy or $50 for urinary cytology. It could be a good marker for high-risk screening groups. Furthermore, it shows a high sensitivity for the diagnosis of low-grade tumours that can escape detection during cytological examination. Results are usually available in 2 to 3 days.

10. Hyaluronidase and hyaluronic acid

Hyaluronidase seems to be directly involved in tumour growth and progression, and recent reports have shown this marker has high accuracy in detecting bladder cancer and evaluating its grade, Hyaluronidase and hyaluronic acid are associated with induction of angiogenesis. It has been shown that Hyaluronic acid (HA), the urinary HAase levels of intermediate (G2) to high- grade (G3) bladder cancer patients are five- to seven-fold elevated as compared to those of normal individuals and patients with other genitourinary conditions or low-grade (G1) bladder cancer. The increase in urinary HAase levels is due to the secretion of a tumour-derived HAase which is elevated eight-fold in G2/G3 tumour tissues. The HAase in bladder tumour tissues is secreted by tumour epithelial cells and is associated with the invasive/ metastatic potential of the tumour cells.[5]
Researchers from Brazil investigated the usefulness of HA for the detection of residual tumours that may remain after incomplete TUR. [10] The authors concluded that HA- in addition to being one of the best markers for the initial evaluation of bladder carcinoma- can be used to determine the presence of a residual tumour. This is associated with poor prognosis. Furthermore, haematuria does not seem to influence the content of urinary HA. Other tumor markers such as FISH (Fluorescence in Situ Hybridization) and NMP22 might be affected by instrumentation and therefore could not be evaluated this early.

11. Low values of urinary HA after TUR indicate a favourable prognosis and could probably avoid the second procedure

The researchers suggest that after more experience and follow-up using this assay in the clinical setting, it might be possible to predict not only the cases with residual tumour, but also those who require early radical surgery or those in whom this can be delayed.
In addition to being a good marker in the initial evaluation of bladder carcinoma thanks to its excellent sensitivity (83.1%) and specificity (90.1%), HA potential uses include follow-up, prognostic evaluation, preventing unnecessary interventions and/or to indicate cases where early radical intervention is necessary.[10]

12. BLCA-4

Robert H. Getzenberg and colleagues at the University of Pittsburgh, USA have identified several components of the nuclear matrix, one of which is called BLCA-4, that differentiate human bladder tumour cells from normal bladder cells. Normal samples from unaffected individuals did not react with the antibody, and importantly, BLCA-4 appears to be present throughout the bladder (i.e., in both normal and tumour areas) in bladder cancer patients. This "field effect" permitted development of a urine immunoassay for BLCA-4 that detects the presence of tumour anywhere in the bladder, regardless of stage or grade. The BLCA-4-urine immunoassay has a specificity of 100% and a sensitivity of 95%. According to Dr. Getzenberg, the assay is currently being tested by the Pittsburgh researchers in a clinical trial of individuals at high risk for bladder cancer. [6]

Using a prospectively determined cut-off, 67 of the 75 samples from patients with bladder cancer were positive for BLCA-4, resulting in an assay sensitivity of 89%. Also, 62 of the 65 samples from individuals without bladder cancer were negative for BLCA-4, resulting in an assay specificity of 95%. The authors concluded that the high sensitivity and specificity of the sandwich BLCA-4 immunoassay may allow for earlier detection and treatment of disease, thus greatly improving patient care. [7]

BLCA-4, appears to be associated with a "field effect" of the disease, and in clinical trials is able to separate individuals with bladder cancer from those without the disease with high sensitivity and specificity. BLCA-4 is a bladder cancer marker that is highly specific and occurs early in the development of the disease. It appears to be a transcription factor that may play a role in the regulation of the gene expression in bladder cancer. BLCA-4 is a marker with significant clinical utility that may have an active role in the disease.

13. Other proposed markers

DD 23 monoclonal antibody recognizes a 185 kDa antigen expressed by bladder cancer cells and has been proposed as an adjunct to cytology for the detection of bladder cancer. Urine fibronectin and chorionic gonadotropin (protein and mRNA transcript) may also be markers for transitional cell carcinoma of the bladder .

14. Role of urine markers in early detection of bladder cancer

Almost all cases of bladder cancer are found during the work-up of patients who present with haematuria (71), but most cases of haematuria are not caused by bladder cancer. Urologic disease is detected in 10% of subjects who present with haematuria, and bladder cancer is detected in fewer than half of these subjects (72,73,74). The work-up of patients with haematuria is costly and often requires cytology, cystoscopy, intravenous urography or computed tomography (75). Thus, tumor markers could be useful in identifying the patients in this high-risk group, which requires more intensive clinical work-up for bladder cancer. Zippe et al reported on the value of the urine NMP22 test in the evaluation of 330 patients with haematuria (76). The NMP22 test when used with a cut-off value of 10.0 u/ml detected all 18 cases of bladder cancer with 45 false positive cases (sensitivity, 100%; specificity, 85%). In this study, 267 unnecessary cystoscopy could have been avoided if cystoscopy had been directed by the NMP22 test. In a clinical trial submitted to the Food and Drug Administration (as Pre-Market Approval Data), the NMP22 test was elevated in 69.6% of 56 bladder cancer that were detected in the high risk group. In this report, the specificity was 67.7% (77). The NMP22 test has been cleared by the FDA for use as an aid to diagnose bladder cancer in individuals with risk factors or who have symptoms of bladder cancer. It is highly likely that other urine markers (e.g. BTA, UroVysion and Immunocyt) may also have value for cancer detection in subjects who present with haematuria. The high false positive rate is the major criticism of the urine-based tests when they are used to assess patients who present with haematuria or are used in patient surveillance. The low false negative rate of these tests is their strength, leading to a high negative predictive value that effectively rules out disease in a significant proportion of patients, thereby eliminating unnecessary clinical work-ups for bladder cancer.

15. Role of tissue markers for prognosis

Considerable research effort continues to be directed towards the identification of markers that predict the aggressive potential of superficial bladder tumors. Such information could lead to more effective surveillance protocols and permit more aggressive treatment of those patients with tumors most likely to progress to invasive or metastatic disease. Stein et al have performed an exhaustive review of a variety of biological markers reported to have prognostic value. More recently, p53 and other cell cycle control genes, chorionic gonadotropin beta gene transcripts, various cell matrix and adhesion proteins and differentially expressed NACB.

16. Role of urine markers for patient surveillance

Many reports have established the value of urine tumor marker tests in the early detection of recurrent bladder tumors, but as yet these urine tests cannot replace routine cystoscopy and cytology in the management of bladder cancer patients. Instead, they may be used as complementary adjuncts that direct more effective utilization of clinical procedures, thus reducing the cost of patient surveillance. Patients with superficial lesions of low grade (Ta, Grade 1 and II) are at lower risk for recurrence than patients with Ta Grade III and T1 tumors, and these lower-risk patients may need less intensive follow-up .

The urine markers used in patient surveillance have on occasion been criticized for their low sensitivity in detecting disease, but in most studies they have significantly improved the detection of bladder cancer when used in conjunction with cytology and cystoscopy. Voided urine cytology has its own limitations in detecting carcinoma in situ (cis) and low-grade bladder tumors. It appears that urine markers can assist in the early detection of recurrence in patients with carcinoma in situ and low-grade superficial tumors.

17. Conclusion

The availability of many new markers for bladder cancer raises the possibility of improving the rate of cancer detection by combined use of selected markers, measured either simultaneously or sequentially. The objective of such panel testing should be to improve both the sensitivity and the specificity for bladder cancer detection. Prospective clinical trials are undoubtedly necessary to prove their clinical value, before such panels could be implemented in routine patient care. It should also be noted that the stability of these tumour marker antigens must be better defined in order to minimize false negative test results. Improved definition of the disease conditions which can produce false positive test results for urine based markers could lead to more effective use of these tests for cancer detection. It seems a long way before these markers replace invasive testing, but at least it can help define those group of patients who need cystoscopic surveillance while sparing the majority of patients who do not need the procedure. This will bring enormous cost saving to the increasing health care cost we face in the presence of dwinding health care budget allocations from other competing needs.

18. References

[1] Bailey MJ. Urinary markers in bladder cancer. BJUI 2003;91:772-773.

[2] Eissa S, Kassim S, El-Ahmady O. Detection of bladder tumours: role of cytology, morphology-based assays, biochemical and molecular markers. Curr Opin Obstet Gynecol 2003;15:395-403.

[3] Fritsche HA. Bladder cancer and urine tumor marker tests. Diamandis EP Fritsche HA Lilja H Chan DW Schwartz MK eds. Tumor markers: physiology, pathobiology, technology and clinical applications 2002:281-286 AACC Press Washington.

[4] Kageyama S, Isono T, Iwaki H, Wakabayashi Y, Okada Y, Kontani K, et al. Identification by proteomic analysis of calreticulin as a marker for bladder cancer and evaluation of the diagnostic accuracy of its detection in urine. Clin Chem 2004;50:857-866.

[5] Celis A, Rasmussen HH, Celis P, Basse B, Lauridsen JB, Ratz G, et al. Short-term culturing of low-grade superficial bladder transitional cell carcinomas leads to changes in the expression levels of several proteins involved in key cellular activities. Electrophoresis 1999;20:355-361.

[6] Bravaccini S, Sanchini MA, Granato AM, Gunelli R, Nanni O, Amadori D, Calistri D, Silvestrini R. Urine telomerase activity for the detection of bladder cancer in females. J Urol. 2007 Jul;178(1):57-61.

[7] Sanchini MA, Gunelli R, Nanni O, Bravaccini S, Fabbri C, Sermasi A, Bercovich E, Ravaioli A, Amadori D, Calistri D. Relevance of urine telomerase in the diagnosis of bladder cancer. JAMA. 2005 Oct 26;294(16):2052-6.

[8] Sanchini MA, Bravaccini S, Medri Urine telomerase: an important marker in the diagnosis of bladder cancer.

[9] Roberta Gunelli, ; Oriana Nanni, ; Sara Bravaccini, ; Carla Fabbri, Alice Sermasi, Eduard Bercovich, Alberto Ravaioli,; Dino Amadori,; Daniele Calistri. JAMA. 2005;294:2052-2056.

[10] Van Le TS, Myers J, Konety BR, Barder T, Getzenberg RH. Functional characterization of the bladder cancer marker, BLCA-4. J.Clin Cancer Res. 2004 ;15;10(4):1384-1391.

[11] Messing EM, Teot L, Korman H, Underhill E, Barker E, Stork B, Qian J, Bostwick DG. J Urol. 2005;174:1238-41.

[12] Oeda T, Manabe D. Nippon Hinyokika Gakkai Zasshi [The usefulness of urinary FDP in the diagnosis of bladder cancer: comparison with NMP22, BTA and cytology]. 2001;92(1):1-5.

[13] Tilki D, Burger M, Dalbagni G, Grossman HB, Hakenberg OW, Palou J, Reich O, Rouprêt M, Shariat SF, Zlotta AR. Urine Markers for Detection and Surveillance of Non-Muscle- Invasive Bladder Cancer. Eur Urol. 2011 Jun 12.

[14] Khadjavi A, Barbero G, Destefanis P, Mandili G, Giribaldi G, Mannu F, Pantaleo A, Ceruti C, Bosio A, Rolle L, Turrini F, Fontana D. Evidence of abnormal tyrosine phosphorylated proteins in the urine of patients with bladder cancer: the road toward a new diagnostic tool? J Urol. 2011 May;185(5):1922-1929.

[15] Sagnak L, Ersoy H, Gucuk O, Ozok U, Topaloglu H. Diagnostic Value of a Urine-Based Tumor Marker for Screening Lower Urinary Tract in Low-Risk Patients with Asymptomatic Microscopic Haematuria. Urol Int. 2011 Jun 3.

[16] Yamada Y, Enokida H, Kojima S, Kawakami K, Chiyomaru T, Tatarano S, Yoshino H, Kawahara K, Nishiyama K, Seki N, Nakagawa M. MiR-96 and miR-183 detection in urine serve as potential tumor markers of urothelial carcinoma: correlation with stage and grade, and comparison with urinary cytology. Cancer Sci. 2011 Mar;102(3):522-529.

[17] Kehinde EO, Al-Mulla F, Kapila K, Anim JT. Comparison of the sensitivity and specificity of urine cytology, urinary nuclear matrix protein-22 and multi-target fluorescence in situ hybridization assay in the detection of bladder cancer. Scand J Urol Nephrol. 2011 Mar;45(2):113-121.

[18] Roobol MJ, Bangma CH, el Bouazzaoui S, Franken-Raab CG, Zwarthoff EC. Urol Oncol. 2010 Nov-Dec;28(6):686-90. Feasibility study of screening for bladder cancer with urinary molecular markers (the BLU-P project).

[19] Costa VL, Henrique R, Danielsen SA, Duarte-Pereira S, Eknaes M, Skotheim RI, Rodrigues A, Magalhães JS, Oliveira J, Lothe RA, Teixeira MR, Jerónimo C, Lind GE. Three epigenetic biomarkers, GDF15, TMEFF2, and VIM, accurately predict bladder cancer from DNA-based analyses of urine samples. Clin Cancer Res. 2010 Dec 1;16(23):5842-51.

[20] Margel D, Pesvner-Fischer M, Baniel J, Yossepowitch O, Cohen IR. Stress proteins and cytokines are urinary biomarkers for diagnosis and staging of bladder cancer. Eur Urol. 2011 Jan;59(1):113-119.

[21] Szarvas T, Singer BB, Becker M, Vom Dorp F, Jäger T, Szendroi A, Riesz P, Romics I, Rübben H, Ergün S. Urinary matrix metalloproteinase-7 level is associated with the presence of metastasis in bladder cancer. BJU Int. 2011 Apr;107(7):1069-73.

[22] Lotan Y, Shariat SF, Schmitz-Dräger BJ, Sanchez-Carbayo M, Jankevicius F, Racioppi M, Minner SJ, Stöhr B, Bassi PF, Grossman HB. Considerations on implementing diagnostic markers into clinical decision making in bladder cancer. Urol Oncol. 2010 Jul-Aug;28(4):441-8.

[23] Yutkin V, Nisman B, Pode D. Can urinary biomarkers replace cystoscopic examination in bladder cancer surveillance? Expert Rev Anticancer Ther. 2010 Jun;10(6):787-90.

[24] Lai Y, Ye J, Chen J, Zhang L, Wasi L, He Z, Zhou L, Li H, Yan Q, Gui Y, Cai Z, Wang X, Guan Z. UPK3A: a promising novel urinary marker for the detection of bladder cancer. Urology. 2010 Aug;76(2):514.6-11.

[25] Horstmann M, Bontrup H, Hennenlotter J, Taeger D, Weber A, Pesch B, Feil G, Patschan O, Johnen G, Stenzl A, Brüning T. Clinical experience with survivin as a biomarker for urothelial bladder cancer.World J Urol. 2010 Jun;28(3):399-404.

[26] Tsui KH, Tang P, Lin CY, Chang PL, Chang CH, Yung BY. Bikunin loss in urine as useful marker for bladder carcinoma. J Urol. 2010 Jan;183(1):339-44.

[27] Mengual L, Burset M, Ars E, Lozano JJ, Villavicencio H, Ribal MJ, Alcaraz A. DNA microarray expression profiling of bladder cancer allows identification of non-invasive diagnostic markers. J Urol. 2009 Aug;182(2):741-748.

[28] Lotan Y, Elias K, Svatek RS, Bagrodia A, Nuss G, Moran B, Sagalowsky AI. Bladder cancer screening in a high risk asymptomatic population using a point of care urine based protein tumour marker. J Urol. 2009 Jul;182(1):52-7; discussion 58.

[29] Svatek RS, Karam J, Karakiewicz PI, Gallina A, Casella R, Roehrborn CG, Shariat SF. Role of urinary cathepsin B and L in the detection of bladder urothelial cell carcinoma. J Urol. 2008 Feb;179(2):478-84; discussion 484.

[30] Cai T, Mazzoli S, Meacci F, Tinacci G, Nesi G, Zini E, Bartoletti R. Interleukin-6/10 ratio as a prognostic marker of recurrence in patients with intermediate risk urothelial bladder carcinoma. J Urol. 2007 Nov;178(5):1906-11;discussion 1911-2.

[31] Yossepowitch O, Herr HW, Donat SM. Use of urinary biomarkers for bladder cancer surveillance: patient perspectives. J Urol. 2007 Apr;177(4):1277-82; discussion 1282.

[32] Shariat SF, Marberger MJ, Lotan Y, Sanchez-Carbayo M, Zippe C, Lüdecke G, Boman H, Sawczuk I, Friedman MG, Casella R, Mian C, Eissa S, Akaza H, Serretta V, Huland H, Hedelin H, Raina R, Miyanaga N, Sagalowsky AI, Roehrborn CG, Karakiewicz PI. Variability in the performance of nuclear matrix protein 22 for the detection of bladder cancer. J Urol. 2006 Sep;176(3):919-26; discussion 926.

[33] Margel D, Pesvner-Fischer M, Baniel J, Yossepowitch O, Cohen IR. Stress proteins and cytokines are urinary biomarkers for diagnosis and staging of bladder cancer. Eur Urol. 2011 Jan;59(1):113-9.

[34] Renard I, Joniau S, van Cleynenbreugel B, Collette C, Naômé C, Vlassenbroeck I, Nicolas H, de Leval J, Straub J, Van Criekinge W, Hamida W, Hellel M, Thomas A, de Leval L, Bierau K, Waltregny D. Identification and validation of the methylated TWIST1 and NID2 genes through real-time methylation-specific polymerase chain reaction assays for the noninvasive detection of primary bladder cancer in urine samples. Eur Urol. 2010 Jul;58(1):96-104.

[35] Tilki D, Singer BB, Shariat SF, Behrend A, Fernando M, Irmak S, Buchner A, Hooper AT, Stief CG, Reich O, Ergün S. CEACAM1: a novel urinary marker for bladder cancer detection. Eur Urol. 2010 Apr;57(4):648-654.

[36] van Rhijn BW. Considerations on the use of urine markers for bladder cancer. Eur Urol. 2008 May;53(5):880-881.

[37] Vrooman OP, Witjes JA. Urinary markers in bladder cancer. Eur Urol. 2008 May;53(5):909-916.

[38] Fernandez-Gomez J, Rodríguez-Martínez JJ, Barmadah SE, García Rodríguez J, Allende DM, Jalon A, Gonzalez R, Alvarez-Múgica M. Urinary CYFRA 21.1 is not a useful marker for the detection of recurrences in the follow-up of superficial bladder cancer. Eur Urol. 2007 May;51(5):1267-74.

[39] Golshani R, Hautmann SH, Estrella V, Cohen BL, Kyle CC, Manoharan M, Jorda M, Soloway MS, Lokeshwar VB. HAS1 expression in bladder cancer and its relation to urinary HA test. Int J Cancer. 2007 Apr 15;120(8):1712-20.

[40] Grossman HB, Blute ML, Dinney CP, Jones JS, Liou LS, Reuter VE, Soloway MS. The use of urine-based biomarkers in bladder cancer. Urology. 2006 Mar;67(3 Suppl 1):62-4.

[41] Simon MA, Lokeshwar VB, Soloway MS. Current bladder cancer tests: unnecessary or beneficial? Crit Rev Oncol Hematol. 2003 Aug;47(2):91-107.

4

Angiogenesis and Lymphangiogenesis in Bladder Cancer

Yasuyoshi Miyata, Hideki Sakai and Shigeru Kanda
Nagasaki University Graduate School of Biomedical Sciences
Japan

1. Introduction

In cancer patients, the majority of deaths occur as a consequence of metastatic diseases. In addition, metastasis is a marker for poor prognosis and low quality of life in many malignancies. Several groups have investigated the mechanism of tumor metastasis. Metastatic lesions are formed through a multi-step complex process and then spread either locally at the site of the primary tumor, or into distant organs through the blood or lymphatic vessels.

Another important feature of cancers is the chaotic behavior of tumor growth and cancer cell cycle progression. To maintain such activities, abundant supply of oxygen and nutrients are necessary. Angiogenesis refers to the formation of new blood vessels and development of new branching vessels from the existing tumor tissue vasculature and this pathological process is important to secure adequate blood supply including oxygen and nutrients to the rapidly dividing malignant cells. In fact, there is a good correlation between tumor growth/cancer cell proliferation and the extent of angiogenesis in almost of all cancers. While there is abundant information on the mechanisms that are involved in the initiation, regulation and maintenance of angiogenesis in cancer tissue, little is known about the mechanisms involved in the formation of new lymphatic vessels (lymphangiogenesis) in cancers. Furthermore, the current knowledge about cancer dissemination through the lymphatics lacks details about the mode of transport of cancer cells within the lymphatic vessels and the mechanisms involved in their exit and seeding into the distant organs.

In this paper, we review the clinical and pathological significance of angiogenesis and lymphangiogenesis in bladder cancer. In addition, the mechanisms that regulate the formation of new vessels in bladder cancer are discussed. Specifically, we focus on the factors that co-regulate these two different vessels and their potential use as predictive marker of outcome in patients with bladder cancer. In addition, we also discuss the limitation of quantification of these vessels in human tissues.

2. Angiogenesis and lymphangiogenesis

2.1 Angiogenesis in cancer tissues

Angiogenesis is defined as the formation of new blood vessels from pre-existing vasculature, and it is an integrated process of tumor growth, maintenance, and progression in solid tumors (Folkmann, 1992). Angiogenesis is a multistep processes involving changes in the extracellular matrix, cell proliferation, cell migration, and tube formation. Blood vessel density (BVD), a surrogate marker for angiogenesis, correlates with the malignant potential and poor prognosis of patients with various types of cancers. In addition, anti-angiogenic therapy that targets the tumor vascular supply and pathways of cancer cell dissemination was first introduced in 1971 (Folkman, 1971). Since then, numerous investigators have focused on the mechanisms of angiogenesis, including molecular mechanisms. At present, there is a general agreement that the regulation of tumor angiogenesis depends on a complex mechanism that dynamically balances angiogenic and anti-angiogenic factors. In this regard, these factors are secreted by both tumor cells and stromal cells in complicated systems. To complicate the issue, the mechanisms and pathological roles of these factors vary according to the type of cancer, its malignant potential, and systemic condition.

2.2 Lymphangiogenesis in cancer tissues

In addition to angiogenesis, many investigators have examined the process of lymphangiogenesis, i.e., the formation of new lymphatic vessels, due to its importance in lymph node metastasis and distant metastasis. Lymph node metastasis occurs in various types of malignancies and its presence is considered a strong predictor of recurrence and poor survival of patients with bladder cancer. However, the clinical role and prognostic value of lymphangiogenesis in cancer patients remain unclear, largely due to the lack of specific endothelial markers for lymphatic vessels as well as the lack of proper imaging procedures for lymphatic vessels in human tissues (Pepper, 2001). In recent years, various specific antibodies for lymphatic endothelial cells have been developed and used to investigate the clinical and pathological significance of lymphangiogenesis in cancer patients. Similar to angiogenesis, evidence suggests that lymphangiogenesis is also regulated by complex mechanisms that include a variety of factors. While various common mechanisms regulate the processes of angiogenesis and lymphangiogenesis, other mechanisms vary according to these processes. For example, in contrast to angiogenesis, no intrinsic anti-lymphangiogenic molecules have yet been isolated.

Thus, to discuss the pathological roles, predictive values, and potential therapeutic targets of angiogenesis and lymphangiogenesis, it is important to understand the various complex mechanisms and cooperative functions involved in these two processes.

2.3 Angiogenesis and lymphangiogenesis in bladder cancer

BVD is often used in the analysis of human cancer tissues as a surrogate and semi-quantitative marker of angiogenesis. Previous studies suggested that BVD provides significant information on prognosis and survival in patients with bladder cancer (Streeter & Harris, 2002; Goddard, 2003). However, other investigators were less supportive for the prognostic value of BVD, especially in patients with non-muscle-invasive bladder cancer (NMIBC) (Korkolopoulou, et al., 2001; Ioachim, et al., 2006; Miyata, et al., 2006). Table 1 provides a summary of the currently held opposing views on BVD.

Such discrepancy could be attributed to differences in methodology, such as methods used for counting, size of the field of view, definition of microvessel, and antibodies used in different assays. For example, measurement at periphery or growth from of the tumor (Stavropoulos et al., 2004) or at highest vascularity "hot spots" (Korkolopoulou et al., 2001). Furthermore, the diameter of the microvessel was no mentioned in some studies; though other provided descriptive terms (the lumen diameter was smaller than approximately eight red blood cells) (Stavropoulos, 2004). More detailed problems are described in the following section.

Patients	Findings	Reference
109 NMIBC	Predictor of muscle invasion in G3 patients, though not an independent factor.	Starvropoulos
66 NMIBC	Independent predictor of recurrence-free survival, particularly in T1G2 tumors	Santos
35 NMIBC + 80 MIBC	Independent predictor for overall survival in MIBC. No significant role in NMIBC	Korkolopoulou
87 NMIBC + MIBC	Independent predictor of lymph node metastasis.	Susuki
104 NMIBC + 22 MIBC	Not significant for recurrence-free, metastasis-free, or cause-specific survival.	Miyata

NMIBC: non-muscle-invasive bladder cancer, MIBC: muscle-invasive bladder cancer

Table 1. Predictive value of blood vessel density (BVD) for progression and survival.

In addition to semi-quantitative measures of BVD, vascular invasion by tumor cells (blood vessel invasion, BVI) has also been identified as a prognostic factor in bladder cancer (Harada et al., 2005). Furthermore, vascular area and various parameters related to the shape, relapse, and/or complexity of the vessels have been suggested as important for more detailed discussion on the relationship between angiogenesis and pathological role, prognosis, and survival. In this regard, several investigators paid special attention to the morphological variability in the vascular pattern (Korkolopoulou et al., 2001; Sharma et al., 2005), and one study reported that the vascular area was an independent predictor of overall survival in patients with T1 disease whereas BVD was not (Korkolopoulou et al., 2001). In contrast to angiogenesis, there is little or no information on the clinical and pathological significance and predictive value of lymphangiogenesis in patients with bladder cancer. Several studies reported that higher LVD correlates significantly with malignant behavior, cancer cell progression, and prognosis (Fernández et al., 2008; Miyata et al., 2006). In addition, one report indicated that the pathological role of lymphangiogenesis was depended on the location of lymphatic vessels, such as intra-tumoral and peri-tumoral area. In other words, intra-tumoral LVD correlated with histological differentiation, and peri-tumoral LVD correlated with lymph node metastasis (Fernández, et al., 2008). Similar to BVI, of lymphatic vessel invasion (LVI) by tumor cells was also identified as a prognostic factor in bladder cancer (Algaba, 2006). In general, however, information on lymphangiogenesis in human bladder cancer is to a large extent scarce, compared to that on angiogenesis.

2.4 Regulation of angiogenesis and/or lymphangiogenesis
Members of the vascular endothelial growth factor (VEGF) family are the most important molecules involved in the processes of angiogenesis and lymphangiogenesis. This family consists of 7 members, including VEGF-A, -B, -C, -D, and -E, svVEGF, and placental growth factor. In addition, three types of receptors have so far been identified: VEGFR-1, -2, and -3 (Takahashi et al., 2005). The angiopoietin (Ang) family also encompasses several pro-angiogenic factors. This family consists of Ang-1 and -2 and Tie2 tyrosine kinase receptors,

and the system is influenced by VEGF family. In addition, several factors, for example, fibroblast growth factor (FGF)-2, hepatocyte growth factor (HGF), and insulin-like growth factor (IGF), are also reported to be involved in the regulation of both angiogenesis and lymphangiogenesis.
Angiostatin and endostatin, which are both produced by proteolytic cleavage of plasminogen and collagen XVIII, respectively, are well characterized anti-angiogenic factors. (O'Reilly, et al., 1994, 1997). In addition, thrombospondins (TSPs) also inhibits angiogenesis (Lawler, 2000). Another report indicated that down-regulation of TSP-1 secretion in bladder cancer tissues was a key event in the change from an anti-angiogenic to an angiogenic phenotype during carcinogenesis (Campbell, et al., 1998). On the other hand, there are conflicting results on the relationship between TSP-1 expression and BVD in human bladder cancer. Specifically, TSP-1 staining correlated negatively with BVD (Grossdfeld et al., 1997), whereas other investigators reported that TSP-1 expression correlated positively with BVD (Ioachim et al., 2006).
We review here in detail two representative pro-angiogenic factors; VEGF family and Ang family. Their selection was based on the finding that they are potential therapeutic targets in various cancers. Actually, targeted therapies based on these factors have been tested already in patients with bladder cancer. Unfortunately, however, anti-angiogenic factor-targeted therapy is still in its infancy and there is little possibility to use such drugs for treatment of bladder cancer in the near future.

2.5 VEGF family

Among the VEGF family members, VEGF-A is a major regulator of angiogenesis. On the other hand, both VEGF-C and VEGF-D have been found to play major roles in lymphangiogenesis. Furthermore, VEGFR-2 and VEGFR-3 are reported to be the major mediators of angiogenic response in blood endothelial cells and lymphangiogenic response in lymphatic endothelial cells, respectively. In other words, VEGF-A signaling through VEGFR-2 is the major pathway that activates angiogenesis by stimulating cell proliferation, survival, and migration of endothelial cells (Shibuya & Claesson-Welsh, 2006). Furthermore, the VEGF-C/D-VEGFR-3 signaling pathway is important for the growth of lymphatic endothelial cells (Skobe et al. 2001; Stacker et al., 2001; Lin, et al., 2005). In support of this notion, blocking the VEGF-C/D-VEGFR-3 signaling pathway was reported to inhibit tumor lymphangiogenesis and lymph node metastasis in several xenograft and transgenic tumor models (He et al., 2002; Lin et al., 2005; Roberts et al., 2006).
In contrast to the above studies, several groups reported that VEGF-A could stimulate lymphangiogenesis *in vivo* (Nagy et al., 2002; Cursiefen et al., 2004). In addition, in an animal model of chemically-induced skin cancer, VEGF-A induced lymphangiogenesis and promoted lymphatic metastasis (Hirakawa et al., 2005). Conversely, VEGF-C and VEGF-D were reported to play important roles in angiogenesis under various physiological and pathological conditions (Cao 1998, Jussila & Alitalo, 2002).
VEGFR-1 has a high affinity for VEGF-A, VEGF-B, and PIGF. However, its tyrosine kinase activity is comparatively weak (Autiero, et al., 2003; Shibutya & Claesson-Welsh, 2006). VEGFR-1 is expressed in endothelial cells. In addition, it is also expressed in monocytes/macrophages, hemopoietic cells, and pericytes. Its tyrosine kinase activity is required for stimulation of hemopoietic cell migration towards VEGFs and PIGFs (Barleon, et al., 1996; Clauss, et al. 1996). Based on these results, VEGF-B, PIGF, and VEGFR-1 are

thought to play minimal roles in angiogenesis. In fact, they do not activate angiogenesis during development. However, they have been reported to exhibit angiogenic activity under a variety of pathological conditions (Fisher et al., 2008). For examples, in animal experiments, PIGF was associated with angiogenesis in various pathological conditions including ischemia, inflammation, and tumor growth (Carmeliet, et al., 2001; Luttun, et al., 2002).

The role of VEGFR-2 in lymphangiogenesis is still controversial. VEHGR-2 is expressed at low levels in lymph vessels, and VEGF-VEGFR-2 signaling can induce lymphatic vessel formation (Hong et al., 2004). On the other hand, evidence suggests that lymphangiogenesis induced by such system involves the recruitment of immune cells producing VEGF-C and – D (Crusiefen, et al., 2004).

The following schematic diagram illustrates the relationship between VEGFs and VEGFRs and angiogenesis and lymphangiogenesis:

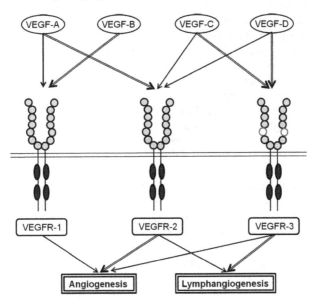

2.6 VEGF family in bladder cancer

Angiogenesis in bladder cancer involves the VEGF-A signaling through the receptor VEGFR-2. The interaction between VEGF-A and VEGFR-2 plays a crucial role in tumor growth, progression, and prognosis via regulation of angiogenesis in patients with bladder cancer.

VEGF-C and –D are highly expressed in cancer cells than in normal urothelial cells (O'Breien, et al., 1995; Zu et al., 2006; Miyata, et al.). Several investigators have reported that the expression of VEGF-C in bladder cancer is closely associated with tumor progression including lymph node metastasis (Suzuki, et al., 2005; Zu, et al., 2006). In addition, the expression of VEGF-C was a significant predictor of poor cause-specific survival in 87 patients. However, multivariate analysis in the same study showed that VEGF-C was not an independent factor and its expression did not correlate with various clinicopathological features (Suzuki, et al, 2005). On the other hand, the same analysis showed that the expression of VEGF-C in bladder cancer was a significant and independent predictor of pelvic lymph node metastasis. Thus, these reports have demonstrated that VEGF-C plays important role in the malignant aggressiveness and its overexpression is associated with poor prognosis of patients with bladder cancer. On the other hand, controversy exists regarding the prognostic value of VEGF-C expression in bladder cancer (Mylona, et al., 2006).

The fact that VEGF-C binds to and stimulates phosphorylation of tyrosine kinase receptor VEGFR-3 is well-known. In addition to VEGFR-3, VEGF-C also binds and activates VEGFR-2, but not VEGFR-1 (Roberts, et al., 2006). Because VEGFR-2 is the major pathway of angiogenesis, it is possible that VEGF-C also correlates with angiogenesis in bladder cancer. One study of 45 patients with bladder cancer reported that VEGF-C expression did not correlate with microvessel density (Zu, et al., 2006). On the other hand, we found that VEGF-C expression correlated positively with both MVD and LVD in 126 patients with bladder cancer. Another group reported that VEGF-C expression correlated with intra-tumoral BVD, but not with overall BVD. They also showed that VEGF-C expression correlated significantly with both intra-tumoral and peri-tumoral LVD (Afonso, et al., 2009). The reasons for these discrepancies are probably related to differences in antibodies used to measure MVD and also differences in sample size.

VEGF-D expression is also reported to be significantly associated with pathological features and prognosis of patients with bladder cancer (Miyata et al, 2006; Herrmann, et al., 2007). In addition, several studies demonstrated that VEGF-D expression also correlated with tumor growth, metastasis, and survival of patients with bladder cancer (Miyata, et al., 2006; Herrmann, et al, 2007). However, in comparison with VEGF-C, information regarding pathological significance and predictive value of VEGF-D in patients with bladder cancer is very limited.

Similarly, there is a little information on VEGF-B expression in bladder cancer. To our knowledge, there is only one study on VEGF-B m-RNA expression in bladder cancer tissues (Fauconett, et al., 2009). These authors used Northern blot analysis and reported the lack of VEGF-B mRNA expression in 37 bladder cancer specimens.

2.7 Ang family in cancers including bladder cancer

Angiopoietin (Ang)-1 and -2 have angiogenic function acting on Tie2 tyrosine kinase receptors (Maisonpierre, et al., 1997; Papapetropoulos, et al., 1999). Ang-1 is known as stabilizing factor because it helps to maintain and stabilize mature vessels by promoting interactions between endothelial cells and neighboring cells including pericytes and smooth muscle cells (Maisonpierre, et al., 1997; Papapetropoulos, et al., 1999, 2000). In contrast, Ang-2 is known as an antagonist to Ang-1 because it is expressed at sites of vascular remodeling and acts to destabilize vessels (Maisonpierre, et al., 1997). Interestingly, Ang-2 is reported to potentiate angiogenesis in the presence of VEGF, but causes regression of this process in the absence of VEGF (Maisonpierre, et al., 1997; Holash, et al., 1999). Thus, the angiopoietin-Tie2 system, comprising Ang-1, Ang-2, Tie2, and VEGF, seems to be regulated by complex mechanisms.

In bladder cancer, there are conflicting results on the clinical and pathological significance of angiopoietin-Tie2 system. One study demonstrated a significant correlation between Ang-2 protein expression and high stage, high grade tumors, and poor prognosis, whereas Ang-1 protein expression did not show the same trend (Oka, et al., 2005). It also showed that Ang-2 expression was an independent predictor of overall survival in patients with bladder cancer. On the other hand, Ang-2 mRNA expression in early stage superficial carcinomas and low grade tumors was reported to be significantly higher than in advanced stage muscle invasive carcinomas and high grade tumors (Quentin, et al., 2004). In comparison, the same study also reported that Ang-1 mRNA was expressed at significantly low levels in low grade and early stage tumors compared to high grade or advanced stage tumors. Other studies on Ang-1 and Ang-2 demonstrated the presence of significantly higher serum levels of Ang-1 in patients with bladder cancer relative to the control; and conversely, Ang-2 and Tie2 levels were significantly lower. (Szarvas, et al., 2009). The same study also showed that high Tie2 serum level was an independent prognostic factor for metastasis in multivariate analysis model that included tumor grade and stage.

2.8 Limitation of quantification of angiogenesis and lymphangiogenesis

BVD is often used as a quantitative marker of angiogenesis. The method used for quantification was first described after antibodies to factor VIII-related antigen became commercially availability; these antibodies were used to immunohistochemically stain blood vessels. Since then, various immunohistochemical pan-endothelial markers, such as CD31, CD34, von-Willebrand factor, have been used to stain and study blood vessels. CD31, also known as PECAM-1 (Platelet Endothelial Cell Adhesion Molecule-1), is a 130 KDa integral membrane protein, and is expressed constitutively on the surface of adult and embryonic endothelial cells. The CD34 protein is a member of a family of single-pass transmembrane proteins expressed on blood vessel endothelial cells (Nielsen & McNagny, 2008). However, these markers cannot distinguish between small and large blood vessels (Hassan, et al., 2002). On the other hand, CD105, also known as endoglin, is a disulphide-linked, proliferation-associated, hypoxia-inducible homodynamic cell membrane glycoprotein, and is known to be over-expressed in proliferating endothelial cells and is strongly up-regulated in endothelial cells of neoplastic tissues compared with normal cells (Fonasanti, et al., 2002; Minhajat, et al., 2006). Based on these properties, many recent studies have recommended the use of CD105 for evaluation of angiogenesis in tumor tissues because it reflects the dynamic status of tumor-related angiogenesis compared to other pan-endothelial markers (Sharma, et al., 2005). In fact, so far, CD105 antibody was demonstrated to have a greater specificity for tumor vasculature than other pan-endothelial markers, such as CD31, CD34, and Factor VIII in a clinical study of colorectal cancer (Saadi, et al., 2004).

In bladder cancer tissues, several antibodies have been used to evaluate angiogenesis. These include factor VIII (Lianes, et al., 1998; Shirotake, et al., 2011), CD31 (Korkolopoulos, et al., 2001; Afonso, et al., 2009), and CD34 (Shirotake, et al., 2011; Stavropoulos, et al., 2004; Ioachim, et al., 2006); whereas CD105 has rarely been used in bladder cancer tissues.

It is suggested that CD31, CD34, and CD105 are more useful because they efficiently recognize small-caliber vessels that are associated with angiogenesis in bladder cancer than factor VIII (Santos, et al., 2003). However, this study did not discuss the difference between these markers. Thus, to date, there is no ideal antibody to truly reflect the clinical and pathological significance of angiogenesis in bladder cancer. To this effect, some investigators have doubted the pathological significance and predictive value of BVD in patients with bladder cancer (Table 2).

Similar to angiogenesis, there is no ideal antibody that reflects the significance of lymphangiogenesis. In general, three different antibodies such as anti-lymphatic vessel endothelial hyaluronan receptor (LYVE)-1 (Yang, et al., 2011), anti-VEGFR-3 (Zhou et al., 2011) and anti-D2-40 (Miyata, et al., 2006; Afonso, et al., 2009,) have been used to detect lymphatic vessels. However, detailed information on the differences and characteristics of each of these factors is not available. Further studies are necessary to discuss the methods of quantification and evaluation of lymphangiogenesis in bladder cancer tissues.

	n	Antibody	Progression	Survival	Reference	year
NMIBC	35	CD31	No	No	Korkolopoulou	2001
NMIBC	66	CD31+CD34+FVIII	Yes*	–	Santos	2003
NMIBC	109	CD34	Yes**	–	Stavropoulos	2004
MIBC	109	FVIII	No	No	Linanes	1998
MIBC	80	CD31	Yes	No	Korkolpoulou	2001
Both	113	CD31+CD34	No	Yes	Bochener	1995
Both	148	CD34	No	No	Ioachim	2006
Both	42	CD31+FVIII	–	–	Gehani	2011

NMIBC, non-muscle invasive bladder cancer; MIBC, muscle invasive bladder cancer; FVIII, factor VIII. * In T1/grade 2 patients. ** In grade 3 patients.

Table 2. Prognostic significance of blood vessel density (BVD)

3. Conclusion

Angiogenesis and lymphangiogensis play important roles for tumor growth and progression in bladder cancer. VEGF family and Ang family are well known to be associated with these phenomenon in bladder cancer. However, other factors and molecules are also speculated to regulate them by complex mechanism. So, detailed mechanism of their regulations is still fully understood. In addition, further studies are necessary to discuss the methods of quantification and evaluation of angiogenesis and lymphangiogenesis in bladder cancer tissues.

4. Acknowledgement

We are grateful to Mr. Takumi Shimogama, Mr. Yoshikazu Tsuji, Mrs. Miki Yoshimoto, and Mrs. Miho M. Kuninaka, for their outstanding support. This manuscript was supported in no funding.

5. References

Afonso, J.; Santos, L.L.; Amaro, T. et al. (2009). The aggressiveness of urothelial carcinoma depends to a large extent on lymphvascular invasion – the prognostic contribution of related molecular markers. Histopathology, Vol.55, No.5, (July), pp. 514-524.

Algaba, F. (2006). Lymphovascular invasion as aprognotic tool for advanced bladder cancer. Curr Opin Urol, Vol.16, No.5 (September), pp. 367-371.

Autiero, M.; Waltenberger, J.; Communi, D. et al. (2003). Role of PIGF in the intra- and intermolecular cross talk between the VEGF receptors Flt1 and Flk1. Nat Med, Vol.9, No.7, (July), pp. 936-943.

Barleon, B.; Sozzani, S.; Zhou, D. et al. (1996). Migration of human monocytes in response to vascular endothelial growth factor (VEGF) is mediated via the VEGF receptor flt-1. Blood, Vol.87, No.8, (April), pp. 3336-3343.

Campbell, SC.; Volpert, O.V.; Ivanovich, M. et al. (1998). Molecular mediators of angiogenesis in bladder cancer. Cancer Res, Vol.58, No.6 (March), pp. 1298-1304.

Cao, Y.; Linden, P.; Famebo, J. et al. (1998). Vascular endothealil growth factor C induceds angiogenesis in vivo. Proc Natl Acd Sci USA, Vol.95, No24. (November), pp. 14389-14394.

Carmeliet, P.; Moons, L.; Luttun, A. et al. (2001). Synergism between vascular endothelial growth factor and placental growth factor contributes to angiognenesis and plasma extravasation in pathological conditions. Nat Med, Vol.7, No.5, (May), pp. 575-583.

Clauss, M.; Weich, H.; Breier, G. et al. (1996). The vascular endothelial growth factor receptor Flt-1 mediates biological activities. Implications for a functional role of placenta growth factor in monocyte activation and chemotaxis. J Biol Chem, Vol.271, No.30, (July), pp.17629-17634.

Cursiefen, C.; Chen, L.; Borges, L.P. (2004). VEGF-A stimulates lymphangiogensis and hemangiogenesis in inflammatory neovasculalization via macrophage recruitment. J Clin Invest, Vol.113, No.7, (April), pp.1040-1050.

Fauconnet, S.; Bernardini, S.; Lascombe, I. et al. (2009). Expression analysis of VEGF-A and VEGF-B: relationship with clinicopathological parameters in bladder cancer. Oncol Rep, Vol.21, No.6, (June), pp. 1495-1504.

Fernández, M.I.; Bolenz, C.; Smith, N.; et al. (2008). Prognostic implications of lymphangiogenesis in muscle-invasive transitional cell carcinoma of the bladder. Eur Urol, Vol.53, No.3, (March), pp. 571-578.

Fischer, C.; Mazzone, M.; Jonckx, B. et al. (2008). Flt1 and its ligands VEGFB and PIGF: during targets for anti-agniogenic therapy? Nat Rev Cancer, Vol.8, No.12, (December), pp. 942-956.

Folkman, J. (1971). Tumor angiogenesis: Thrapeutic implications. N Engl J Med, Vol.285, No.21, (November), pp. 285: 1182-1186.

Folkman, J. (1992). The role of angiogenesis in tumor growth. Semin Cancer Biol Vol.3, No.2, (April), pp. 65-71.

Fonsatti, E.; Altomonte, M.; Nicotra, M.R. et al. (2003). Endoglin (CD105): a powerful therapeutic target on tumor-associated angiognenenic blood vessels. Oncogene, Vol.22, No.42, (May), pp. 6557-6563.

Goddard, J.C.; Sutton, C.D.; Furness, P.N.; et al. (2003). Microvessel density at presentation predicts subsequent muscle invasion in superficial bladder cancer. Clin Cancer Res 2003, Vol.9, No.7, (July), pp. 2583-2586.

Grossfeld, G.D.; Ginsberg, D.A.; Stein, J.P. et al. (1997). Thrombospondin-1 expression in bladder cancer: association with p53 alternations, tumor angiogenesis, and tumor progression. J Natl Cancer Inst, Vol.89, No.3, (February), pp. 219-227.

Harada, K.; Sakai, I, Hara, I.; et al. (2005). Prognostic significance of vascular invasion in patients with bladder cancer who underwent radical cystectomy. J Urol. Vol.12, No.3, (March), pp.250-255.

Hasan, J.; Byers, R. & Jayson, GC. (2002). Intra-tumoural microvessel density in human solid tumours. Br J Cancer, Vol.86, No. 1566 – 1577.

He, Y.; Kozaki, K.; Karpanen, T. et al. (2002). Suppression of tumor lymphangiogensis and lymph node metastasis by blocking vascular endothelial growth factor 3 signaling. J Natl Cancer Inst, Vol.94, No.11, (June), pp. 819-825.

Herrmann, E.; Eltze, E.; Bierer, S. et al. (2007). VEGF-C, VEGF-D, and Flt-4 in transitional bladder cancer: relationships to clinicopathological parameters and long-term survival. Anticancer Res, Vol.27, No.5A, (September-October), pp. 3127-3133.

Hirakawa, S.; Kodama, S.; Kunstfeld, R. et al. (2005). VEGF-A induces tumor and sentinel lymph node lymphangiogensis and promotes lymphatic metastasis. J Exp Med, Vol.201, No.7, (April), pp. 1089-1099.

Hong, Y.K.; Lange-Asschenfeldt, B.; Velasco, P. et al. VEGF-A promotes tissue repair-associated lymphatic vessel formation via VEGFR-2 and the alpha1beta1 and alpha2beta1 integrins. FASEB J, Vol.18, No.10, (July), pp. 1111-1113.

Holash, J.; Maisonpierre, P.C.; Olsson, L.E. et al. (1999). Vessel cooption, regression, and growth in tumors mediated by angiogenesis and VEGF. Science, Vol.284, No.5422 : pp. 1994-1998.

Jussila, L. & Alitalo, K. (2002). Vascular growth factors and lymphangiogensis. Physiol Rev, Vol.82, No.3, (July), pp. 673-700.

Ioachim, E.; Michael M.C.; Salmas, M.; et al. (2006) Thrombospondin-1 expression in urothelial carcinoma: prognostic significance and association with p53 alterations, tumour angiogenesis and extracellular matrix components. BMC Cancer Vol. 29, No.6, (May), p140.

Korkolopoulou, P.; Konstantinidou, A.E.; Kavantzas, N.; et al. (2001). Morphometric microvascular characteristics predict prognosis in superficial and invasive bladder cancer. Virchow Arch (2001) Vol.438, No. 6, (June): 603-611.

Lawler, J. (2000). The functions of thromboospondin-1 and -2. Curr Opin Cell Biol, Vol.12, No.5, (October), pp. 634-640.

Lianes, P.; Chartytonowicz, E.; Cordon-Cardo, C. et al. (1998). Biomarker study of primary nonmetastatic versus metastatic invasive bladder cancer. Clin Cancer Res, Vol.4, No.5, (May), pp. 1267-1271.

Lin, J.; Lalani, A.S.; Harding, T.C., et al. (2005). Inhibition of lymphogenous metastasis using adeno-associated virus-mediated gene transfer of a soluble VEGFR-3 decoy receptor. Cancer Res, Vol.65, No.15, (August), pp. 6901-6909.

Luttun, A.; Tjwa, M,; Moons, L. et al. (2002). Revascularization of ischemic tissues by PIGF treatment, and inhibition of tumor angiogenesis, arthritis, and atherosclerosis by anti-Flt1. Nat Med, Vol.8, No.8, (August), pp. 831-840.

Maisonpierre, P.C.; Suri, C.; Jones, P.F. et al. (1997). Angiopoietin-2, a natural antagonists for Tie 2 that discupts in vivo angiongeensis. Science, Vol.227, No.5322, (July), pp. 55-60.

Miyata, Y.; Kanda, S.; Ohba, K.; et al. (2006). Lymphangiogenesis and angiogenesis in bladder cancer: prognostic implications and regulation by vascular endothelial growth factors-A, -C, and -D. Clin Cancer Res Vol.12, No.3 pt 1, (February), pp. 300-306.

Mylona, E.; Magkou, C.; Gorantonakis, G. et al. (2006). Evaluation of the vascular endothelial growth factor (VEGF)-C role in urothelial carcinomas of the bladder. Anticancer Res, Vol.26, No.5A, (Deptember-October), pp. 3567-3571.

Nagy, J.A.; Vasile, E.; Feng, D. et al. (2002). Vascular permeability factor/vascular endothelial growth factor induces lymphangiogenesis as well as angiogenesis. J Exp Med, Vol.196, No.11, (December), pp. 1497-1506.

Nielsen, J.S. & McNagny, K.M. (2008). Novel functions of the CD34 family. J of Cell Science, Vol.121, Vol.Pt 22, (November), pp. 3682-3692

O'Brien, T.; Cranston, D.; Fuggle, S. et al. (1995). Different angiogenic pathways characterize superficial and invasive bladder cancer. Cancer Res, Vol.55, No3, (February), pp. 510-513.

Oka, N.; Yamamoto, Y.; Takahashi, M. et al. (2005). Expression of angiopoietin-1 and -2, and its clinical significance in human bladder cancer. BJU Int, Vol.95, No.4, (March), pp. 660-773.

O'Reilly, M.S.; Holmgren, L.; Shing, Y. et al. (1994). Angiostatin: a novel angiogenesis inhibitor that medicates the suppression of metastases by a Lewis lung carcinoma. Cell, Vol.79, No.2, (October), pp. 315-328.

O'Reilly, M.S.; Boehm, T.; Shing, Y.; et al. (1997). Endostatin: an endogenous inhibitor of angiogenesis and tumor growth. Cell 1997, Vol.88, No.2 (January), pp277-285.

Papapetropoulos, A.; Garcia-Cardena, G.; Dengler, T.J. et al. (1999), Direct actions of angiopoietin-1 on human endothelium: evidence for network stabilization, cell survival, and interaction with other angiogenic growth factors. Lab Invest, Vol.79, No.2, (February), pp. 213-223.

Papapetropoulos, A.; Fulton, D.; Mahboubi, K. et al. (2000). Angiopoietin-1 inhibits endothelial cell apoptosis via the Akt/survival pathway. J Biol Chem, Vol.275, No.13, (March), pp. 9102-9105.

Pepper, M.S. (2001). Lymphangiogenesis and tumor metastasis: myth or reality? Clin Cancer Res, Vol.7, No.3, (March): pp.462-468.

Roberts, N.; Kloos, B.; Cassella, M. et al. (2006). Inhibition of VEGFR-3 activation with the antagonistic antibody more potentially suppresses lymph node and distant metastases than inactivation of VEGFR-2. Cancer Res, Vol.66, No.5, (March), pp. 2650-2657.

Quentin, T.; Schlott, T.; Korabiowska, M. et al. (2004). Alternation of the vascular endothelial growth factor and angiopoientin-1 and -2 pathways in transitional cell carcinoma of the urinary bladder asscoaited with tumor progression. Anticancer Res, Vol.24, No.5A, (September-October), pp. 2745-2756.

Santos, L.; Costa, C.; Pereira, S. et al. (2003). Neovascularisation is a prognostic factor of early recurrence in T1/G2 urothelial bladder cancer. Ann Oncol, Vol.14, No.9, (September): pp.1419-1424.

Sharma, S.; Sharma, M.C. & Sarkar, C. (2005). Morphology of angiogenesis in human cancer: a conceptual overview, histoprognostic perspective and significance of neoangiogenesis. Histopathology, Vol.46, No.5, pp. 481-489.

Shibuya, M. & Claesson-Welsh L. (2006). Sinal transduction by VEGF receptors in regulation of angiogenesis and lymphangiogensis. Exp Cell Res, Vol.312, No.5, (March), pp. 549-560.

Shirotake, S.; Miyajima, A.; Kosaka, T. et al. (2011). Angiotensin II type 1 receptor expression and microvessel density in human bladder cancer. Urology, Vol.77, No.4, (April), 1009.e19pe25.

Skobe, M.; Hawighorst, T.; Jackson, D.G., et al. (2001). Induction of tumor lymphangiogensis by VEGF-C promotes breast cancer metastasis. Nat Med, Vol.7, No.2, (February), pp. 192-198.

Stacker SA, Caesar C, Baldwin ME, et al. (2001). VEGF-D promotes the metastatic spread of tumor cells via the lymphatics. Nat Med, Vol.7, No.2, (February), pp. 186-191.

Stavropoulos, N.E.; Bouropoulos, C.; Ioachim, I.E.; et al. (2004). Prognostic significance of angiogenesis in superficial bladder cancer. Int Urol Nephrol Vol.36, No.2, : pp. 163-167.

Streeter, E.H. & Harris, A.L. (2002). Angiogenesis in bladder cancer – prognostic marker and target for further therapy. Surg Oncol Vol.11, No.1-2 (March): pp. 85-100.

Szarvas, T.; Jäger, T.; Droste, F. et al. (2009). Serum levels of angiogenic factors and their prognostic releavance in bladder cancer. Pathol Oncol Res, Vol.15, No.2, (June), pp. 193-201.

Takahashi, H. & Shibuya, M. (2005). The vascular endothelial growth factor (VEGF)/VEGF receptor system and its role under physiological and pathological conditions. Clin Sci (Lond), Vol.109, No. 3, pp. 227-241.

Yang, H.; Kim, C.; Kim, M-J. et al. (2011). Soluble vascular endothelial growth factor receptor-3 suppresses lymphangiogensis and lymphatic metastasis in bladder cancer. Mol Cancer, Vol.10, No.10, (April), pp. 36-48.

Zhou, M.; He, L.; Zu, X. et al. Lymphatic vessel density as a predictor of lymph node metastasis and its relationship with prognosis in urothelial carcinoma of the bladder. BJU Int, in press.

Zu, X.; Tang, Z.; Li, Y. et al. (2006). Vascular endothelial growth factor-C expression in bladder transitional cell cancer and its relationship to lymph node metastasis. BJU Int, Vol.98, No.5, (November), pp. 1090-1093.

5

UHRF1 is a Potential Molecular Marker for Diagnosis and Prognosis of Bladder Cancer

Motoko Unoki

Division of Epigenomics, Department of Molecular Genetics,
Medical Institute of Molecular Genetics, Kyushu University,
Japan

1. Introduction

Bladder cancer is the second most common cancer of the urinary system. An estimated 386,300 new cases and 150,200 deaths from bladder cancer occurred in 2008 worldwide (Jemal et al., 2011). The highest rates of bladder cancer incidence are found in industrially developed countries, particularly in North America and Western Europe (Parkin et al., 2005). Bladder cancer is more common in males. The cancer is the 7th most common cancer in males worldwide and 4th most common cancer in males in industrially developed countries, while the cancer is not ranked in the top 10 most common cancers in females even in industrially developed countries (Jemal et al., 2011). In industrially developed countries, approximately 90% of the cancers are transitional cell carcinomas (TCCs), while the remaining 10% are squamous cell carcinomas and adenocarcinomas (Stein et al., 2001). There are several potential biomarkers for diagnosis and prognosis for bladder cancer, including Nuclear matrix protein-22 (NMP-22), human complement factor H related protein, telomerase, fibrin degradation product, and hyaluronic acid (Dey, 2004). Among these, only two biomarkers, NMP-22 and human complement factor H related protein, are in clinical use in Japan. Although these two markers are in clinical use, sensitivity and specificity of these markers are not perfect (van Rhijn et al., 2005); NMP-22 staining shows false positivity reactions in patients with hematuria, and the BTA (bladder tumour antigen) stat/BTA TRAK assay, which detects human complement factor H related protein, shows false positivity reactions in patients with urinary tract inflammation, recent genitourinary tumours and in cases of bladder stone (Dey, 2004). Cytology is still the most accurate diagnosis method, although sensitivity is not enough high (van Rhijn et al., 2005). Thus, discovery of a novel biomarker, which is sensitive and specific for bladder cancer, is an urgent subject.

2. UHRF1 is a potential molecular marker for diagnosis and prognosis of bladder cancer

UHRF1 (ubiquitin-like with PHD and ring finger domains 1), also known as ICBP90 (Inverted CCAAT box-binding protein of 90 kDa), was identified as a protein, whose expression is only detectable in proliferating cells, not in quiescent cells (Hopfner et al., 2000; Unoki et al., 2004). UHRF1 plays a central role in transferring DNA methylation status from mother cells to daughter cells. Its SET and RING finger-associated (SRA) domain recognizes hemi-methylated DNA that appears in newly synthesized daughter DNA strands during duplication of DNA strands through the S phase (**Arita et al., 2008; Avvakumov et al., 2008; Hashimoto et al., 2008**). UHRF1 recruits DNA methyltransferase 1 (DNMT1) to the site with proliferating cell nuclear antigen (PCNA) and methylates the newly synthesized strands (**Achour et al., 2008; Sharif et al., 2007**). UHRF1 also recognizes tri/di-methylated H3K9, and recruits the H3K9 methyltransferase G9a, the histone deacetylase 1 (HDAC1), and the histone acetylase Tip60 (**Achour et al., 2009; Hashimoto et al., 2009; Karagianni et al., 2008; Kim et al., 2009; Unoki et al., 2004**), indicating that UHRF1 links DNA methylation and histone modification status (Fig. 1).

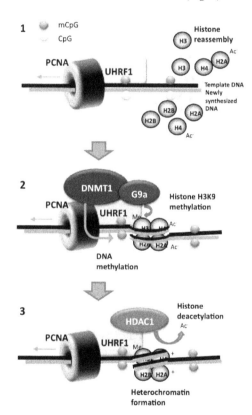

Fig. 1. Proposed mechanism of heterochromatin formation through UHRF1 at DNA replication fork or DNA repair site. 1) UHRF1 binds to PCNA and the SRA domain of UHRF1 recognizes hemi-methylated CpG on newly synthesized DNA. Then histones are reassembled. 2) UHRF1 recruits DNMT1 to methylate both DNA strands to transfer methylation status. UHRF1 also recruits G9a to methylate histone H3K9. Methylated histone H3K9 interacts with the Tudor-PHD domain of UHRF1. 3) UHRF1 recruits HDAC1 to the site and deacetylates histones. Then, histones become charged positively and bind to negatively charged DNA tightly, causing heterochromatin formation. This figure is cited from our article (**Unoki et al., 2009a**).

UHRF1 promotes G1/S transition (**Arima et al., 2004; Jeanblanc et al., 2005**) and is a direct target of E2F transcription factor 1 (E2F1) (**Abbady et al., 2005; Mousli et al., 2003; Unoki et al., 2004**). The tumour suppressor p53, which is deficient in 50% of all human cancers (**Hussain & Harris, 2000**), indirectly down-regulates UHRF1 through up-regulation of p21/WAF1 and subsequent deactivation of E2F1 (**Arima et al., 2004**) (Fig. 2).

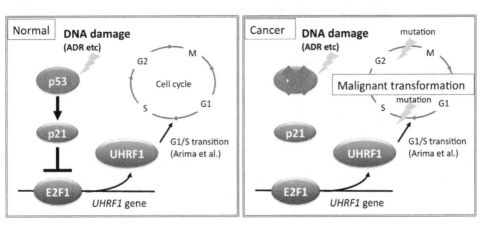

Fig. 2. Proposed p53-UHRF1 pathway model.

Expression of UHRF1 is up-regulated in various cancers, including breast cancer (Fig. 3), lung cancer (Fig. 4), prostate cancer, astrocytoma, pancreatic cancer, cervical cancer, and poorly differentiated thyroid carcinoma (**Crnogorac-Jurcevic et al., 2005; Jenkins et al., 2005; Lorenzato et al., 2005; Mousli et al., 2003; Oba-Shinjo et al., 2005; Pita et al., 2009; Unoki et al., 2010; Unoki et al., 2004**). Overexpression of UHRF1 in these cancers could be partially due to the inactivation of p53, although there could be several pathways, which regulate expression of UHRF1. Knock down of UHRF1 expression in cancer cells suppressed cell growth, indicating that UHRF1 is essential for progression of cancers and thus could be an anticancer drug target (**Tien et al., 2011; Unoki, 2011; Unoki et al., 2009a; Unoki et al., 2004; Yan et al., 2011**). Moreover, knockdown or inactivation of UHRF1 is reported to enhance sensitivity against current chemotherapies and radiation therapy *in vitro* (**Alhosin et al., 2010; Jenkins et al., 2005; Jin et al., 2010; Li, X. et al., 2011; Li, X. L. et al., 2009; Muto et al., 2002**). Therefore, UHRF1 is also an attractive target of cancer combination therapies (**Bronner et al., 2007; Unoki, 2011; Unoki et al., 2009a**).

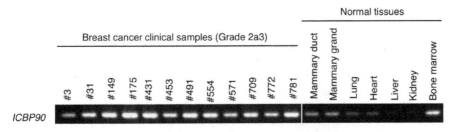

Fig. 3. Expression of *UHRF1* in breast cancer clinical samples detected by semi-quantitative RT-PCR. This figure is cited from our article (**Unoki et al., 2004**).

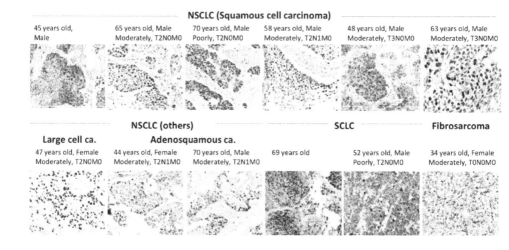

Fig. 4. Expression of UHRF1 in lung cancer clinical samples detected by immunohistochemistry. Representative data of UHRF1 staining in small cell lung carcinoma (SCLC), fibrosarcoma, and non-adenocarcinoma (ADC) histological types of non-small-cell lung carcinoma including squamous cell carcinoma (SCC), large cell carcinoma, and adenosquamous carcinoma (x 200). This figure is cited from our article (**Unoki et al., 2010**).

2.1 UHRF1 is overexpressed in bladder cancer

Considering these features of UHRF1, we thought that UHRF1 could be also important for bladder carcinogenesis, and examined expression of UHRF1 in bladder cancer specimens obtained from 124 UK cases (Table 1) and 36 Japanese cases (**Unoki et al., 2009b**). As a result, we found that UHRF1 was significantly overexpressed in bladder cancers at the mRNA and protein level (Fig. 5 and Fig. 6).

Because overexpression of UHRF1 in the cancer was detected both in UK cases and also in Japanese cases, the overexpression of UHRF1 could be common worldwide. Recently, another group showed that UHRF1 is also overexpressed in superficial, non-muscle-invasive bladder cancer of Chinese cases (**Yang et al., 2011**). Their result supports our observation. We also examined correlation between expression of UHRF1, p53, and *p21/WAF1*, and observed accumulation of stabilized p53 protein, which is probably mutated, in cancer tissues at grade II-III. However, we did not observe any accumulation of p53 in cancer tissues at grade I, although overexpression of UHRF1 was observed in this grade (Fig. 7). There was no relationship between expression levels of *UHRF1* and *p21* mRNA. Therefore, UHRF1 seems to be superior to p53 as a potential diagnostic marker of bladder cancer. This result is concordant with the fact that p53 is mutated only in 10-30 % of bladder cancer cases (**Berggren et al., 2001; Lorenzo Romero et al., 2004**).

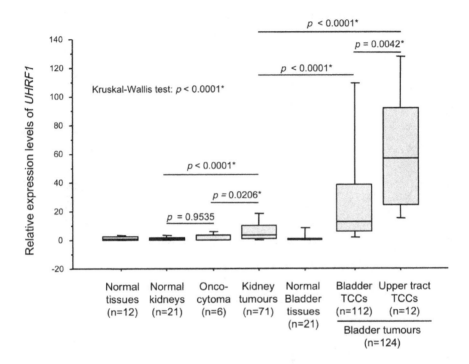

Fig. 5. Expression levels of *UHRF1* mRNA in urinary system tumours and normal tissues detected by TaqMan qRT-PCR. Expression of *UHRF1* in 12 different normal tissues, 21 normal kidneys, 6 oncocytomas, 71 kidney tumours, 21 normal bladders, and 124 bladder tumours, including 112 bladder located transitional cell carcinomas (TCCs) and 12 TCCs occurred in upper tract, were compared. Expression of *UHRF1* differed among the seven groups ($p<0.0001$, Kruskal-Wallis' test). Expression of *UHRF1* in the kidney cancers was higher than that in the normal kidneys and also in the oncocytomas significantly ($p<0.0001$, and $p=0.0206$, respectively, Mann-Whiteney's U-test), but expression levels of *UHRF1* in the bladder cancers were much higher than those in the kidney cancers ($p<0.0001$, Mann-Whiteney's U-test). Among the bladder cancers, expression of *UHRF1* was significantly high in upper tract TCCs (n=12) compared with the bladder-origin bladder tumours (n=112) (Mann-Whiteney's U-test; $p=0.0042$). *β2-microgloblin* was used for normalization. Asterisk indicates statistically significant *p*-values. This figure is cited from our article **(Unoki et al., 2009b)**.

Characteristics	[a]n (%)	Characteristics	n (%)
Total numbers of patients	124	Sex	
Anatomic site		Male	75 (72%)
Bladder	112 (90%)	Female	29 (28%)
Upper tract	12 (10%)	Numbers of tumours	
Type		<4	53 (85%)
TCC	122 (>99%)	>4	9 (15%)
Others	1 (<1%)	Tumour size	
Invasiveness		<5	38 (66%)
Superficial	71 (63%)	>5	20 (34%)
Invasive	41 (37%)	Growth pattern	
T-category		[c]CIS	1 (2%)
Ta	40 (35%)	Papillary	32 (52%)
T1	32 (28%)	Solid	19 (31%)
T2	24 (21%)	Solid/Papillary	9 (15%)
T3	14 (12%)	Recurrence	
T4	4 (4%)	No	19 (29%)
WHO grading		Yes	46 (71%)
Grade 1	9 (8%)	5-years survival	
Grade 2	59 (51%)	Alive	46 (49%)
Grade 3	47 (41%)	Dead	48 (51%)
Risk after [b]TURBT		Smoking	
Low	7 (13%)	Non-smoker	22 (35%)
Intermediate	26 (46%)	Smoker	40 (65%)
High	23 (41%)		

[a]Total numbers of the patients are not always 124, because not all patients have all the clinical information; [b]TURBT, transurethral resection of the bladder tumour; [c]CIS, carcinoma *in situ*.

Table 1. Base line characteristics of bladder cancer patients used for our analyses (Unoki et al., 2009b).

We also examined expression of UHRF1 in kidney cancer, another urinary system tumour, together with the bladder cancer by immunohistochemistry. Although overexpression of *UHRF1* is significant at mRNA level (Fig. 5), expression of UHRF1 in kidney cancer was not detected at protein level (Fig. 8A). Therefore, immunohistochemical staining of UHRF1 in the cancer seems not to be useful. However, overexpression of *UHRF1* at the mRNA level was associated with several characteristics of kidney cancer patients including 5-year survival rates, pathological staging and histological grade (Fig. 8B-D). Thus, detection of

UHRF1 mRNA overexpression in surgical specimen might be useful as a prognosis tool in kidney cancer.

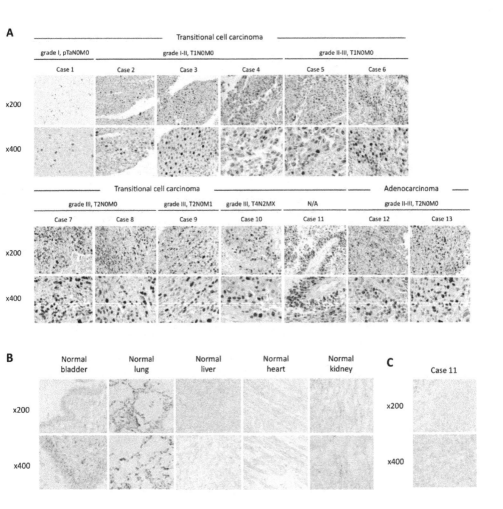

Fig. 6. Immunohistochemical staining of UHRF1 in 13 bladder tumour cases. A. Expression of UHRF1 in 11 transitional cell carcinomas and two adenocarcinomas with the different stage and grade. High expression of UHRF1 was detected only in nucleus of cancer cells, not in stromal cells. B. Expression of UHRF1 in normal tissues including bladder, lung, liver, heart, and kidney. No expression was observed in these normal tissues. Original magnifications, x 200 (top), and x 400 (bottom). C. Representative images of normal IgG staining as a negative control (Case 11 used for Fig. 6A). Original magnifications, x 200 (top), and x 400 (bottom). This figure is cited from our article (Unoki et al., 2009b).

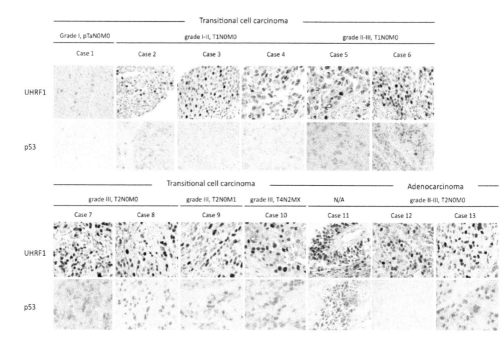

Fig. 7. Expression of p53 and UHRF1 in bladder cancers detected by immunohistochemistry. This figure is cited from our article (**Unoki et al., 2009b**).

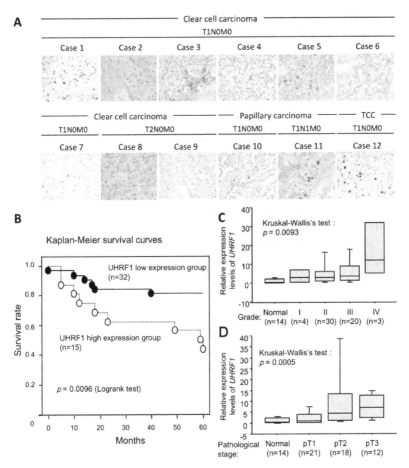

Fig. 8. Expression of UHRF1 in kidney cancer. A. UHRF1 expression in kidney cancers examined by immunohistochemistry. Magnification level is x400. B. Expression levels of *UHRF1* correlate with 5-years' survival rate of kidney tumours detected by TaqMan qRT-PCR. Patients were categorized into two groups by expression levels of *UHRF1*. The *UHRF1* high expression group is a group, which expresses *UHRF1* eight or more (≥8) and the low expression group is a group, which expresses *UHRF1* less than eight fold (<8) compared with average of *UHRF1* expression level in normal kidney from 21 individuals as 1.0. In the result of Kaplan-Meier survival analysis, the *UHRF1* high expression group showed significantly poor survival rate compared with the *UHRF1* low expression group (p=0.0096: Logrank test). *β2-microgloblin* was used for normalization. C. Expression levels of *UHRF1* correlated with histological grade of kidney tumours detected by TaqMan qRT-PCR. Patients were categorized into four groups by histological grade (I to IV). High expression of *UHRF1* correlated with advanced grade (p=0.0093: Kruskal-Wallis's test). *β2-microgloblin* was used for normalization. D. Expression levels of *UHRF1* correlated with pathological staging and histological grade of renal cancers detected by TaqMan qRT-PCR. Patients were categorized into three groups with pathological stages, pT1 to pT3. High expression of

UHRF1 correlated with advanced stage (*p*=0.0005: Kruskal-Wallis's test). *β2-microgloblin* was used for normalization. This figure is cited from our article (Unoki et al., 2009b).

2.2 Expression level of *UHRF1* correlates with malignancy of bladder cancer

We examined correlations between *UHRF1* expression in bladder cancer and various clinical features of the patients (Table 1). Among these features, the expression of *UHRF1* correlated with the T-category and the WHO histological grading significantly (Fig. 9A and 9B). Expression level of *UHRF1* in superficial bladder cancers (T-category: Ta and T1) and invasive bladder cancers (T-category classification: T2, T3 and T4) was both significantly higher than that in normal bladders. This result is concordant with data from the another group (**Yang et al., 2011**). In addition, expression of *UHRF1* in invasive bladder cancers was higher than that in superficial cancers, when we compared the three groups, normal bladders, invasive bladder cancers (pTa, pT1), and superficial bladder cancers (pT2-4), by Kruskal-Wallis's test (Fig. 9A). In addition, expression level of *UHRF1* in cancers with grade-II and -III was up-regulated compared with that in normal bladders (Fig. 9B). Therefore, up-regulation level of *UHRF1* reflects progression level of bladder cancer.

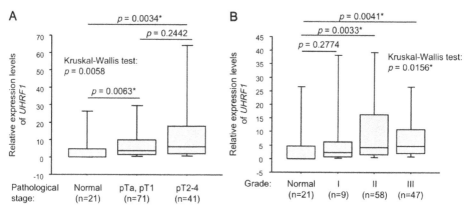

Fig. 9. Expression of *UHRF1* correlated with the stage, and grade. A. Expression of *UHRF1* in 21 normal bladders, 71 superficial bladder tumours (T-category is pTa and pT1), and 41 invasive bladder tumours (T-category is pT2, pT3, and pT4) detected by TaqMan qRT-PCR. Expression levels of *UHRF1* in superficial bladder tumours and in invasive tumours were significantly higher compared with those in normal bladders by Mann-Whiteney's U-test (*p*=0.0063 and *p*=0.0034, respectively). Although its expression in superficial tumours and invasive tumours did not differ (*p*=0.2442, Mann-Whiteney's U-test), it differed among the three different groups (*p*=0.0058, Kruskal-Wallis' test). *β2-microgloblin* was used for normalization. B. Expression of *UHRF1* differed among four groups with the different grade (*p*=0.0156, Kruskal-Wallis' test) detected by TaqMan qRT-PCR. Expression of *UHRF1* in grade II, and III tumour was higher than that in the normal bladders (*p*=0.0033 and *p*=0.0041). *β2-microgloblin* was used for normalization.

In our result, expression of *UHRF1* was not associated with difference of gender, numbers of tumour, tumour size, growth pattern (papillary or solid), incidence of recurrence, survival status after five years from surgery, and smoking history (Fig. 10), although the another group showed an association between UHRF1 expression levels and tumour recurrence in superficial bladder cancer of Chinese cases (**Yang et al., 2011**). Therefore, UHRF1 could be a molecular marker for predicting the recurrence of superficial bladder cancers in some ethnic groups.

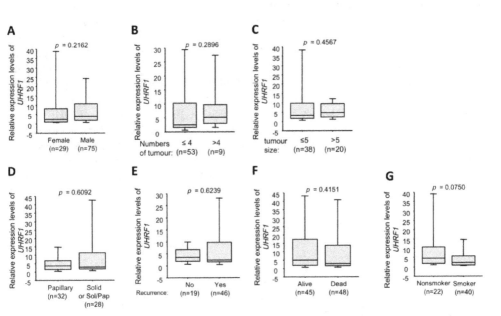

Fig. 10. Expression of *UHRF1* detected by TaqMan qRT-PCR and many characteristics of patients were compared by Mann-Whiteney's U-test. A. Expression levels of *UHRF1* in female patients (n=29) and male patients (n=75). Gender was not associated with expression levels of *UHRF1* (p=0.2162). B. Expression levels of *UHRF1* in patients with tumours four and less (n=53) and more than four (n=9) were not different (p=0.2896). C. Expression levels of *UHRF1* in patients with ≤ 5cm tumours (n=38) and with >5 cm tumours (n=20) were not different (p=0.4567). D. Expression levels of *UHRF1* in patients with papillary type tumours (n=32) and with solid or solid/papillary tumours (n=28) were not different (p=0.4567). E. Expression levels of *UHRF1* in patients who did not have a recurrence (n=19) and have a recurrence (n=46) were not different (p=0.6239). F. Expression levels of *UHRF1* in patients who survived 5 years after surgery (n=45) and died within 5 years (n=48) were not different (p=0.4151). G. Expression levels of *UHRF1* in non-smoker patients (n=22) and smoker patients including 4 ex-smokers (n=40) was not different (p=0.0750). *β2-microgloblin* was used for normalization.

2.3 Expression *UHRF1* can be used for predicting recurrence risk after TURBT

Over 75% bladder cancer patients have one or more superficial bladder cancers, and two thirds of them will develop recurrent disease (**Lutzeyer et al., 1982**), with 10–20% progressing to an invasive phenotype (**Torti & Lum, 1984**). The outcome of patients with invasive tumours remains still poor, with distant metastasis occurring in over 50% within 2 years and an average 5-year survival of only 50% (**Raghavan et al., 1990**). Currently, superficial bladder cancers are resected by a procedure called TURBT (TransUrethral

Resection of Bladder Tumour), and patients are treated differently based on estimated recurrence risk after TURBT. Thus, diagnosis of bladder cancer at non-advanced stage and also precise estimation of the risk after the TURBT, are very important for prognosis of patients. Currently, the risk after the surgery is estimated by a scoring system and risk tables developed by European Organization for Research and Treatment of Cancer (EORTC). The EORTC scoring system was developed based on the six most significant clinical and pathological factors, which are tumour stage, tumour grade, numbers of tumour, tumour size, prior recurrence rate, and presence of carcinoma *in situ* (CIS). Bladder cancer patients with pTaG1 tumours (50% of all patients) are at very low risk, and those with CIS or with pT1G3 tumours are at the highest risk (15% of all patients). Intermediate risk patients are those with pTa/pT1 G1/G2 disease who develop multiple recurrent cancers (35% of all patients). Our TaqMan qRT-PCR result showed that high expression of *UHRF1* was associated with high risk after TURBT (Fig. 11), probably because reflecting the association between high expression of *UHRF1* and stage, and/or grade (Fig. 9A and 9B). Based on these results, detection of *UHRF1* in tissue samples after TURBT will be a prognostic marker of future recurrence and may help to determine the risk together with the current prognostic factors.

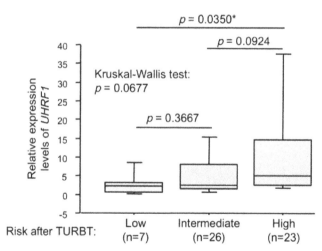

Fig. 11. Expression of *UHRF1* correlated with the recurrence risk after TURBT. Significant high expression of *UHRF1* in the high risk group after TURBT (n=23) was observed compared with that in the low risk group (n=7) by Mann-Whiteney's U-test (p=0.0350). Asterisk indicates statistically significant p-values. *β2-microglobin* was used for normalization. This figure is cited from our article (Unoki et al., 2009b).

2.4 UHRF1 is a possible marker of bladder cancers and upper tract TCCs

Because *UHRF1* was significantly overexpressed in bladder cancers and upper tract TCCs (Fig. 5), UHRF1 might be a useful diagnostic marker especially for upper tract TCCs. Upper tract TCCs are often very malignant when it is diagnosed, partially because it is relatively difficult to find at an early stage. If the cancer is found at an early stage, the prognosis of patients is improved. The development of a sensitive urine based detection marker is still being sought. Examination of voided urine or bladder barbotage for exfoliated cancer cells is useful for diagnosis of urothelial tumours anywhere in the urinary tract, from the calyx, through the ureters, into bladder and urethra. However, cytological interpretation can be problematic; low cellular yields, atypia, degenerative changes, urinary tract infections, stones and intravesical instillations hamper a correct diagnosis. Because the current two biomarker tests in clinical use, NMP-22 detection and BTA stat/BTA TRAK assay, can be hampered by existence of bleeding, inflammation, recent genitourinary tumours, and bladder stone (**Dey, 2004**), these markers have not improved the traditional cytology-based bladder cancer diagnosis largely. Thus, cytology is still the mainstay for diagnosing bladder cancer. Because the expression of *UHRF1* in peripheral blood mononuclear cells (PBMCs) was under detection limit of qRT-PCR (Fig. 12), the presence of these cells in urine would not impede the diagnosis. Additionally, expression of UHRF1 was not detected in adjacent normal bladder tissues by immunohistochemistry (Fig. 6A and 6B). Thus, contamination of these stromal cells also would not disturb the diagnosis, either. Therefore, an immunohistochemistry or Enzyme-Linked ImmunoSorbent Assay (ELISA)-based UHRF1 detection in urine sediment can be a sensitive and cancer-specific diagnostic method, and may greatly improve the current diagnosis based on cytology.

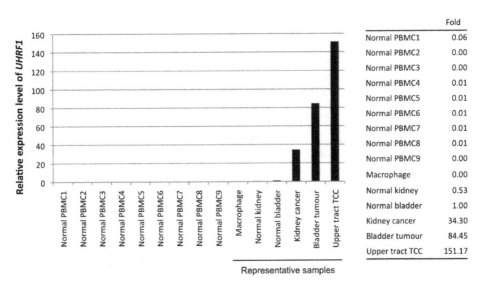

Fig. 12. Relative expression levels of *UHRF1* in peripheral blood mononuclear cells (PBMCs) were examined by TaqMan qRT-PCR. Almost no expression of *UHRF1* was detected in PBMCs.

3. Conclusion

Although UHRF1 expression in muscle invasive cancer was greater than in non-invasive (pTa) or superficially invasive (pT1) cancers, UHRF1 could still be detected by immunohistochemistry in the early stage bladder cancers. In addition, overexpression of *UHRF1* was associated with increased risk of progression after TURBT. Therefore, our result indicates that detection of UHRF1 may be a useful marker for early stage bladder cancers, and also for estimation of risk after TURBT, although it should be tested in larger series to determine if it can improve current strategies for diagnosis and prognosis of bladder cancer.

4. Acknowledgement

I thank Professor Yusuke Nakamura for his continuous support of my research, Dr. Ryuji Hamamoto, Professor John D. Kelly, Professor David E. Neal, and Professor Sir Bruce A. J. Ponder for providing us UK bladder cancer specimens and for helpful discussion, Professor Tomoaki Fujioka for providing us Japanese bladder cancer specimens, and Drs. Ryo Takata, Hitoshi Zembutsu, and Yoichiro Kato for very useful advice and discussion.

5. References

Abbady, A. Q.; Bronner, C.; Bathami, K.; Muller, C. D.; Jeanblanc, M.; Mathieu, E.; Klein, J. P.; Candolfi, E. & Mousli, M. (2005). TCR pathway involves ICBP90 gene down-regulation via E2F binding sites. *Biochem Pharmacol*, Vol.70, No.4, (Aug 2005), pp.570-579, ISSN 0006-2952

Achour, M.; Jacq, X.; Ronde, P.; Alhosin, M.; Charlot, C.; Chataigneau, T.; Jeanblanc, M.; Macaluso, M.; Giordano, A.; Hughes, A. D.; Schini-Kerth, V. B. & Bronner, C. (2008). The interaction of the SRA domain of ICBP90 with a novel domain of DNMT1 is involved in the regulation of VEGF gene expression. *Oncogene*, Vol.27, No.15, (Apr 2008), pp.2187-2197, ISSN 1476-5594

Achour, M.; Fuhrmann, G.; Alhosin, M.; Ronde, P.; Chataigneau, T.; Mousli, M.; Schini-Kerth, V. B. & Bronner, C. (2009). UHRF1 recruits the histone acetyltransferase Tip60 and controls its expression and activity. *Biochem Biophys Res Commun*, Vol.390, No.3, (Oct 2009), pp.523-528, ISSN 1090-2104

Alhosin, M.; Abusnina, A.; Achour, M.; Sharif, T.; Muller, C.; Peluso, J.; Chataigneau, T.; Lugnier, C.; Schini-Kerth, V. B.; Bronner, C. & Fuhrmann, G. (2010). Induction of apoptosis by thymoquinone in lymphoblastic leukemia Jurkat cells is mediated by a p73-dependent pathway which targets the epigenetic integrator UHRF1. *Biochem Pharmacol*, Vol.79, No.9, (May 2010), pp.1251-1260, ISSN 1873-2968

Arima, Y.; Hirota, T.; Bronner, C.; Mousli, M.; Fujiwara, T.; Niwa, S.; Ishikawa, H. & Saya, H. (2004). Down-regulation of nuclear protein ICBP90 by p53/p21Cip1/WAF1-dependent DNA-damage checkpoint signals contributes to cell cycle arrest at G1/S transition. *Genes Cells*, Vol.9, No.2, (Feb 2004), pp.131-142, ISSN 1356-9597

Arita, K.; Ariyoshi, M.; Tochio, H.; Nakamura, Y. & Shirakawa, M. (2008). Recognition of hemi-methylated DNA by the SRA protein UHRF1 by a base-flipping mechanism. *Nature*, Vol.455, No.7214, (Oct 2008), pp.818-821, ISSN 1476-4687

Avvakumov, G. V.; Walker, J. R.; Xue, S.; Li, Y.; Duan, S.; Bronner, C.; Arrowsmith, C. H. & Dhe-Paganon, S. (2008). Structural basis for recognition of hemi-methylated DNA by the SRA domain of human UHRF1. *Nature*, Vol.455, No.7214, (Oct 2008), pp.822-825, ISSN 1476-4687

Berggren, P.; Steineck, G.; Adolfsson, J.; Hansson, J.; Jansson, O.; Larsson, P.; Sandstedt, B.; Wijkstrom, H. & Hemminki, K. (2001). p53 mutations in urinary bladder cancer. *Br J Cancer*, Vol.84, No.11, (Jun 2001), pp.1505-1511, ISSN 0007-0920

Bronner, C.; Achour, M.; Arima, Y.; Chataigneau, T.; Saya, H. & Schini-Kerth, V. B. (2007). The UHRF family: oncogenes that are drugable targets for cancer therapy in the near future? *Pharmacol Ther*, Vol.115, No.3, (Sep 2007), pp.419-434, ISSN 0163-7258

Crnogorac-Jurcevic, T.; Gangeswaran, R.; Bhakta, V.; Capurso, G.; Lattimore, S.; Akada, M.; Sunamura, M.; Prime, W.; Campbell, F.; Brentnall, T. A.; Costello, E.; Neoptolemos, J. & Lemoine, N. R. (2005). Proteomic analysis of chronic pancreatitis and pancreatic adenocarcinoma. *Gastroenterology*, Vol.129, No.5, (Nov 2005), pp.1454-1463, ISSN 0016-5085

Dey, P. (2004). Urinary markers of bladder carcinoma. *Clin Chim Acta*, Vol.340, No.1-2, (Feb 2004), pp.57-65, ISSN 0009-8981

Hashimoto, H.; Horton, J. R.; Zhang, X.; Bostick, M.; Jacobsen, S. E. & Cheng, X. (2008). The SRA domain of UHRF1 flips 5-methylcytosine out of the DNA helix. *Nature*, Vol.455, No.7214, (Oct 2008), pp.826-829, ISSN 1476-4687

Hashimoto, H.; Horton, J. R.; Zhang, X. & Cheng, X. (2009). UHRF1, a modular multi-domain protein, regulates replication-coupled crosstalk between DNA methylation and histone modifications. *Epigenetics*, Vol.4, No.1, (Jan 2009), pp.8-14, ISSN 1559-2308

Hopfner, R.; Mousli, M.; Jeltsch, J. M.; Voulgaris, A.; Lutz, Y.; Marin, C.; Bellocq, J. P.; Oudet, P. & Bronner, C. (2000). ICBP90, a novel human CCAAT binding protein, involved in the regulation of topoisomerase IIalpha expression. *Cancer Res*, Vol.60, No.1, (Jan 2000), pp.121-128, ISSN 0008-5472

Hussain, S. P. & Harris, C. C. (2000). Molecular epidemiology and carcinogenesis: endogenous and exogenous carcinogens. *Mutat Res*, Vol.462, No.2-3, (Apr 2000), pp.311-322, ISSN 0027-5107

Jeanblanc, M.; Mousli, M.; Hopfner, R.; Bathami, K.; Martinet, N.; Abbady, A. Q.; Siffert, J. C.; Mathieu, E.; Muller, C. D. & Bronner, C. (2005). The retinoblastoma gene and its product are targeted by ICBP90: a key mechanism in the G1/S transition during the cell cycle. *Oncogene*, Vol.24, No.49, (Nov 2005), pp.7337-7345, ISSN 0950-9232

Jemal, A.; Bray, F.; Center, M. M.; Ferlay, J.; Ward, E. & Forman, D. (2011). Global cancer statistics. *CA Cancer J Clin*, (Feb 2011), ISSN 1542-4863

Jenkins, Y.; Markovtsov, V.; Lang, W.; Sharma, P.; Pearsall, D.; Warner, J.; Franci, C.; Huang, B.; Huang, J.; Yam, G. C.; Vistan, J. P.; Pali, E.; Vialard, J.; Janicot, M.; Lorens, J. B.; Payan, D. G. & Hitoshi, Y. (2005). Critical role of the ubiquitin ligase activity of

UHRF1, a nuclear RING finger protein, in tumor cell growth. *Mol Biol Cell*, Vol.16, No.12, (Dec 2005), pp.5621-5629, ISSN 1059-1524

Jin, W.; Liu, Y.; Xu, S. G.; Yin, W. J.; Li, J. J.; Yang, J. M. & Shao, Z. M. (2010). UHRF1 inhibits MDR1 gene transcription and sensitizes breast cancer cells to anticancer drugs. *Breast Cancer Res Treat*, Vol.124, No.1, (Nov 2010), pp.39-48, ISSN 1573-7217

Karagianni, P.; Amazit, L.; Qin, J. & Wong, J. (2008). ICBP90, a novel methyl K9 H3 binding protein linking protein ubiquitination with heterochromatin formation. *Mol Cell Biol*, Vol.28, No.2, (Jan 2008), pp.705-717, ISSN 1098-5549

Kim, J. K.; Esteve, P. O.; Jacobsen, S. E. & Pradhan, S. (2009). UHRF1 binds G9a and participates in p21 transcriptional regulation in mammalian cells. *Nucleic Acids Res*, Vol.37, No.2, (Feb 2009), pp.493-505, ISSN 1362-4962

Li, X.; Meng, Q.; Rosen, E. M. & Fan, S. (2011). UHRF1 confers radioresistance to human breast cancer cells. *Int J Radiat Biol*, Vol.87, No.3, (Mar 2011), pp.263-273, ISSN 1362-3095

Li, X. L.; Meng, Q. H. & Fan, S. J. (2009). Adenovirus-mediated expression of UHRF1 reduces the radiosensitivity of cervical cancer HeLa cells to gamma-irradiation. *Acta Pharmacol Sin*, Vol.30, No.4, (Apr 2009), pp.458-466, ISSN 1745-7254

Lorenzato, M.; Caudroy, S.; Bronner, C.; Evrard, G.; Simon, M.; Durlach, A.; Birembaut, P. & Clavel, C. (2005). Cell cycle and/or proliferation markers: what is the best method to discriminate cervical high-grade lesions? *Hum Pathol*, Vol.36, No.10, (Oct 2005), pp.1101-1107, ISSN 0046-8177

Lorenzo Romero, J. G.; Salinas Sanchez, A. S.; Gimenez Bachs, J. M.; Sanchez Sanchez, F.; Escribano Martinez, J.; Hernandez Millan, I. R.; Segura Martin, M. & Virseda Rodriguez, J. A. (2004). p53 Gene mutations in superficial bladder cancer. *Urol Int*, Vol.73, No.3, (2004), pp.212-218, ISSN 0042-1138

Lutzeyer, W.; Rubben, H. & Dahm, H. (1982). Prognostic parameters in superficial bladder cancer: an analysis of 315 cases. *J Urol*, Vol.127, No.2, (Feb 1982), pp.250-252, ISSN 0022-5347

Mousli, M.; Hopfner, R.; Abbady, A. Q.; Monte, D.; Jeanblanc, M.; Oudet, P.; Louis, B. & Bronner, C. (2003). ICBP90 belongs to a new family of proteins with an expression that is deregulated in cancer cells. *Br J Cancer*, Vol.89, No.1, (Jul 2003), pp.120-127, ISSN 0007-0920

Muto, M.; Kanari, Y.; Kubo, E.; Takabe, T.; Kurihara, T.; Fujimori, A. & Tatsumi, K. (2002). Targeted disruption of Np95 gene renders murine embryonic stem cells hypersensitive to DNA damaging agents and DNA replication blocks. *J Biol Chem*, Vol.277, No.37, (Sep 2002), pp.34549-34555, ISSN 0021-9258

Oba-Shinjo, S. M.; Bengtson, M. H.; Winnischofer, S. M.; Colin, C.; Vedoy, C. G.; de Mendonca, Z.; Marie, S. K. & Sogayar, M. C. (2005). Identification of novel differentially expressed genes in human astrocytomas by cDNA representational difference analysis. *Brain Res Mol Brain Res*, Vol.140, No.1-2, (Oct 2005), pp.25-33, ISSN 0169-328X

Parkin, D. M.; Bray, F.; Ferlay, J. & Pisani, P. (2005). Global Cancer Statistics, 2002. *CA-Cancer J Clin*, Vol.55, No.2, (Mar-Apr 2005), pp.74-108, ISSN 0007-9235

Pita, J. M.; Banito, A.; Cavaco, B. M. & Leite, V. (2009). Gene expression profiling associated with the progression to poorly differentiated thyroid carcinomas. *Br J Cancer,* Vol.101, No.10, (Nov 2009), pp.1782-1791, ISSN 1532-1827

Raghavan, D.; Shipley, W. U.; Garnick, M. B.; Russell, P. J. & Richie, J. P. (1990). Biology and management of bladder cancer. *N Engl J Med,* Vol.322, No.16, (Apr 1990), pp.1129-1138, ISSN 0028-4793

Sharif, J.; Muto, M.; Takebayashi, S.; Suetake, I.; Iwamatsu, A.; Endo, T. A.; Shinga, J.; Mizutani-Koseki, Y.; Toyoda, T.; Okamura, K.; Tajima, S.; Mitsuya, K.; Okano, M. & Koseki, H. (2007). The SRA protein Np95 mediates epigenetic inheritance by recruiting Dnmt1 to methylated DNA. *Nature,* Vol.450, No.7171, (Dec 2007), pp.908-912, ISSN 1476-4687

Stein, J. P.; Lieskovsky, G.; Cote, R.; Groshen, S.; Feng, A. C.; Boyd, S.; Skinner, E.; Bochner, B.; Thangathurai, D.; Mikhail, M.; Raghavan, D. & Skinner, D. G. (2001). Radical cystectomy in the treatment of invasive bladder cancer: long-term results in 1,054 patients. *J Clin Oncol,* Vol.19, No.3, (Feb 2001), pp.666-675, ISSN 0732-183X

Tien, A. L.; Senbanerjee, S.; Kulkarni, A.; Mudbhary, R.; Goudreau, B.; Ganesan, S.; Sadler, K. C. & Ukomadu, C. (2011). UHRF1 depletion causes a G2/M arrest, activation of DNA damage response and apoptosis. *Biochem J,* Vol.435, No.1, (Apr 1 2011), pp.175-185, ISSN 1470-8728

Torti, F. M. & Lum, B. L. (1984). The biology and treatment of superficial bladder cancer. *J Clin Oncol,* Vol.2, No.5, (May 1984), pp.505-531, ISSN 0732-183X

Unoki, M.; Nishidate, T. & Nakamura, Y. (2004). ICBP90, an E2F-1 target, recruits HDAC1 and binds to methyl-CpG through its SRA domain. *Oncogene,* Vol.23, No.46, (Oct 2004), pp.7601-7610, ISSN 0950-9232

Unoki, M.; Brunet, J. & Mousli, M. (2009a). Drug discovery targeting epigenetic codes: The great potential of UHRF1, which links DNA methylation and histone modifications, as a drug target in cancers and toxoplasmosis *Biochem Pharmacol.,* Vol.78, No.10, (Nov 2009a), pp.1279-1288, ISSN 1873-2968

Unoki, M.; Kelly, J. D.; Neal, D. E.; Ponder, B. A. J.; Nakamura, Y. & Hamamoto, R. (2009b). UHRF1 is a novel molecular marker for diagnosis and the prognosis of bladder cancer. *Br J Cancer,* Vol.101, No.1, (Jul 2009b), pp.98-105, ISSN 1532-1827

Unoki, M.; Daigo, Y.; Koinuma, J.; Tsuchiya, E.; Hamamoto, R. & Nakamura, Y. (2010). UHRF1 is a novel diagnostic marker of lung cancer. *Br J Cancer,* Vol.103, No.2, (Jul 2010), pp.217-222, ISSN 1532-1827

Unoki, M. (2011). Current and potential anticancer drugs targeting members of the UHRF1 complex including epigenetic modifiers. *Recent Pat Anticancer Drug Discov,* Vol.6, No.1, (Jan 2011), pp.116-130, ISSN 1574-8928

van Rhijn, B. W.; van der Poel, H. G. & van der Kwast, T. H. (2005). Urine markers for bladder cancer surveillance: a systematic review. *Eur Urol,* Vol.47, No.6, (Jun 2005), pp.736-748, ISSN 0302-2838

Yan, F.; Tan, X. Y.; Geng, Y.; Ju, H. X.; Gao, Y. F. & Zhu, M. C. (2011). Inhibition Effect of siRNA-Downregulated UHRF1 on Breast Cancer Growth. *Cancer Biother Radiopharm,* Vol.26, No.2, (Apr 2011), pp.183-189, ISSN 1557-8852

Yang, G. L.; Zhang, L. H.; Bo, J. J.; Chen, H. G.; Cao, M.; Liu, D. M. & Huang, Y. R. (2011). UHRF1 is associated with tumor recurrence in non-muscle-invasive bladder cancer. *Med Oncol*, (May 25 2011), ISSN 1559-131X

6

Angiogenesis, Lymphangiogenesis and Lymphovascular Invasion: Prognostic Impact for Bladder Cancer Patients

Julieta Afonso[1,2,3], Lúcio Lara Santos[4,5] and Adhemar Longatto-Filho[1,3,6]

[1]Life and Health Sciences Research Institute - ICVS, University of Minho
[2]ICVS/3B's - PT Government Associate Laboratory
[3]Alto Ave Superior Institute of Health - ISAVE
[4]Portuguese Institute of Oncology - IPO
[5]University Fernando Pessoa - UFP
[6]Faculty of Medicine, São Paulo State University
[1,2,3,4,5]Portugal
[6]Brazil

1. Introduction

Bladder cancer is the second most common tumor of the urogenital tract. Urothelial carcinoma is the most frequent histologic type, being unique among epithelial carcinomas in its divergent pathways of tumorigenesis. Surgery continues to have a predominant role in the management of urothelial bladder cancer (Kaufman et al., 2009). However, the debate about the best treatment approach for T1G3 and muscle invasive tumors continually challenges all urologic surgeons and oncologists. This debate involves several aspects. First, a significant number of T1G3 tumors recurs and progresses rapidly after transurethral resection and BCG treatment (Wiesner et al., 2005). Second, half of patients with invasive tumors have a dismal outcome despite an effective treatment by radical cystectomy (Sternberg et al., 2007). Third, the extension of lymphadenectomy remains an issue of controversy, although clinical evidence suggests that an extended lymph node dissection may not only provide prognostic information, but also a significant therapeutic benefit for both lymph node-positive and lymph node-negative patients undergoing radical cystectomy (May et al., 2011). In muscle invasive bladder cancer, the presence of tumor foci in lymph nodes is an early event in progression, and the lymphatic vessels within or in the proximity to the primary tumor serve as the primary conduits for tumor dissemination (Youssef et al., 2011). Fourth, although urothelial bladder cancer is a chemo-sensitive tumor (Kaufman et al., 2000; von der Maase et al., 2000), adjuvant systemic chemotherapy does not reveal benefits (Walz et al., 2008), and neoadjuvant chemotherapy is not yet accepted as the best approach in invasive bladder cancer (Clark, 2009). Therefore, in order to solve the aforementioned problems, it is crucial to improve the knowledge about tumor microenvironment, regulation of cancer metabolism and neovascularization.

Blood and lymphatic neovascularization are essential for tumor progression and metastasis, by promoting oxygenation and fluid drainage, and establishing potential routes of dissemination (Adams and Alitalo, 2007). Therefore, the inhibition of tumor-induced neovascularization represents a powerful option for target therapy, in order to restrain the most efficient pathway of cancer spread.

2. Angiogenesis and lymphangiogenesis: Molecular regulation of vasculature development

During embryogenesis, the formation of the blood vascular system initiates by vasculogenesis: haemangioblasts proliferate, migrate and differentiate into endothelial cells, which in turn will organize a primitive vascular plexus. In parallel, angiogenesis promotes the remodeling and expansion of the primary capillary network, originating a hierarchical structure of different sized vessels that will mature into functional capillaries, veins and arteries (Risau, 1997). The lymphatic vascular system develops latter, when a group of blood endothelial cells differentiates into a lymphatic endothelium that subsequently sprouts to form the primary lymph sacs. By lymphangiogenesis, the lymphatic endothelial cells from the lymph sacs will further sprout, originating the peripheral lymphatic system (Sabin, 1902, as cited by Oliver & Detmar, 2002).

During postnatal life, blood and lymphatic vascular systems are, normally, in a quiescent state. Physiological angiogenesis and/or lymphangiogenesis occur to maintain or restore the integrity of tissues, namely during wound healing and the ovarian cycle. Conversely, the neovascularization machinery may be activated in pathological processes such as cancer and inflammatory diseases (reviewed in Lohela et al., 2009).

Similarly to physiological neovascularization, tumor-induced angiogenesis and/or lymphangiogenesis occur to satisfy the metabolic demands of a new tissue – the malignant tissue. Therefore, the molecular factors involved in the formation of the vascular systems during embryogenesis are newly recruited by the growing tumor (Papetti & Herman, 2002).

2.1 From angiogenesis to lymphangiogenesis in the embryo

The proliferation, sprouting and migration of endothelial cells during vasculogenesis and angiogenesis is mainly guided by the vascular endothelial growth factor (VEGF) signaling through VEGF receptor-2 (VEGFR-2) (Risau, 1997).

VEGF (or VEGF-A), initially termed as vascular permeability factor (VPF) (Senger et al., 1983), is a specific mitogen and pro-survival factor for blood endothelial cells, also stimulating vascular permeability. It binds and activates two tyrosine kinase receptors primarily found on the blood endothelium: VEGFR-1 (or Flt-1, fms-like tyrosine kinase 1) and VEGFR-2 (or KDR/Flk-1, human kinase insert domain receptor/mouse foetal liver kinase 1) (reviewed in Carmeliet, 2005). Interaction of VEGF with VEGFR-1 negatively regulates vasculogenesis and angiogenesis during early embryogenesis (Fong et al., 1999). On the contrary, VEGFR-2 is the earliest marker for endothelial cell development: mouse embryos lacking VEGFR-2 die at embryonic day 8.5-9.5 due to no development of blood vessels as well as very low hematopoiesis (Shalaby et al., 1995). Regarding the ligand, even heterozygote mice for *Vegf* deficiency die at embryonic day 11-12: blood islands, endothelial cells and vessel-like tubes fail to develop (Carmeliet et al., 1996; Ferrara et al., 1996).

In humans, five weeks after fertilization, certain blood endothelial cells become responsive to lymphatic inducing-signals. The lymphatic vessel endothelial hyaluronan receptor-1 (LYVE-1), a CD44 homologous transmembrane protein, is the first marker of lymphatic endothelial commitment. Initially, it is evenly expressed by the blood endothelium of the cardinal vein, which causes the blood endothelium to acquire the ability to differentiate in lymphatic endothelium (Banerji et al., 1999). The polarized expression of the prospero related homeobox gene-1 (Prox-1) transcription factor in a subpopulation of blood endothelial cells determines the establishment of the lymphatic identity and initiates the formation of the lymphatic vascular system. In mice, Prox-1 expressing cells are first observed at embryonic day 10 in the jugular vein (Wigle & Oliver, 1999). *Prox1* deletion leads to a complete absence of the lymphatic vasculature (Wigle et al., 2002). The expression of the transcription factor Sox18 [SRY (sex determining region Y) box 18] acts as a molecular switch to induce differentiation of lymphatic endothelial cells: it activates Prox-1 transcription by binding to its proximal promoter. Sox18-null embryos show a complete blockade of lymphatic endothelial cell differentiation (François et al., 2008). Later, the sprouting, migration and survival of the newly formed lymphatic endothelial cells depends on the expression of VEGF-C by the mesenchymal cells surrounding the cardinal veins (Karkkainen et al., 2004) (Fig. 1).

VEGF-C, like VEGF, is a member of the VEGF family of growth factors and a mitogen for lymphatic endothelial cells. VEGF-D is also a pro-lymphangiogenic factor, although its deletion does not affect the development of the primitive lymphatic vessels (Baldwin et al. 2001). Conversely, in *Vegfc-/-* mice, Prox-1 positive cells appear in the cardinal veins, but fail to migrate and proliferate to form primary lymph sacs (Karkkainen et al., 2004). VEGF-C and VEGF-D interact with VEGFR-3 (of Flt-4, fms-like tyrosine kinase 4). Their affinity to VEGFR-3 is increased by proteolytic cleavage; the fully processed forms can also bind to VEGFR-2 (reviewed in Lohela et al., 2009).

VEGFR-3 is widely expressed at the early stages of embryonic blood vasculature, becoming virtually restricted to lymphatic endothelium in the later stages of embryonic development, (after the lymphatic commitment mediated by Prox-1 expression), and during adult life (Kaipainen et al., 1995). In mice, inhibition of VEGFR-3 expression at embryonic day 15 induces regression of the developing lymphatic vasculature by apoptosis of lymphatic endothelial cells (Makinen et al., 2001).

The subsequent development of the lymphatic vasculature involves the separation of the blood and lymphatic vascular systems, the maturation of lymphatic vessels and the formation of secondary lymphoid organs. The molecular regulation of these processes involves the coordinated expression of distinct genes from those involved in the early events of lymphangiogenesis (reviewed in Alitalo et al., 2005) (Fig. 1). Moreover, several other growth factors, namely cyclooxygenase-2 (COX-2) fibroblast growth factor-2 (FGF-2), hepatocyte growth factor (HGF), insulin-like growth factors (IGFs) and platelet-derived growth factor-B (PDGF-B) have been shown to induce lymphangiogenesis and/or angiogenesis in experimental models (reviewed in Cao, 2005). These are mainly protein tyrosine kinases, which play central roles in signal transduction networks and regulation of cell behavior. In the lymphatic endothelium, these tyrosine kinases are collectively involved in processes such as the maintenance of existing lymphatic vessels, growth and maturation of new vessels and modulation of their identity and function (Williams et al., 2010).

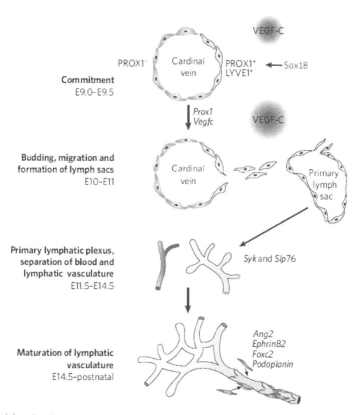

Fig. 1. Model for the development of mouse lymphatic vasculature (E- embryonic day; Syk-protein-tyrosine kinase SYK; Slp76- SH2 domain-containing leucocyte protein, 76-kDa; Ang2- angiopoietin 2; Foxc2- Forkhead Box C2) (adapted by permission from © 2005 Nature Publishing Group. Originally published in *Nature*. 438: 946-953)

2.2 Promotion of angiogenesis and lymphangiogenesis in the malignancy context

The major cause of cancer mortality is the metastatic spread of tumor cells that can occur via multiple routes, including blood and lymphatic vasculatures. For metastasis to occur, selected clones of malignant cells must be able to invade the newly formed vessels and disseminate. Induction of angiogenesis and/or lymphangiogenesis is, therefore, one of the first steps of the metastatic cascade (Alitalo & Carmeliet, 2002; Tobler & Detmar, 2006).

During the pre-vascular phase, the malignant tumor remains small (up to 1 or 2 mm³); the preexistent surrounding blood vessels ensure the supply of oxygen and nutrients necessary for its survival. However, the expansion of the tumor mass is angiogenesis-dependent. As a compensatory response to hypoxia, proangiogenic factors such as VEGF are released by the malignant cells and infiltrating immune cells, namely monocytes. As a result, angiogenesis occurs and the tumor acquires its own blood supply. Neoplastic growth is thus promoted, as well as the potential for invasion and haematogenic metastasis (Kerbel, 2000).

Vegf is upregulated in hypoxia via the oxygen sensor hypoxia-inducible factor (HIF)-1α (Pugh & Ratcliffe, 2003). Another recently described VEGF activation mechanism is the induction of the transcriptional coactivator peroxisoma proliferator-activated receptor-gamma coactivator-1α (PGC-1α) in response to the lack of nutrients and oxygen (Arany et al., 2008). Additionally, VEGF gene expression can be upregulated by oncogene signaling, several growth factors, inflammatory cytokines and hormones (reviewed in Ferrara, 2004). Tumor cells secrete VEGF mainly in a paracrine manner, although it can also act in an autocrine manner to promote a protective/survival effect to endothelial cells, among other cell types (Brusselmans et al., 2005). The mechanisms underlying tumor lymphangiogenesis are not clearly defined. Inflammation seems to promote lymphatic neovascularization: inflammatory cells that infiltrate in the growing tumor produce lymphangiogenic growth factors. Another lymphangiogenesis trigger mechanism may be the high interstitial pressure generated inside the tumors due to the excessive production of interstitial fluid (reviewed in Cao, 2005). On the other hand, the extracellular matrix is of central importance for the generation of new lymphatic vessels as a response to the pathological stimulus. Integrins, a superfamily of cell adhesion molecules, are able to influence cell migration: integrin α9β1 is a target gene for Prox1, and its direct binding to VEGF-C and VEGF-D stimulates cell migration (reviewed in Wiig, 2010).

VEGF-C and VEGF-D, via signaling through VEGFR-3, appear to be essential for tumor-associated lymphangiogenesis, leading to lymphatic vessel invasion, lymph node involvement and distant metastasis (reviewed in Achen & Stacker, 2008). Moreover, VEGF interaction with VEGFR-2 may also promote lymphatic neovascularization, namely inside the regional draining lymph nodes, even before lymph node metastasis occurrence. This probably corresponds to a pathophysiologic strategy of "soil" preparation by the primary tumor to ensure the success of its future dissemination (Hirakawa et al., 2005). In fact, sentinel lymph node metastasis is the first step in the spreading of many cancer types.

Preexisting blood and lymphatic vessels in the vicinity of the malignant mass may contribute to tumor spread. However, de novo formed vessels by tumor-induced angiogenesis and lymphangiogenesis seem to be the preferential routes for dissemination (reviewed in Cao, 2005). This is a consequence of the ultra-structure of the tumor-associated blood and lymphatic vessels.

2.3 Ultra-structure of tumor-associated blood and lymphatic vessels

Blood vessels present in malignant tissues show remarkable differences with vessels present in normal tissues. Tumor blood vessels are highly disorganized: they are tortuous, excessively branched and dilated. The basement membrane and the muscular coverage are incomplete or absent. The endothelial cells, abnormal in shape, overlap and are projected into the lumen rather than organizing a pavement layer below the basement membrane. Blood vessel invasion is facilitated by this aberrant structure, but the extravasation rate is high, and blood flow is variable. As a result, interstitial tumor hypertension occurs, and delivery of therapeutic agents into tumors is compromised (Jain & Carmeliet, 2001; reviewed in Cao, 2005). The intratumoral edema is pernicious to malignant cells; therefore, homeostasis needs to be re-established. The formation of a tumoral lymphatic vasculature could potentially resolve this problem.

The key function of lymphatic vessels is to collect the excessive amount of interstitial fluid back to the blood circulation for immune surveillance in lymph nodes. Unlike normal blood capillaries, lymphatic capillaries have a discontinuous or fenestrated basement membrane and are not ensheathed by pericytes or smooth muscle cells; the endothelial cells are arranged in a slightly overlapping pattern and lack tight interendothelial junctions. Specialized anchoring filaments of elastic fibers connect the endothelial cells to the extracellular matrix, which causes the vessels to dilate rather than to collapse when hydrostatic pressure rises (Alitalo et al., 2005; Tobler & Detmar, 2006). This structure facilitates the collection of interstitial fluid and is ideal for malignant cells' entry into the lymphatic flow.

A highly debated question is whether there are functional lymphatic vessels inside tumors (reviewed in Alitalo & Carmeliet, 2002; reviewed in Detmar & Hirakawa, 2002). On one hand, the elevated interstitial pressure generated by the proliferation of the malignant cells and by the high extravasation rate compromises the infiltration of new lymphatic vessels in the tumor stroma. Although intratumoral lymphangiogenesis may occur, the newly formed vessels are compressed and nonfunctional (Jain & Fenton, 2002). To compensate the lack of an intratumoral draining mechanism, the peritumoral lymphatic vessels enlarge due to an excess of pro-lymphangiogenic factors in that area. Therefore, in this model, the peritumoral lymphatic vessels passively collect interstitial fluid and, eventually, malignant cells (Carmeliet & Jain, 2000) (Fig. 2, A). However, some studies have demonstrated a relationship between the existence of functional intratumoral lymphatics, with cycling lymphatic endothelial cells and tumor emboli, and lymph node involvement (reviewed in Da et al., 2008). Additionally, peritumoral lymphangiogenesis occurs, and the new vessels actively contribute to metastatic spread (Padera et al., 2002) (Fig. 2, B). Probably, there are some organ-specific determinants that influence the occurrence of peritumoral and/or intratumoral lymphangiogenesis, as well as the function of the newly formed vessels.

2.4 Lymphovascular invasion and metastasis

Tumor metastasis involves a coordinated series of complex events that include promotion of angiogenesis and lymphangiogenesis, detachment of malignant cells from the primary tumor, microinvasion of the surrounding stroma, blood and/or lymphatic vessel invasion, survival of the malignant cells in the blood and/or lymphatic flow, and extravasion and growth in secondary sites. Because the large lymphatic vessels reenter the blood vascular system, malignant cells spread via the lymphatic system to the regional lymph nodes and, from this point, to distant organs (Alitalo & Carmeliet, 2002; Tobler & Detmar, 2006) (Fig. 3). Follow-up data have shown that 80% of the tumors, mainly those of epithelial origin, disseminate through the lymphatic vasculature; the remaining 20% use the blood circulation to colonize secondary organs (reviewed in Saharinen et al., 2004; reviewed in Wilting et al., 2005).

The blood vessels are not the best route for the success of malignant dissemination. Although their disorganized structure may contribute to the intravasion of malignant cells or emboli, in the bloodstream these cells experience serum toxicity, high shear stresses and mechanical deformation. Consequently, the viability of the tumor cells is seriously compromised (reviewed in Swartz, 2001). Conversely, the success rate of lymphogenous spread is high. As previously referred, the structure and function of the lymphatic capillaries facilitates intravasion of tumor cells or emboli. On the other hand, the composition of the lymph is similar to interstitial fluid, which provides an optimal medium for the survival of malignant cells. In collecting lymphatic vessels, muscle fibers assure lymph propulsion, that flows slowly, and valves prevent its backflow. Lymph nodes are areas of flow stagnation that represent ideal "incubators" for malignant cells' growth. Some cells exit the lymph node through the efferent channels or high endothelial venules. Other cells may remain mechanically entrapped for long periods of time, originating

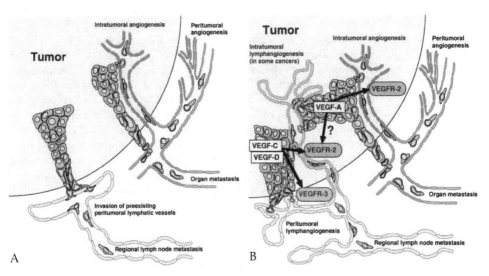

Fig. 2. (A) Traditional model of tumor metastasis via lymphatic and blood vessels. (B) Active lymphangiogenesis model of tumor metastasis (reprinted by permission from © 2002 Rockefeller University Press. Originally published in *J. Exp. Med.* 196: 713-718)

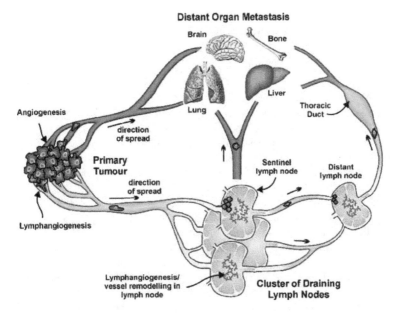

Fig. 3. Pathways of dissemination of malignant cells (reprinted by permission from © 2008 John Wiley & Sons, Inc. Originally published in *Ann. N. Y. Acad. Sci.* 1131: 225-234)

micrometastases (Swartz, 2001; Van Trapen & Pepper, 2002). Martens and colleagues described the expression of a gene signature of scavenger and lectin-like receptors in the lymph node sinus, which are known mediators of tumour cell adhesion and, therefore, can contribute to selective metastasis in an organ-specific context (Martens et al., 2006). Probably, tumor-cell-specific characteristics, microenvironmental factors and crosstalk between tumor and host cells have a pivotal role in determining survival and growth of micrometastasis. Moreover, lymph node lymphangiogenesis may provide an additional mechanism to facilitate further metastatic spread throughout the lymphatic system (Ji, 2009). The occurrence of lymphangiogenesis prior to arrival of tumor cells indicates that signals derived from the primary tumor are transported to the draining lymph nodes (Hirakawa et al., 2005).

Different tumors metastasize preferentially to different organs, suggesting that tumor spread is a guided process. It has been reported that malignant cells may use chemokine receptor ligand interactions to guide the colonization of target organs (reviewed in Saharinen et al., 2004; reviewed in Achen & Stacker, 2008). Chemokines are a family of chemoattractant cytokines that bind to G protein-coupled receptors expressed on target cells, namely malignant cells (Laurence, 2006). For instance, breast cancer cells, that normally choose regional lymph nodes, bone marrow, lung and liver as their first sites of destination, overexpress CCR7 (chemokine, CC motif, receptor 7) and CXCR4 (chemokine, CXC motif, receptor 4). Their ligands, SLC/CCL2 (secondary lymphoid chemokine / CC-type chemokine ligand 21) and SDF-1 CXCL12/ (stromal cell-derived factor 1 / chemokine, CXC motif, ligand 12) are expressed at high levels by isolated lymphatic endothelial cells and lymphatic endothelium from vessels present in the preferred sites of metastasis (Muller et al., 2001). This guides chemoattraction and migration of tumor cells, and characterizes lymphatic vessel invasion as an active event.

3. Angiogenesis, lymphangiogenesis and lymphovascular invasion in urothelial bladder cancer

The metastatic profile of urothelial bladder carcinoma implies, as in most malignant tumors, the dissemination of tumor cells through the lymphatic vasculature, and the colonization of regional lymph nodes is an early event in progression. Smith & Whitmore reported the involvement of the internal iliac and obturator groups of lymph nodes in about 74% of patients who underwent radical cystectomy; the external iliac nodes were involved in 65% of the patients, and the common iliac were involved in 20% of the cases (Smith & Whitmore, 1981). As already referred, controversy exists regarding the optimal extent of lymphadenectomy and the number of lymph nodes to be retrieved at radical cystectomy. An extended pelvic lymph node dissection (encompassing the external iliac vessels, the obturator fossa, the lateral and medial aspects of the internal iliac vessels, and at least the distal half of the common iliac vessels together with its bifurcation) has been suggested as potentially curative in patients with metastasis or micrometastasis to a few nodes (Karl et al., 2009; Abol-Enein et al., 2011). Wright and colleagues observed that an increased number of lymph nodes removed at the time of radical cystectomy associates with improved survival in patients with lymph node-positive bladder cancer (Wright et al., 2008). The recommendation from the Bladder Cancer Collaboration Group is that ten to fourteen lymph nodes should be removed at the time of radical cystectomy (Herr et al., 2004). The concept of lymph node density (the number of positive lymph nodes divided by the total number of lymph nodes) was introduced by Stein and colleagues and helps to select lymph node-positive patients after radical cystectomy for adjuvant treatment (Stein et al., 2003). However, the lymph node density threshold is a debatable question (Gilbert, 2008). In large series, the median number of total lymph nodes removed was nine, with high lymph node density (25%), which can lead to misleading N0 staging (Wright et al., 2008). Therefore, in this subgroup of patients (lymph nodes removed ≤ 9 and N0), another prognostic factor is needed to better select patients for adjuvant treatment. Moreover, according to Malmström, extending the boundaries of surgery will not drastically improve survival. The focus should be on exploring biomarkers that predict extravesical dissemination and improving on the systemic treatment concept (Malmström, 2011). In this line of investigation, angiogenesis, lymphangiogenesis and lymphovascular invasion occurrence have been implicated in bladder cancer progression, invasion and metastasis, and represent potential targets for guided therapy.

Several studies reported a significant association between VEGF overexpression — both in tumor tissue (Crew et al., 1997; O'Brien et al., 1995) and urine (Crew et al., 1999; Jeon et al., 2001) —, high blood vessel density (Goddard et al., 2003; Santos et al., 2003) and the occurrence of recurrence and progression in patients with non-muscle invasive bladder cancer. In this group of patients, it has been observed that angiotensin II type 1 receptor (AT1R) expression associates with high blood vessel density and is related to early intravesical recurrence (Shirotake et al., 2011). AT1R supports tumor-associated macrophage infiltration, which results in enhanced tissue VEGF protein levels (Egami et al., 2009). These results suggest that AT1R is involved in bladder tumor angiogenesis and may become a new molecular target and a prognostic factor for urothelial bladder cancer patients

In the subset of invasive urothelial bladder cancer, most studies also reported the association between angiogenesis occurrence and unfavorable prognosis. High blood vessel density was identified as an independent prognostic factor by several authors (Bochner et al., 1995; Chaudhary et al., 1999; Dickinson et al., 1994; Jaeger et al., 1995). Moreover, overexpression of VEGF associates with high blood vessel density (Sato et al., 1998; Yang et al., 2004). Analysis of serum levels of VEGF has demonstrated its optimal sensitivity and specificity for predicting metastatic disease (Bernardini et al., 2001). Inoue and colleagues reported the importance of measuring blood vessel density and VEGF immunoexpression in identifying patients with invasive tumors who are at high risk of recurrence and development of metastasis after radical cystectomy and neoadjuvant systemic chemotherapy. The author highlighted the role of VEGF as a cell survival factor, not only by protecting the malignant cells in situations of hypoxia, but also during the occurrence of chemotherapy-induced apoptosis (Inoue et al., 2000).

Beyond VEGF signaling, other angiogenesis-related molecules have been implicated in bladder cancer recurrence, progression and metastasis, namely several proangiogenic factors — matrix metalloproteinases, fibroblast growth factors, platelet derived-growth factors, cyclooxygenases, integrins, angiopoietins, Notch signaling — and several antiangiogenic factors — thrombospondin-1, angiostatin-endostatin, platelet factor-4 (Chikazawa et al., 2008; Durkan et al., 2001; Grossfeld et al., 1997; Patel et al., 2006; reviewed in Pinto et al., 2010; Shariat et al., 2010).

The relevance of lymphangiogenesis in bladder cancer setting has gained recent attention. A few articles suggest that lymphangiogenesis occurrence, detected using specific lymphatic markers, is associated with poor prognosis (Fernández et al., 2008; Ma et al., 2010; Miyata et al., 2006; Zhou et al., 2011; Zu et al., 2006). VEGF-C, VEGF-D and VEGFR-3 are overexpressed in bladder cancer and promote tumor-induced lymphangiogenesis. This correlates with tumor upstaging and lymph node involvement, and results in a worse prognosis (Afonso et al., 2009; Miyata et al., 2006; Suzuki et al., 2005; Herrmann et al., 2007; Zhou et al., 2011; Zu et al., 2006). Interestingly, VEGF-C overexpression also associates with angiogenic events, probably by interaction of the fully processed form with VEGFR-2 (Afonso et al., 2009; Miyata et al., 2006). On the other hand, tumor associated macrophages play an important role in promoting lymphangiogenesis by producing VEGF-C and VEGF-D, mainly in peritumoral areas (Schoppmann et al., 2002). The blockade of VEGF-C/D with a soluble VEGF receptor-3 markedly inhibited lymphangiogenesis and lymphatic metastasis in an orthotopic urinary bladder cancer model. In addition, the depletion of tumor associated macrophages exerted similar effects (Yang et al. 2011).

Lymphovascular invasion has been identified as an independent prognostic factor for bladder cancer patients in several studies (Cho et al., 2009; Leissner et al., 2003; Lotan et al., 2005; Quek et al., 2005). In patients with newly diagnosed T1 urothelial bladder cancer, lymphovascular invasion in transurethral resection of bladder tumor specimens predicts disease progression and metastasis (Cho et al., 2009). Lotan and colleagues observed that blood and lymphatic vessel invasion (accessed by Haematoxylin-eosin stain) is an independent predictor of recurrence and low overall survival in patients who undergo radical cystectomy for invasive urothelial bladder cancer and are lymph node negative. They emphasized that these patients represent a high risk group that may benefit from neoadjuvant or adjuvant treatments. However, in this study, the mean number of lymph nodes removed per patient at the time of radical cystectomy was 20,1±10,2 (Lotan et al., 2005).

The prognostic impact of lymphovascular invasion in patients with lymph node-negative urothelial bladder cancer treated by radical cystectomy has been recently validated in large multicentre trials (Bolenz et al., 2010; Shariat et al, 2010). May and colleagues emphasized that, besides the importance of performing extended lymphadenectomies, the information resulting from an assessment of lymphovascular invasion is critical for stratification of risk groups and identification of patients who might benefit from adjuvant treatments (May, 2011). Algaba underlined that, in this field, it would be necessary to reach a consensus on strict diagnostic criteria as soon as possible, to be able to incorporate this prognostic factor in clinical practice (Algaba, 2006). Leissner and colleagues endorsed that blood and lymphatic vessel invasion should be commented on separately in the pathology report (Leissner et al., 2003).

Afonso and colleagues reported the prognostic contribution of molecular markers of blood vessels (like CD31) (Fig. 4, A) and lymphatic vessels (like D2-40) (Fig. 4, B) to accurately assess the occurrence of blood and/or lymphatic vessel invasion. The use of endothelial markers is encouraged because immunohistochemistry antibodies are significantly more sensitive in detecting invasive events than the standard Haematoxylin-eosin staining method and, additionally, facilitate the discrimination between blood and lymphatic vessel invasion. This is particularly important in identifying isolated malignant cells invading lymphatic vessels, because their viability is more probable in the lymphatic flow than in the blood circulation. Conversely, emboli of malignant cells are better suited to survive in the bloodstream, and are more easily identified, even by the traditional Haematoxylin-eosin staining method. This advocates the use of lymphatic markers for purposes of counting invaded lymphatic vessels. In this study, blood vessel invasion by malignant emboli assessed by CD31 staining (Fig. 5, A), and lymphatic vessel invasion by isolated malignant cells assessed by D2-40 staining (Fig. 5, B) significantly affected patients' prognosis; blood vessel invasion remained as an independent prognostic factor (Afonso et al., 2009). When included in a model of bladder cancer aggressiveness, these parameters contributed to a clear separation between low and high aggressiveness groups (Afonso et al., 2011).

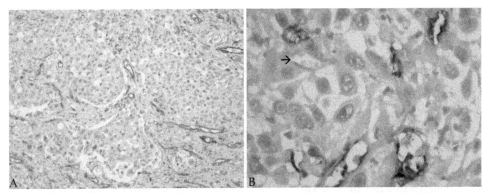

Fig. 4. Intratumoral blood vessels highlighted by CD31 (A), and intratumoral lymphatic vessels highlighted by D2-40 (B), in invasive urothelial bladder carcinoma. Evidence of internal negative control in A (D2-40 negative blood vessel →) (original magnification x100) (reprinted by permission from © 2009 John Wiley & Sons, Inc. Originally published in *Histopathol.* 55: 514-524)

Both peritumoral and intratumoral lymphatic vessels seem to be functional for urothelial cells' dissemination. Some articles reported the existence of intratumoral lymphatic vessels in bladder tumors, and their possible participation in metastatic events. No intratumoral edema has been observed, which is consistent with the occurrence of efficient lymphatic neovascularization (Afonso et al., 2009; Fernández et al., 2008; Ma et al., 2010; Miyata et al. 2006). Lymphatic vessel invasion occurrence correlates with high lymphatic vessel density values, mainly in the intratumoral areas. Although most of the invaded lymphatic vessels were distorted and collapsed, single malignant cells were significantly observed in the well-preserved intratumoral lymphatic vessels (Fig. 5, B). Moreover, the absence of intratumoral edema is a surrogate marker of an efficient lymphatic flow (Afonso et al., 2009).

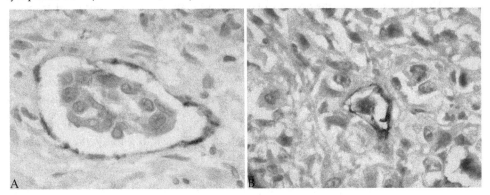

Fig. 5. Intratumoral blood vessel highlighted by CD31 invaded by a small malignant embolus (A), and intratumoral lymphatic vessel highlighted by D2-40 invaded by an isolated malignant cell (B), in invasive urothelial bladder carcinoma (original magnification x100) (reprinted by permission from © 2009 John Wiley & Sons, Inc. Originally published in *Histopathol.* 55: 514-524)

4. Angiogenesis and Lymphangiogenesis as therapeutic targets in urothelial bladder cancer

Our current understanding of the importance of tumor-induced angiogenesis and lymphangiogenesis for the occurrence of haematogenous and lymphogenous metastasis suggests that, by blocking the activity of key molecules involved in these processes, it should be possible to suppress the onset of metastasis following diagnosis of cancer and its subsequent therapy. Moreover, prophylactic suppression of metastasis would be useful for patients who are at risk of recurrence (Thiele & Sleeman, 2006). Therefore, clinical trials evaluating novel agents and combinations including chemotherapeutic drugs, as well as targeted inhibitors, are desperately needed (Iyer et al., 2010).

Two types of neovascularization inhibitors have been described. The direct inhibitors refer to compounds that function directly on endothelial cells by blocking a common pathway of vessel growth. Indirect inhibitors are molecules that neutralize the functions of angiogenic and lymphangiogenic growth factors; due to their mode of action, these are preferred over the direct inhibitors (Cao, 2005; Folkman, 2003). The main strategies that have been tested focus on modulating the signaling of VEGF family of growth factors and receptors, and are based on the use of monoclonal antibodies or soluble versions of receptors to neutralize the ligand-receptor interaction, and the inhibition of the kinase activity of the receptors (Achen et al., 2006; Thiele & Sleeman, 2006).

In 2004, the U.S. Food and Drug Administration (FDA) has approved bevacizumab (Avastin®), a humanized monoclonal antibody that binds to VEGF-A, as the first drug developed solely for antiangiogenesis anticancer use in humans. Antiangiogenic drugs are presently approved in a wide number of tumor types, namely in breast, colorectal, lung, liver, glioblastoma and kidney cancer. Other compounds are currently in preclinical development, with many of them now entering the clinic and/or achieving approval (reviewed in Boere et al., 2010; reviewed in Cook & Figg, 2010; reviewed in Pinto et al., 2010).

In anticancer therapy, an angiogenesis inhibitor may prevent the growth of new blood vessels. This should decrease the delivery of oxygen and nutrients – the "starving therapy" – which are indispensable elements for the support of uncontrolled cell division and tumor expansion. Angiogenesis inhibitors are predicted to be cytostatic, stabilizing tumors and perhaps preventing metastasis, rather than being curative (Zhi-chao & Jie, 2008). Therefore, there is the need to administrate this type of therapy for long periods of time. As a consequence, problems with bleeding, blood clotting, heart function and depletion of the immune system are common (Cohen et al., 2007). Nevertheless, inhibition of circulating VEGF reduces vascular permeability and thus tumoral interstitial pressure, permitting easier penetration of the tumor by conventional chemotherapeutic targets (Ferrara, 2005).

A second concern of anti-angiogenesis therapy is the approach to objectify the response to anti-angiogenic drugs. Chan and colleagues found that targeted contrast enhanced micro-ultrasound imaging enables investigators to detect and monitor vascular changes in orthotopic bladder tumors. Therefore, this technique may be useful for direct, noninvasive and in vivo evaluation of angiogenesis inhibitors (Chan et al., 2011). Lassau and colleagues demonstrated that dynamic ultrasound can be used to quantify dynamic changes in tumor vascularity as early as three days after the administration of the anti-angiogenic drug. These changes may be potential surrogate measures of the effectiveness of antiangiogenic therapy, namely by predicting progression-free survival and overall survival (Lassau et al., 2011).

Regarding antilymphangiogenic strategies, numerous compounds that could be used to block lymphangiogenesis already exist, although there is some delay in the translation to the clinic. These act mainly by targeting lymphangiogenic protein tyrosine kinases (Williams et al., 2010) (Table 1) or other indirect regulators of lymphangiogenic events. For instance, rapamycin (sirolimus), a classical immunosuppressant drug used to prevent rejection in organ transplantation, and a known inhibitor of the mTOR (mammalian target of rapamycin) signaling, has demonstrated potent antilymphangiogenic properties (Huber et al., 2007), and may suppress lymphatic metastasis (Kobayashi et al., 2007). mTOR is a member of the phosphoinositide-3-kinase-related kinase family, and is centrally involved in growth regulation, proliferation control and cancer cell metabolism (Rosner et al., 2008). Its inhibition impairs downstream signaling of VEGF-A as well as VEGF-C via mTOR to the ribosomal p70S6 kinase (a regulator of protein translation, and a major substrate of mTOR) in lymphatic endothelial cells (Huber et al., 2007). Other derivative compounds of rapamycin, like everolimus (RAD001) and temsirolimus (Torisel), have also demonstrated anti-tumor properties, namely by inhibiting tumor neovascularization (reviewed in Garcia & Danielpour, 2008). Recently, in patients with lymphangioleiomyomatosis (LAM, a progressive, cystic lung disease in women, which is associated with inappropriate activation of mTOR) sirolimus stabilized lung function, reduced serum VEGF-D levels, and was associated with a reduction in symptoms and improvement in the quality of life (McCormack et al., 2011).

Inhibition of lymphangiogenesis has been shown to block lymphatic metastasis by 50-70% in preclinical animal models, with good safety profiles, which suggests that anti-lymphangiogenic therapy could possibly be used safely in cancer patients, without disrupting normal lymphatic function (reviewed in Holopainen et al., 2011). Optimally, the gold-standard strategy would be the one that could inhibit both angiogenic and lymphangiogenic cascades, in order to compromise the success of haematogenous and lymphogenous dissemination. Some potential compounds are being investigated (reviewed in Boere et al., 2010; reviewed in Cook & Figg, 2010; reviewed in Pinto et al., 2010; reviewed in Stacker & Achen, 2008).

Urothelial bladder carcinoma has experienced very few therapeutic successes, regarding antineovascularization therapy, in the last years. Compounds like bevacizumab (Avastin®), aflibercept (VEGF-Trap, AVE0005), sunitinib malate (Sutent, SU11248), sorafenib (BAY 43-9006), vandetanib (Zactima, ZD6474) and pazopanib (Votrient, GW786034) are being tested in preclinical and clinical trials (reviewed in Pinto et al., 2010) (Table 2). Bevacizumab, as has been already referred, is a monoclonal antibody that binds and neutralizes VEGF in the serum. Aflibercept is a soluble fusion protein of the human extracellular domains of VEGFR-1 and VEGFR-2, and the Fc portion of human immunoglobulin G. It binds, with a higher affinity than other monoclonal antibodies, to VEGF and additional VEGF-family members, namely VEGF-B and placental growth factor (PIGF). Sunitinib is an oral multi-targeted receptor tyrosine kinase inhibitor, with activity against VEGF receptors and PDGF receptors, among others. Sorafenib is a small, oral molecule that inhibits various targets along the EGFR/MAPK (epidermal growth factor receptor / mitogen-activated protein kinase) signal transduction pathway, and also through VEGFR and PDGFR families. Vandetanib is a tyrosine kinase inhibitor, antagonist of VEGFR and EGFR. Pazopanib is a multitargeted tyrosine kinase inhibitor against VEGF receptors, c-kit, and PDGF receptors (Cook & Figg, 2010).

Gene	Role in lymphatic vessels	Inhibitors available	Effect of pathway inhibition
VEGFR-2	Receptor for the VEGF family of ligands. Can also heterodimerize with VEGFR-3.	Yes	Secreted VEGFR-2 is a naturally occurring inhibitor of lymphatic vessel growth; however, Sorafenib[†] did not block VEGF-C/D induced tumor lymphangiogenesis.
VEGFR-3	Predominant receptor for VEGF-C and VEGF-D. Transduces survival, proliferation and migration signals.	Yes	Cediranib[‡] blocks VEGFR-3 activity and inhibits lymphangiogenesis. Anti-VEGFR-3 antibody prevented tumor lymphangiogenesis with no effect on preexisting vessels.
Tie1	Not critical for lymphatic cell commitment during development, and no ligand has been shown.	None reported.	Tie1 knockout mouse has lymphatic vascular abnormalities that precede the blood vessel phenotype.
Tie2	Receptor for Ang-1 and Ang-2. Appears to control vessel maturation.	Yes	Tie2-/- mice are embryonic lethal due to vascular defects. Inhibition of Ang-2 leads to tumor blood vessel normalization.
EphB4	Expressed on lymphatic capillary vessels. Involved in vascular patterning. Binds to the ephrinB2 ligand.	Yes	Mice expressing a mutant form of ephrinB2 lacking the PDZ binding domain show major lymphatic defects in capillary vessels and collecting vessel valve formation.
FGFR3	The ligands FGF-1 and FGF-2 promote proliferation, migration, and survival of cultured lymphatic endothelial cells. FGFR3 is a direct transcriptional target of Prox1.	Yes	Knockdown of FGFR3 reduced lymphatic endothelial cells' proliferation.
IGF1R	Both of the IGF1R ligands, IGF-1 and IGF-2, significantly stimulated proliferation and migration of primary lymphatic endothelial cells.	Yes	None reported.
PDGFRβ	The ligand PDGF-BB stimulated MAP kinase activity and cell motility of isolated lymphatic endothelial cells.	Yes	None reported.

Gene	Role in lymphatic vessels	Inhibitors available	Effect of pathway inhibition
MET	The ligand for c-Met, hepatocyte growth factor, has lymphangiogenic effect, but it is unclear if c-Met is expressed on lymphatic endothelial cells.	Yes	May be indirect effect.

†Sorafenib inhibits B-Raf, PDGFRb, VEGFR-2 and c-Kit. ‡Cediranib inhibits VEGFR-1, -2, -3, PDGFRb and c-Kit.

Table 1. Protein tyrosine kinases involved in lymphatic biology, and available inhibitors (Tie- tyrosine kinase with immunoglobulin and EGF homology domain; EphB4- ephrin type-B receptor 4) (reprinted by permission from © 2010 BioMed Central Ltd. Originally published in *J. Ang. Res.* 2: 1-13)

Principal investigator/ organization	Regimen	Patient population	Phase
Siefker-Radtke/MDACC	Methotrexate + vinblastine + doxorubicin+ cisplatin + bevacizumab	Neoadjuvant (muscle-invasive)	II
Kraft/MUSC	Gemcitabine + cisplatin + bevacizumab → cystectomy → paclitaxel + bevacizumab	Neoadjuvant/adjuvant (muscle-invasive)	II
Hahn/HOG	Gemcitabine + cisplatin + bevacizumab	First-line metastatic	II
Bajorin/MSKCC	Gemcitabine + carboplatin + bevacizumab	First-line metastatic (cisplatin-ineligible)	II
Rosenberg/CALGB	Gemcitabine + cisplatin ± bevacizumab	First-line metastatic	III
Garcia/Cleveland Clinic	Sunitinib	Neoadjuvant (muscle-invasive)	II
Sonpavde/HOG	Gemcitabine + cisplatin + sunitinib	Neoadjuvant (muscle-invasive)	II
Bellmunt	Sunitinib	First-line metastatic (cisplatin-ineligible)	II
Galsky/US Oncology	Gemcitabine + cisplatin + sunitinib	First-line metastatic	II
Hussain/University of Michigan	Sunitinib versus placebo	Maintenance after first-line chemotherapy	II
Gallagher/MSKCC	Sunitinib	Second-line metastatic	II
Milowsky/MSKCC	Gemcitabine + cisplatin + sorafenib	First-line metastatic	II
Kelly/Yale	Gemcitabine + carboplatin + sorafenib	First-line metastatic (cisplatin-ineligible)	II

Principal investigator/ organization	Regimen	Patient population	Phase
Sternberg/EORTC	Gemcitabine + carboplatin ± sorafenib	First-line metastatic	II
Dreicer/ECOG	Sorafenib	Second-line metastatic	II
Choueiri/DFCI	Docetaxel ± vandetanib	Second-line metastatic	II
Vaishampayan/Mayo Clinic	Pazopanib	Second-line metastatic	II

MDACC = MD Anderson Cancer Center; MUSC = Medical University of South Carolina; HOG = Hoosier Oncology Group; MSKCC = Memorial Sloan-Kettering Cancer Center; CALGB = Cancer and Leukemia Group B; EORTC = European Organization for Research and Treatment of Cancer; ECOG = Eastern Cooperative Oncology Group; DFCI = Dana-Farber Cancer Institute

Table 2. Selected ongoing or recently completed trials exploring antiangiogenic therapies in urothelial bladder carcinoma (reprinted by permission from © 2010 Elsevier. Originally published in *Commun. Oncol.* 7: 500-504)

4.1 Preclinical studies

In the preclinical scenario, Videira and colleagues studied the effect of bevacizumab on autocrine VEGF stimulation in bladder cancer cell lines, and concluded that, at clinical bevacizumab concentrations, cancer cells compensate the VEGF blockade, by improving the expression of VEGF and related genes. This highlights the need to follow the patient's adaptation response to bevacizumab treatment (Videira et al., 2011). The antiangiogenic treatment of tumours may restore vascular communication and, thereby, normalize flow distribution in tumour vasculature. The use of antiangiogenic drugs leads to improved tumour oxygenation and chemotherapy drug delivery (Pries et al., 2010). However, these mechanisms may be also the cause of malignant dissemination, because tumours elicit evasive resistance. Caution is recommended, due to the divergent effects that VEGF inhibitors can induce on primary tumor growth and metastasis (Loges et al., 2009).

Yoon and colleagues, when exposing six human bladder cancer cell lines to an escalating dose of sunitinib alone or in combination with cisplatin/gemcitabine, demonstrated that sunitinib malate has a potent antitumor effect and may synergistically enhance the known antitumor effect of gemcitabine (Yoon et al, 2011).

The first study with vandetanib in bladder cancer cell lines demonstrated its potential to sensitize tumor cells to cisplatin. At vandetanib concentrations of ≤2microM, the combination with cisplatin was synergistic, especially when given sequentially after cisplatin , and additive with vandetanib followed by cisplatin (Flaig et al., 2009).

Li and colleagues studied the efficacy of pazopanib, both alone and in combination with docetaxel, in bladder cancer cell lines. They demonstrated that single-agent pazopanib has modest activity, but when given in combination with docetaxel, acted synergistically in docetaxel-resistant bladder cancer cells, with the potential of improved toxicity (Li et al., 2001).

Urothelial bladder carcinoma expresses mTOR signaling molecules, providing a rationale for clinical trials evaluating agents targeting this pathway (Tickoo et al., 2011). In fact, some studies using bladder cancer cell lines have demonstrated that sirolimus and related drugs inhibit the growth of cancer cells and decrease their viability (Fechner et al., 2009; Hansel et al., 2010; Pinto-Leite et al., 2009; Schedel et al., 2011). Similar results were obtained when treating bladder cancer animal models with sirolimus or everolimus (Chiong et al., 2011; Oliveira et al., 2011; Parada et al., 2011; Seager et al., 2009; Vasconcelos-Nóbrega et al., 2011).

4.2 Phase II studies

The results of a phase II trial of cisplatin, gemcitabine, and bevacizumab (CGB) as first-line therapy for metastatic urothelial carcinoma revealed that CGB may improve overall survival — with a median follow-up of 27.2 months, overall survival time was 19.1 months. However, the rate of side effects was high, namely neutropenia, thrombocytopenia, anemia, and deep vein thrombosis/pulmonary embolism (Hahn et al., 2011).

In a phase II trial of gemcitabine, carboplatin, and bevacizumab in patients with advanced/metastatic urothelial carcinoma, Balar and colleagues concluded that addition of bevacizumab does not improve the response rate. However, bevacizumab can be safely added to gemcitabine and carboplatin, because the rate of venous thromboembolisms is similar to the one observed with gemcitabine and carboplatin alone (Balar et al., 2011). Moreover, in a pooled analysis of cancer patients in randomized phase II and III studies, the addition of bevacizumab to chemotherapy did not statistically significantly increase the risk of venous thromboembolisms *versus* chemotherapy alone. Probably, the risk for venous thromboembolisms is driven predominantly by tumor and host factors (Hurwitz et al., 2011). This type of side effect is primarily prevented by using anticoagulants simultaneously with cytotoxic chemotherapy (Riess et al., 2010). However, anticoagulant use during bevacizumab therapy may increase the risk of serious hemorrhage, although it is generally well tolerated (Bartolomeo et al., 2010). This controversial issue is still under scrutiny and more data are needed to clarify the optimal regime to reduce venous thromboembolisms in bladder cancer patients, particularly in those who are being treated with antiangiogenic drugs.

Patients with recurrent or metastatic urothelial carcinoma who had received a prior platinum-containing regimen were entered in a phase II trial with aflibercept as a second-line therapy. Aflibercept was well tolerated, but it had limited single agent activity in platinum-pretreated bladder cancer patients (Twardowski et al., 2009).

In a phase II study of sunitinib in patients with metastatic urothelial cancer designed to assess the efficacy and tolerability of this drug in patients with advanced, previously treated urothelial cancer, anti-tumour responses were observed. However, sunitinib did not achieve the predetermined threshold of ≥20% activity defined by the Response Evaluation Criteria in Solid Tumors, and side effects such as embolic events were reported (Gallagher et al., 2010).

In a multicenter phase II trial with sunitinib as first-line treatment in patients with metastatic urothelial cancer ineligible for cisplatin, on intention-to-treat analysis revealed that 38% of the patients showed partial responses (PRs), and 50% presented with stable disease (SD), the majority more than 3 months. Clinical benefit (PR + SD) was 58%. Median time to progression was 4.8 months and median overall survival 8.1 months (Bellmunt et al., 2011).

In a multicentre phase II trial of sorafenib as second-line therapy in patients with metastatic urothelial carcinoma, there were no objective responses to therapy. The 4-month progression-free survival rate was 9.5%, and the overall survival was 6.8 months (Dreicer et al., 2009).

Choueiri and colleagues conducted a double-blind randomized trial in which patients with metastatic bladder cancer and as many as three previous chemotherapy regimens received intravenous docetaxel with or without vandetanib. The results demonstrated that the

addition of vandetanib to second-line docetaxel did not result in significant improvements in progression-free survival, overall survival or response rates (Choueiri et al., 2011). The final results of a phase II study of everolimus in metastatic urothelial cell carcinoma have been presented at 2011 ASCO (American Society of Clinical Oncology) Annual Meeting. It was demonstrated that everolimus has clinical activity in patients with advanced urothelial bladder cancer. For the thirty-seven evaluable patients, the median progression-free survival was 3.3 months, and the median overall-survival was 10.5 months. Some side effects possibly related to everolimus were observed, namely anemia, infection, hyperglycemia, lymphopenia, hypophosphatemia and fatigue (Milowsky et al., 2011).
Dovitinib (TKI258) is an oral investigational drug that inhibits angiogenic factors, including FGFR and VEGFR. A multicenter, open-label phase II trial of dovitinib in advanced urothelial carcinoma patients with either mutated or wild-type FGFR3 is currently underway (Milowsky et al., 2011).

4.3 Phase III studies
A randomized double-blinded phase III study comparing gemcitabine, cisplatin, and bevacizumab to gemcitabine, cisplatin, and placebo in patients with advanced urothelial carcinoma is open to enrollment. The primary end point is to compare the overall survival of patients with advanced urothelial carcinoma treated with gemcitabine hydrochloride, cisplatin, and bevacizumab *versus* gemcitabine hydrochloride, cisplatin, and placebo. The secondary end points are to compare the progression-free survival, the objective response rate and the grade 3 and greater toxicities of these regimens in the patients (Cancer and Leukemia Group B, 2011).

5. Conclusion

Bladder cancer represents a significant health problem, and the costliest type of cancer to treat. Although the majority of cases present as non-muscle invasive disease, the recurrence and progression rates are high, which demands for long-term follow-up and repeated interventions. Moreover, patients with advanced tumors treated by neoadjuvant or adjuvant regiments frequently progress and may develop chemotherapy resistance. Therefore, biomarkers of tumour aggressiveness and response to therapy are urgently needed, since the classical formulae based on stage and grade classification are insufficient to characterize bladder cancer. In this sense, angiogenesis, lymphangiogenesis and lymphovascular invasion have been described as surrogate markers of bladder cancer progression, invasion and metastasis, and represent potential fields of intervention. On one hand, the combined analysis of these biological parameters in tumor samples with the classical clinicopathological parameters may improve the individual characterization of bladder cancer, in what concerns to its clinical and prognostic course, and should allow therapeutic adequacy. On the other hand, the knowledge and modulating of biological phenomena related with bladder cancer progression may represent a significant improvement in the development of new drugs and in the pathological response to therapy, which ultimately will lead to an increase in disease-free survival and overall survival rates.
Targeted therapy has caused dramatic changes in the treatment of other types of tumors. However, in bladder cancer setting, clinical trials with molecularly targeted agents have been few in number and largely unsuccessful. Regarding antiangiogenic and

antilymphangiogenic agents, these are still considered an investigational option for urothelial bladder cancer patients, and more results are needed to establish their roles in the treatment armamentarium. Research studies with anti-neovascularization drugs should not only provide effective agents to treat bladder cancer patients, but also predictive biomarkers for response to anti-neovascularization therapy, in order to implement the concept of personalized therapy.

6. Acknowledgements

We thank Nuno Sousa, from the Department of Medical Oncology of the Portuguese Institute of Oncology – IPO, for a critical review of the chapter.

7. References

Abol-Enein, H.; Tilki, D.; Mosbah, A. et al. (2011). Does the Extent of Lymphadenectomy in Radical Cystectomy for Bladder Cancer Influence Disease-Free Survival? A Prospective Single-Center Study. *European Urology*, (June 2011), [Epub ahead of print], ISSN 0302-2838.

Achen, M.G. & Stacker, S. (2008). Molecular Control of Lymphatic Metastasis. *Annals of the New York Academy of Sciences*, Vol.1131, pp. 225-234, ISSN 0077-8923.

Achen, M.G.; Mann, G.B. & Stacker, S.A. (2006). Targeting lymphangiogenesis to prevent tumor metastasis. *British Journal of Cancer*, Vol.94, No.10 (May 2006), pp.1355-1360.

Adams, R.H. & Alitalo, K. (2007). Molecular regulation of angiogenesis and lymphangiogenesis. *Nature Reviews Cancer*, Vol.8, No.6 (June 2007), pp. 464-478, ISSN 1474-175X.

Afonso, J.; Santos, L.L.; Amaro, T.; Lobo, F. & Longatto-Filho, A. (2009). The aggressiveness of urothelial carcinoma depends to a large extent on lymphovascular invasion – the prognostic contribution of related molecular markers. *Histopathology*, Vol.55, No.5 (November 2009), pp: 514-524, ISSN 1365-2559.

Afonso, J.; Longatto-Filho, A.; Baltazar, F. et al. (2011). CD147 overexpression allows an accurate discrimination of bladder cancer patients' prognosis, *European Journal of Surgical Oncology*, (July 2011), doi:10.1016/j.ejso.2011.06.006, ISSN 0748-7983.

Algaba, F. (2006). Lymphovascular invasion as a prognostic tool for advanced bladder cancer. *Current Opinion in Urology*, Vol.16, No.5 (September 2006), pp. 367-371, ISSN 1473-6586.

Alitalo, K. & Carmeliet, P. (2002). Molecular mechanisms of lymphangiogenesis in health and disease. *Cancer Cell*. Vol.1, No.3 (April 2002), pp. 219-227, ISSN 1535-6108.

Alitalo, K.; Tammela, T. & Petrova, T. (2005). Lymphangiogenesis in development and human disease. *Nature*, Vol.438, No.7070 (December 2005), pp. 946-953, ISSN 0028-0836.

Arany, Z.; Foo, S.Y.; Ma, Y. et al. (2008). HIF-independent regulation of VEGF and angiogenesis by the transcriptional coactivator PGC-1alpha. *Nature*, Vol.451, No.7181 (February 2008), pp. 1008-1012, ISSN 0028-0836.

Balar, A.V.; Milowsky, M.I.; Apolo, A.B. et al. (2011). Phase II trial of gemcitabine, carboplatin, and bevacizumab in chemotherapy-naive patients with advanced/metastatic urothelial carcinoma. *Proceedings of the 2011 Genitourinary Cancers Symposium*, Abstract No 248, Orlando, Florida, USA, February 17-19, 2011.

Baldwin, M.E.; Halford, M.M.; Roufail, S. et al. (2005). Vascular Endothelial Growth Factor D is dispensable for Development of the Lymphatic System. *Molecular and Cellular Biology*, Vol.25, No.6 (March 2005), pp. 2441-2449, ISSN 1098-5549.

Banerji, S.; Ni, J.; Wang, S.X. et al. (1999). LYVE-1, a new homologue of the CD44 glycoprotein, is a lymph-specific receptor for hyaluronan. *The Journal of Cell Biology*, Vol.144, No.4 (February 1999), pp. 789-801, ISSN 1540-8140.

Bartolomeo, J.; Norden, A.D.; Drappatz, J. et al. (2010). Safety of concurrent bevacizumab therapy and anticoagulation in high-grade glioma patients. *Proceedings of the 2010 ASCO Annual Meeting*, Abstract No 2043, Chicago, Illinois, USA, June 4-8, 2010.

Bellmunt, J.; González-Larriba, J.L.; Prior, C. et al. (2011). Phase II study of sunitinib as first-line treatment of urothelial cancer patients ineligible to receive cisplatin-based chemotherapy: baseline interleukin-8 and tumor contrast enhancement as potential predictive factors of activity. *Annals of Oncology*, (March 2011), [Epub ahead of print], ISSN 1569-8041.

Bernardini, S.; Fauconnet, S.; Chabannes, E. et al. (2001). Serum levels of vascular endothelial growth factor as a prognostic factor in bladder cancer. *The Journal of Urology*, Vol.166, No.4 (October 2001), pp. 1275-1279, ISSN 0022-5347.

Bochner, B.H.; Cote, R.J.; Weidner, N. et al. (1995). Angiogenesis in bladder cancer: relationship between microvessel density and tumor prognosis. *Journal of the National Cancer Institute*, Vol.87, No.21 (November 1995), pp. 1603-1612, ISSN 1460-2105.

Boere, I.A.; Hamberg, P. & Sleijfer, S. (2010). It takes two to tango: combinations of conventional cytotoxics with compounds targeting the vascular endothelial growth factor-vascular endothelial growth factor receptor pathway in patients with solid malignancies. *Cancer Science*, Vol.101, No.1 (January 2010), pp. 7-15, ISSN 1349-7006.

Bolenz, C.; Herrmann, E.; Bastian, P.J. et al. (2010). Lymphovascular invasion is an independent predictor of oncological outcomes in patients with lymph node-negative urothelial bladder cancer treated by radical cystectomy: a multicentre validation trial. *British Journal of Urology International*, Vol.106, No.4 (August 2010), pp. 493-499, ISSN 2042-2997.

Brusselmans, K.; Bono, F.; Collen, D. et al. (2005). A novel role for vascular endothelial growth factor as an autocrine survival factor for embryonic stem cells during hypoxia. *The Journal of Biological Chemistry*, Vol.280, No.5 (February 2005), pp. 3493-3499, ISSN 1083-351X.

Cancer and Leukemia Group B (2011). CALGB90601 A Randomized Double-Blinded Phase III Study Comparing Gemcitabine, Cisplatin, and Bevacizumab to Gemcitaine, Cisplatin, and Placebo in Patients with Advanced Transitional Cell Carcinoma, In: University of Colorado Hospital, 08.07.2010, Available from: http://www.uch.edu/ClinicalTrials/clinical-trials-detail/?id=117

Cao, Y. (2005). Emerging mechanisms of tumour lymphangiogenesis and lymphatic metastasis. *Nature Reviews Cancer*, Vol.5, No.9 (September 2005), pp. 735-743, ISSN 1474-175X.

Carmeliet, P. & Jain, R.K. (2000). Angiogenesis in cancer and other diseases. *Nature*, Vol.407, No.6801 (September 2000), pp. 249-257, ISSN 0028-0836.

Carmeliet, P. (2005). VEGF as a Key Mediator of Angiogenesis in Cancer. *Oncology*, Vol.69, No.3 (November 2005) pp. 4-10, ISSN 1423-0232.

Carmeliet, P.; Ferreira, V.; Breier, G. et al. (1996). Abnormal blood vessel development and lethality in embryos lacking a single VEGF allele. *Nature*, Vol.380, No.6573 (April 1996), pp. 435-439, ISSN 0028-0836.

Chan, E.S.; Patel, A.R.; Larchian, W.A. & Heston, W.D. (2011). In vivo targeted contrast enhanced micro-ultrasound to measure intratumor perfusion and vascular endothelial growth factor receptor 2 expression in a mouse orthotopic bladder cancer model. *The Journal of Urology*, Vol.185, No.6 (June 2011), pp. 2359-2365, ISSN 0022-5347.

Chaudhary, R.; Bromley, M.; Clarke, N.W. et al. (1999). Prognostic relevance of micro-vessel density in cancer of the urinary bladder. *Anticancer Research*, Vol.19, No.4C (July-August 1999), pp. 3479-3484, ISSN 1791-7530.

Chikazawa, M.; Inoue, K.; Fukata, S.; Karashima, T. & Shuin, T. (2008). Expression of angiogenesis-related genes regulates different steps in the process of tumor growth and metastasis in human urothelial cell carcinoma of the urinary bladder. *Pathobiology*, Vol.75, No.6 (December 2008), pp.335-345, ISSN 1423-0291.

Chiong, E.; Lee, I.L.; Dadbin, A. et al. Effects of mTOR inhibitor everolimus (RAD001) on bladder cancer cells. *Clinical Cancer Research*, Vol.17, No.9 (May 2011), pp. 2863-2873, ISSN 1557-3265.

Cho, K.S.; Seo, H.K.; Joung, J.Y. et al. (2009). Lymphovascular invasion in transurethral resection specimens as predictor of progression and metastasis in patients with newly diagnosed T1 bladder urothelial cancer. *The Journal of Urology*, Vol.182, No.6 (December 2009), pp.2625-2630, ISSN 0022-5347.

Choueiri, T.K.; Vaishampayan U.N.; Yu, E.Y. et al. (2011). A double-blind randomized trial of docetaxel plus vandetanib versus docetaxel plus placebo in platinum-pretreated advanced urothelial cancer. *Proceedings of the 2011 Genitourinary Cancers Symposium*, Abstract LBA239, Orlando, Florida, USA, February 17-19, 2011.

Clark, P.E. (2009). Neoadjuvant versus adjuvant chemotherapy for muscle-invasive bladder cancer. *Expert Review of Anticancer Therapy*, Vol.9, No.6 (June 2009), pp. 821-830, ISSN 1473-7140.

Cohen, M.H.; Gootenberg, J.; Keegan, P. & Pazdur, R. (2007). FDA drug approval summary: Bevacizumab plus FOLFOX4 as second-line treatment of colorectal cancer. *The Oncologist*, Vol.12, No.3 (March 2007), pp. 356-361, ISSN 1549-490X.

Cook, K.M. & Figg, W.D. (2010). Angiogenesis inhibitors: current strategies and future prospects. *CA: A Cancer Journal for Clinicians*, Vol.60, No.4 (July-August 2010), pp. 222-243, ISSN 1542-4863.

Crew, J.P.; O'Brien, T.; Bicknell, R. et al. (1999). Urinary vascular endothelial growth factor and its correlation with bladder cancer recurrence rates. *The Journal of Urology*, Vol.161, No.3 (March 1999), pp. 799-804, ISSN 0022-5347.

Crew, J.P.; O'Brien, T.; Bradburn, M. et al. (1997). Vascular endothelial growth factor is a predictor of relapse and stage progression in superficial bladder cancer. *Cancer Research*, Vol.57, No.23 (December 1997), pp. 5281-5285, ISSN 1538-7445.

Da, M.X.; Wu, Z. & Tian, H.W. (2008). Tumor lymphangiogenesis and lymphangiogenic growth factors. *Archives of Medical Research*, Vol.39, No.4 (May 2008), pp. 365-372, ISSN 0188-4409.

Detmar, M. & Hirakawa, S. (2002). The Formation of Lymphatic Vessels and Its Importance in the Setting of Malignancy. *The Journal of Experimental Medicine*, Vol.196, No.6 (September 2002), pp. 713-718, ISSN 1540-9538.

Dickinson, A.J.; Fox, S.B.; Persad, R.A. et al. (1994). Quantification of angiogenesis as an independent predictor of prognosis in invasive bladder carcinomas. *British Journal of Urology International*, Vol.74, No.6 (December 1994), pp. 762-766, ISSN 2042-2997.

Dreicer, R.; Li, H.; Stein, M. et al. (2009). Phase 2 trial of sorafenib in patients with advanced urothelial cancer: a trial of the Eastern Cooperative Oncology Group. *Cancer*, Vol.115, No.18 (September 2009), pp. 4090-4095, ISSN 1097-0142.

Durkan, G.C.; Nutt, J.E.; Rajjayabun, P.H. et al. (2001). Prognostic significance of matrix metalloproteinase-1 and tissue inhibitor of metalloproteinase-1 in voided urine samples from patients with transitional cell carcinoma of the bladder. *Clinical Cancer Research*, Vol.7, No.11 (November 2001), pp. 3450-3456, ISSN 1557-3265.

Egami, K.; Murohara, T.; Shimada, T. et al. (2003). Role of host angiotensin II type 1 receptor in tumor angiogenesis and growth. *The Journal of Clinical Investigation*, Vol.112, No.1 (July 2003), pp. 67-75, ISSN 0021-9738.

Fechner, G.; Classen, K.; Schmidt, D.; Hauser, S. & Müller, S.C. (2009). Rapamycin inhibits in vitro growth and release of angiogenetic factors in human bladder cancer. *Urology*, Vol.73, No.3 (March 2009), pp. 665-668 (discussion 668-669), ISSN 0090-4295.

Fernández, M.I.; Bolenz, C.; Trojan, L. et al. (2007). Prognostic Implications of Lymphangiogenesis in Muscle-Invasive Transitional Cell Carcinoma of the Bladder. *European Urology*, Vol.53, No.3 (March 2008), pp.571-578, ISSN 0302-2838.

Ferrara, N. (2004). Vascular endothelial growth factor: basic science and clinical progress. *Endocrine Reviews*, Vol.25, No.4 (August 2004), pp. 581-611, ISSN 1945-7189.

Ferrara, N. (2005). VEGF as a Therapeutic Target in Cancer. *Oncology*, Vol. 69, No.3 (November 2005), pp. 11-16, ISSN 1423-0232.

Ferrara, N.; Carver-Moore, K.; Chen, H. et al. (1996). Heterozygous embryonic lethality induced by targeted inactivation of the VEGF gene. *Nature*, Vol.380, No.6573 (April 1996), pp. 439-442, ISSN 0028-0836.

Flaig, T.W.; Su, L.J.; McCoach, C. et al. (2009). Dual epidermal growth factor receptor and vascular endothelial growth factor receptor inhibition with vandetanib sensitizes bladder cancer cells to cisplatin in a dose- and sequence-dependent manner. *British Journal of Urology International*, Vol.103, No.12 (June 2009), pp. 1729-1737, ISSN 2042-2997.

Folkman, J. (2003). Angiogenesis inhibitors: a new class of drugs. *Cancer Biology & Therapy*, Vol.2, No.4 Suppl 1 (July-August 2003), pp. S127-S133, ISSN 1555-8576.

Fong, G.H.; Zhang, L.; Bryce, D.M. & Peng, J. (1999). Increased hemangioblast commitment, not vascular disorganization, is the primary defect in flt-1 knock-out mice. *Development*, Vol.126, No.13 (July 1999), pp. 3015-3025, ISSN 1477-9129.

François, M.; Caprini, A.; Hosking, B. et al. (2008). Sox18 induces development of the lymphatic vasculature in mice. *Nature*, Vol.456, No.7222 (December 2008), pp. 643-647, ISSN 0028-0836.

Gallagher, D.J.; Milowsky, M.I.; Gerst, S.R. et al. (2010). Phase II study of sunitinib in patients with metastatic urothelial cancer. *Journal of Clinical Oncology*, Vol.28, No.8 (March 2010), pp. 1373-1379, ISSN 1527-7755.

Galsky, M.D. (2010). Integrating antiangiogenic therapy for advanced urothelial carcinoma: rationale for a phase II study of gemcitabine, cisplatin, and sunitinib. *Community Oncology*, Vol.7, No.11 (November 2010), pp. 500-504, ISSN 1548-5315.

Garcia, J.A. & Danielpour, D. (2008). Mammalian target of rapamycin inhibition as a therapeutic strategy in the management of urologic malignancies. *Molecular Cancer Therapeutics*, Vol.7, No.6 (June 2008), pp. 1347-1354, ISSN 1538-8514.

Gilbert, S.M. (2008). Separating surgical quality from causality-gaining perspective in the debate on lymph node count and extent of lymphadenectomy. *Cancer*, Vol.112, No. (June 2008), pp. 2331-2233, ISSN 1097-0142.

Goddard, J.C.; Sutton, C.D.; Furness, P.N.; O'Byrne, K.J. & Kockelbergh, R.C. (2003). Microvessel Density at Presentation Predicts Subsequent Muscle Invasion in Superficial Bladder Cancer. *Clinical Cancer Research*, Vol.9, No.7 (July 2003), pp. 2583-2586, ISSN 1557-3265.

Grossfeld, G.D.; Ginsberg, D.A.; Stein, J.P. et al. (1997). Thrombospondin-1 expression in bladder cancer: association with p53 alterations, tumor angiogenesis, and tumor progression. *Journal of the National Cancer Institute*, Vol.89, No.3 (February 1997), pp. 219-227, ISSN 1460-2105.

Hahn, N.M.; Stadler, W.M.; Zon, R.T. et al. (2011). Phase II trial of cisplatin, gemcitabine, and bevacizumab as first-line therapy for metastatic urothelial carcinoma: Hoosier Oncology Group GU 04-75. *Journal of Clinical Oncology*, Vol.29, No.12 (April 2011), pp. 1525-1530, ISSN 1527-7755.

Hansel, D.E.; Platt, E.; Orloff, M. et al. (2010). Mammalian target of rapamycin (mTOR) regulates cellular proliferation and tumor growth in urothelial carcinoma. *American Journal of Pathology*, Vol.176, No.6 (June 2010), pp. 3062-3072, ISSN 0002-9440.

Herr, H.; Lee, C.; Chang, S.; Lerner, S. & Bladder Cancer Collaborative Group (2004). Standardization of radical cystectomy and pelvic lymph node dissection for bladder cancer: a Collaborative Group report. *The Journal of Urology*, Vol.171, No.5 (May 2004), pp. 1823-1828, ISSN 0022-5347.

Herrmann, E.; Eltze, E.; Bierer, S. et al. (2007). VEGF-C, VEGF-D and Flt-4 in transitional bladder cancer: relationships to clinicopathological parameters and long-term survival. *Anticancer Research*, Vol.27, No.5A (September-October 2007), pp. 3127-3133, ISSN 1791-7530.

Hirakawa, S.; Kodama, S.; Kunstfeld, R. et al. (2005). VEGF-A induces tumor and sentinel lymph node lymphangiogenesis and promotes lymphatic metastasis. *The Journal of Experimental Medicine*, Vol.201, No.7 (April 2005), pp. 1089-1099, ISSN 1540-9538.

Holopainen, T.; Bry, M.; Alitalo, K. & Saaristo, A. (2011). Perspectives on lymphangiogenesis and angiogenesis in cancer. *Journal of Surgical Oncology*, Vol.103, No.6 (May 2011), pp. 484-488, ISSN 1096-9098.

Huber, S.; Bruns, C.J.; Schmid, G. et al. (2007). Inhibition of the mammalian target of rapamycin impedes lymphangiogenesis. *Kidney International*, Vol.71, No.8 (April 2007), pp. 771-777, ISSN 0085-2538.

Hurwitz, H.I.; Saltz, L.B.; Van Cutsem, E. et al. (2011). Venous thromboembolic events with chemotherapy plus bevacizumab: a pooled analysis of patients in randomized phase II and III studies. *Journal of Clinical Oncology*, Vol.29, No.13 (May 2011), pp. 1757-1764, ISSN 1527-7755.

Inoue, K.; Slaton, J.W.; Karashima, T. et al. (2000). The prognostic value of angiogenesis factor expression for predicting recurrence and metastasis of bladder cancer after neoadjuvant chemotherapy and radical cystectomy. *Clinical Cancer Research*, Vol.6, No.12 (December 2000), pp. 4866-4873, ISSN 1557-3265.

Iyer, G.; Milowsky, M.I. & Bajorin, D.F. (2010). Novel strategies for treating relapsed/ refractory urothelial carcinoma. *Expert Review of Anticancer Therapy*, Vol.10, No.12 (December 2010), pp. 1917-1932, ISSN 1473-7140.

Jaeger, T.M.; Weidner, N. & Chew, K. (1995). Tumor angiogenesis correlates with lymph node metastases in invasive bladder cancer. *The Journal of Urology*, Vol.154, No.1 (July 1995), pp. 69-71, ISSN 0022-5347.

Jain, R.K. & Carmeliet, P.F. (2001). Vessels of death or life. *Scientific American*, Vol. 285, No.6 (December 2001), pp. 38-45, ISSN 0036-8733.

Jain, R.K. & Fenton, B.T. (2002). Intratumoral lymphatic vessels: a case of mistaken identity or malfunction? *Journal of the National Cancer Institute*, Vol.94, No.6 (March 2002), pp. 417-421, ISSN 1460-2105.

Jeon, S.H.; Lee, S.J. & Chang, S.G. (2001). Clinical significance of urinary vascular endothelial growth factor in patients with superficial bladder tumors. *Oncology Reports*, Vol.8, No.6 (November-December 2001), pp. 1265-1267, ISSN 1791-2431.

Ji, R.C. (2009). Lymph node lymphangiogenesis: a new concept for modulating tumor metastasis and inflammatory process. *Histology and Histopathology*, Vol.24, No.3 (March 2009), pp. 377-384, ISSN 1699-5848.

Kaipainen, A.; Korhonen, J.; Mustonen, T. et al. (1995). Expression of the fms-like tyrosine kinase 4 gene becomes restricted to lymphatic endothelium during development. *Proceedings of the National Academy of Sciences USA*, Vol.92, No.8 (April 1995), pp. 3566-3570, ISSN 0027-8424.

Karkkainen, M.J.; Haiko, P.; Sainio, K. et al. (2004). Vascular endothelial growth factor C is required for sprouting of the first lymphatic vessels from embryonic veins. *Nature Immunology*, Vol.5, No.1 (January 2004), pp.74-80, ISSN 1529-2908.

Karl, A.; Carroll, P.R.; Gschwend, J.E. et al. (2009). The impact of lymphadenectomy and lymph node metastasis on the outcomes of radical cystectomy for bladder cancer. *European Urology*, Vol.55, No.4 (April 2009), pp. 826-35, ISSN 0302-2838.

Kaufman, D.; Raghavan, D.; Carducci, M. et al. (2000). Phase II trial of gemcitabine plus cisplatin in patients with metastatic urothelial cancer. *Journal of Clinical Oncology*, Vol.18, No.9 (May 2000), pp. 1921-1927, ISSN 1527-7755.

Kaufman, D.S.; Shipley, W.U. & Feldman, A.S. (2009). Bladder Cancer. *The Lancet*, Vol.374, No 9685, (July 2009), pp. 239-49, ISSN 0140-6736.

Kerbel, R.S. (2000). Tumor angiogenesis: past, present and the near future. *Carcinogenesis*, Vol.21, No.3 (March 2000), pp. 505-515, ISSN 1460-2180.

Kobayashi, S.; Kishimoto, T.; Kamata, S. et al. (2007). Rapamycin, a specific inhibitor of the mammalian target of rapamycin, suppresses lymphangiogenesis and lymphatic metastasis. *Cancer Science*, Vol.98, No.5 (May 2007), pp. 726-733, ISSN 1349-7006.

Lassau, N.; Koscielny, S.; Chami, L. et al. (2011). Advanced hepatocellular carcinoma: early evaluation of response to bevacizumab therapy at dynamic contrast-enhanced US with quantification - preliminary results. *Radiology*, Vol.258, No.1 (January 2011), pp. 291-300, ISSN 1527-1315.

aurence A.D. (2006). Location, movement and survival: the role of chemokines in haematopoiesis and malignancy. *British Journal of Haematology*, Vol. 132, No.3 (February 2006), pp. 255-267, ISSN 0007-1048.

eissner, J.; Koeppen, C. & Wolf, H.K. (2003). Prognostic significance of vascular and perineural invasion in urothelial bladder cancer treated with radical cystectomy. *The Journal of Urology*, Vol.169, No.3 (March 2003), pp. 955-960, ISSN 0022-5347.

i, Y.; Yang, X.; Su, L.J. & Flaig, T.W. (2011). Pazopanib synergizes with docetaxel in the treatment of bladder cancer cells. *Urology*, Vol.78, No.1 (July 2011), pp. 233.e7-233.e13, ISSN 0090-4295.

oges, S.; Mazzone, M.; Hohensinner, P. & Carmeliet, P. (2009). Silencing or fueling metastasis with VEGF inhibitors: antiangiogenesis revisited. *Cancer Cell*, Vol.15, No.3 (March 2009), pp. 167-70, ISSN 1535-6108.

ohela, M.; Bry, M.; Tammela, T. & Alitalo, K. (2009). VEGFs and receptors involved in angiogenesis versus lymphangiogenesis. *Current Opinion in Cell Biology*, Vol.21, No.2, (February 2009), pp. 154-165, ISSN 0955-0674.

otan, Y.; Gupta, A.; Shariat, S.F. et al. (2005). Lymphovascular invasion is independently associated with overall survival, cause-specific survival, and local and distant recurrence in patients with negative lymph nodes at radical cystectomy. *Journal of Clinical Oncology*, Vol.23, No.27 (September 2005), pp. 6533-6539, ISSN 1527-7755.

Ma, Y.; Hou, Y.; Liu, B. et al. (2010). Intratumoral lymphatics and lymphatic vessel invasion detected by D2-40 are essential for lymph node metastasis in bladder transitional cell carcinoma. *Anatomical Record (Hoboken)*, Vol.293, No.11 (November 2010), pp. 1847-1854, ISSN 1932-8494.

Mäkinen, T.; Jussila, L.; Veikkola, T. et al. (2001). Inhibition of lymphangiogenesis with resulting lymphedema in transgenic mice expressing soluble VEGF receptor-3. *Nature Medicine*, Vol.7, No.2 (February 2001), pp.199-205, ISSN 1078-8956.

Malmström, P.U. (2011). Bladder tumours: time for a paradigm shift? *British Journal of Urology International*, Vol.107, No.10 (May 2011), pp.1543-1545, ISSN 2042-2997.

Martens, J-H.; Kzhyshkowska, J.; Falkowski-Hansen, M. et al. (2006). Differential expression of a gene signature for sacavanger/lectin receptors by endothelial cells and macrophages in human lymph node sinuses, the primary sites of regional metastasis. *The Journal of Pathology*, Vol.208, No.4 (March 2006), pp. 574-589, ISSN 1096-9896

May, M.; Herrmann, E.; Bolenz, C. et al. (2011). Association Between the Number of Dissected Lymph Nodes During Pelvic Lymphadenectomy and Cancer-Specific Survival in Patients with Lymph Node-Negative Urothelial Carcinoma of the Bladder Undergoing Radical Cystectomy. *Annals of Surgical Oncology*, Vol.18, No.7 (July 2011), pp. 2018-2025, ISSN 1534-4681.

McCormack, F.X.; Inoue, Y.; Moss, J. et al. (2011). Efficacy and safety of sirolimus in lymphangioleiomyomatosis. *The New England Journal of Medicine*, Vol.364, No.17 (April 2011), pp. 1595-1606, ISSN 1533-4406.

Milowsky, M.I.; Carlson, L.; Shi, M.M. et al. (2011). A multicenter, open-label phase II trial of dovitinib (TKI258) in advanced urothelial carcinoma patients with either mutated or wild-type FGFR3. *Proceedings of the 2011 Genitourinary Cancers Symposium*, Abstract TPS186, Orlando, Florida, USA, February 17-19, 2011.

Milowsky, M.I.; Regazzi, A.M.; Garcia-Grossman, I.R. et al. (2011). Final results of a phase II study of everolimus (RAD001) in metastatic transitional cell carcinoma (TCC) of the urothelium. *Proceedings of the 2011 Genitourinary Cancers Symposium*, Abstract 4606, Orlando, Florida, USA, February 17-19, 2011.

Miyata, Y.; Kanda, S.; Ohba, K. et al. (2006). Lymphangiogenesis and Angiogenesis in Bladder Cancer: Prognostic implications and Regulation by Vascular Endothelial Growth Factors-A, -C and -D. *Clinical Cancer Research*, Vol.12, No.3Pt1 (February 2006), pp. 800-806, ISSN 1557-3265.

Muller, A.; Homey, B.; Soto, H. et al. (2001). Involvement of chemokine receptors in breast cancer metastasis. *Nature*, Vol.410, No.6824 (March 2001), pp. 50-56, ISSN 0028-0836.

O'Brien, T.; Cranston, D.; Fuggle, S.; Bicknell, R. & Harris, A.L. (1995). Different Angiogenic Pathways Characterize Superficial and Invasive Bladder Cancer. *Cancer Research*, Vol.55, No.3 (February 1995), pp. 510-513, ISSN 1538-7445.

Oliveira, P.A.; Arantes-Rodrigues, R.; Sousa-Diniz, C. et al. (2009). The effects of sirolimus on urothelial lesions chemically induced in ICR mice by BBN. *Anticancer Research*. Vol.29, No.8 (August 2009), pp. 3221-3226, ISSN 1791-7530.

Oliver, G. & Detmar, M. (2002). The rediscovery of the lymphatic system: old and new insights into the development and biological function of the lymphatic vasculature. *Genes & Development*, Vol.16, No.7 (April 2002), pp. 773-783, ISSN 1549-5477.

Padera, T.P.; Kadambi, A. & di Tomaso, E. (2002). Lymphatic metastasis in the absence of functional intratumor lymphatics. *Science*, Vol.296, No.5574 (June 2002), pp. 1883-1886, ISSN 1095-9203.

Papetti, M. & Herman, I.M. (2002). Mechanisms of normal and tumor-derived angiogenesis. *American Journal of Physiology – Cell Physiology*, Vol. 282, No.5 (May 2002), pp. 947-970, ISSN 1522-1563.

Parada, B.; Reis, F.; Figueiredo, A. et al. (2011). Inhibition of bladder tumour growth by sirolimus in an experimental carcinogenesis model. *British Journal of Urology International*, Vol.107, No.1 (January 2011), pp. 135-143, ISSN 2042-2997.

Patel, N.S.; Dobbie, M.S.; Rochester, M. et al. (2006). Up-regulation of endothelial delta-like 4 expression correlates with vessel maturation in bladder cancer. *Clinical Cancer Research*, Vol.12, No.16 (August 2006), pp. 4836-4844, ISSN 1557-3265.

Pinto, A.; Redondo, A.; Zamora, P.; Castelo, B. & Espinosa, E. (2010). Angiogenesis as a therapeutic target in urothelial carcinoma. *Anticancer Drugs*, Vol.21, No.10 (November 2010), pp. 890-896, ISSN 1473-5741.

Pinto-Leite, R.; Botelho, P.; Ribeiro, E.; Oliveira, P.A. & Santos, L. (2009). Effect of sirolimus on urinary bladder cancer T24 cell line. *Journal of Experimental & Clinical Cancer Research*, Vol.28, No.3 (January 2009), ISSN 1557-3265.

Pries, A.R.; Höpfner, M.; le Noble, F.; Dewhirst, M.W. & Secomb, T.W. (2010). The shunt problem: control of functional shunting in normal and tumour vasculature. *Nature Reviews Cancer*, Vol.10, No.8 (August 2010), pp. 587-593, ISSN 1474-175X.

Pugh, C.W. & Ratcliffe, P.J. (2003). Regulation of angiogenesis by hypoxia: role of the HIF system. *Nature Medicine*, Vol.9, No.6 (June 2003), pp. 677-684, ISSN 1078-8956.

Quek, M.L.; Stein, J.P.; Nichols, P.W. et al. (2005). Prognostic significance of lymphovascular invasion of bladder cancer treated with radical cistectomy. *The Journal of Urology*, Vol.174. No.1 (July 2005), pp. 103-106, ISSN 0022-5347.

Riess, H.; Pelzer, U.; Opitz, B. et al. (2010). A prospective, randomized trial of simultaneous pancreatic cancer treatment with enoxaparin and chemotherapy: Final results of the CONKO-004 trial. *Proceedings of the 2010 ASCO Annual Meeting*, Abstract No 4033, Chicago, Illinois, USA, June 4-8, 2010.

Risau W. (1997). Mechanisms of angiogenesis. *Nature*, Vol.386, No.6626 (April 1997), pp. 671-674, ISSN 0028-0836.

Rosner, M.; Hanneder, M.; Siegel, N. et al. (2008). The mTOR pathway and its role in human genetic diseases. *Mutation Research*, Vol.659, No.3 (September-October 2008), pp. 284-292, ISSN 1383-5742.

Saharinen, P.; Tammela, T.; Karkkainen, M. & Alitalo, K. (2004). Lymphatic vasculature: development, molecular regulation and role in tumor metastasis and inflammation. *TRENDS in Immunology*, Vol.25, No.7 (July 2004), pp. 387-395, ISSN 1471-4906.

Santos, L.; Costa, C.; Pereira, S. et al. (2003). Neovascularization is a prognostic factor for early recurrence in T1/G2 urothelial bladder tumours. *Annals of Oncology*. Vol.14, No.9 (September 2003), pp. 1419-1424, ISSN 1569-8041.

Sato, K.; Sasaki, R.; Ogura, Y. et al. (1998). Expression of vascular endothelial growth factor gene and its receptor (flt-1) gene in urinary bladder cancer. *The Tohoku Journal of Experimental Medicine*, Vol.185, No.3 (July 1998), pp. 173-184, ISSN 1349-3329.

Schedel, F.; Pries, R.; Thode, B. et al. (2011). mTOR inhibitors show promising in vitro activity in bladder cancer and head and neck squamous cell carcinoma. *Oncology Reports*, Vol.25, No.3 (March 2011), pp. 763-768, ISSN 1791-2431.

Schoppmann, S.F.; Birner, P.; Stockl, J. et al. (2002). Tumor-associated macrophages express lymphatic endothelial growth factors and are related to peritumoral lymphangiogenesis. *The American Journal of Pathology*, Vol.161, No.3 (September 2002), pp. 947-956, ISSN 0002-9440.

Seager, C.M.; Puzio-Kuter, A.M.; Patel, T. et al. (2009). Intravesical delivery of rapamycin suppresses tumorigenesis in a mouse model of progressive bladder cancer. *Cancer Prevention Research (Philadelphia, Pa.)*, Vol. 2, No.12 (December 2009), pp.1008-1014, ISSN 1940-6215.

Senger, D.R.; Galli, S.J.; Dvorak, A.M. et al. (1983). Tumor cells secrete a vascular permeability factor that promotes accumulation of ascites fluid. *Science*, Vol. 219, No. 4587 (February 1983), pp. 983-985, ISSN 1095-9203.

Shalaby, F.; Rossant, J.; Yamaguchi, T.P. et al. (1995). Failure of blood-island formation and vasculogenesis in Flk-1-deficient mice. *Nature*, Vol. 376, No. 6535 (July 1995), pp. 62-66, ISSN 0028-0836.

Shariat, S.F.; Svatek, R.S.; Tilki, D. et al. (2010). International validation of the prognostic value of lymphovascular invasion in patients treated with radical cystectomy. *British Journal of Urology International*, Vol.105, No.10 (May 2010), pp. 1402-1412, ISSN 2042-2997.

Shariat, S.F.; Youssef, R.F.; Gupta, A. et al. (2010). Association of angiogenesis related markers with bladder cancer outcomes and other molecular markers. *The Journal of Urology*, Vol.183, No.5 (May 2010), pp. 1744-1750, ISSN 0022-5347.

Shirotake, S.; Miyajima, A.; Kosaka, T. et al. (2011). Angiotensin II type 1 receptor expression and microvessel density in human bladder cancer. *Urology*, Vol.77, No.4 (April 2011), pp. 1009.e19-25, ISSN 0090-4295.

Si, Z.C. & Liu, J. (2008). What "helps" tumors evade vascular targeting treatment? *Chinese Medical Journal (English)*, Vol.121, No.9 (May 2008), pp.844-849, ISSN 0366-6999.

Smith, J.A. & Whitmore, W.F.Jr. (1981). Regional lymph node metastasis from bladder cancer. *The Journal of Urology*. Vol.126, No.5 (November 1981), pp. 591-593, ISSN 0022-5347.

Stacker, S.A. & Achen, M.G. (2008). From anti-angiogenesis to anti-lymphangiogenesis: emerging trends in cancer therapy. *Lymphatic Research and Biology*, Vol.6, No.3-4, pp. 165-172, ISSN 1557-8585.

Stein, J.P.; Cai, J.; Groshen, S. & Skinner, D.G. (2003). Risk factors for patients with pelvic lymph node metastasis following radical cystectomy with en bloc pelvic lymphadenectomy: concept of lymph node density. *The Journal of Urology*, Vol.170, No.1 (July 2003), pp. 35-41, ISSN 0022-5347.

Sternberg, C.N.; Donat, S.M.; Bellmunt, J. et al. (2007). Chemotherapy for bladder cancer: treatment guidelines for neoadjuvant chemotherapy, bladder preservation, adjuvant chemotherapy, and metastatic cancer. *Urology*, Vol.69, No.1 (January 2007), pp. 62-79, ISSN 0090-4295.

Suzuki, K.; Morita, T. & Tokue, A. (2005). Vascular endothelial growth factor-C (VEGF-C) expression predicts lymph node metastasis of transitional cell carcinoma of the bladder. *International Journal of Urology*, Vol.12, No.2 (February 2005), pp. 152-158, ISSN 1442-2042.

Swartz, M.A. (2001). The physiology of the lymphatic system. *Advanced Drug Delivery Reviews*, Vol.50, No1-2 (August 2001), pp. 3-20, ISSN 0169-409X.

Thiele, W. & Sleeman, J.P. (2006). Tumor-induced lymphangiogenesis: a target for cancer therapy? *Journal of Biotechnology*, Vol.124, No.1 (June 2006), pp. 224-241, ISSN 0168-1656.

Tickoo, S.K.; Milowsky, M.I.; Dhar, N. et al. (2011). Hypoxia-inducible factor and mammalian target of rapamycin pathway markers in urothelial carcinoma of the bladder: possible therapeutic implications. *British Journal of Urology International*, Vol.107, No.5 (March 2011), pp. 844-849, ISSN 2042-2997.

Tobler, N.E. & Detmar, M. (2006). Tumor and lymph node lymphangiogenesis – impact on cancer metastatis. *Journal of Leukocyte Biology*, Vol.80, No.4 (October 2006), pp. 691-696, ISSN 0741-5400.

Twardowski, P.; Stadler, W.M.; Frankel, P. et al. (2010). Phase II study of Aflibercept (VEGF-Trap) in patients with recurrent or metastatic urothelial cancer, a California Cancer Consortium Trial. *Urology*, Vol.76, No.4 (October 2010), pp.923-926, ISSN 0090-4295.

Van Trappen, P.O. & Pepper, M.S. (2002). Lymphatic dissemination of tumour cells and the formation of micrometastases. *Lancet Oncology*, Vol.3, No.1 (January 2002), pp. 44-52. ISSN 1470-2045.

Vasconcelos-Nóbrega, C.; Colaço, A.; Santos, L. et al. Experimental study of the anticancer effect of gemcitabine combined with sirolimus on chemically induced urothelial lesions. *Anticancer Research*, Vol.31, No.5 (May 2011), pp. 1637-1642, ISSN 1791-7530.

Videira, P.A.; Piteira, A.R.; Cabral, M.G. et al. (2011). Effects of bevacizumab on autocrine VEGF stimulation in bladder cancer cell lines. *Urologia Internationalis*, Vol.86, No.1 (February 2011), pp. 95-101, ISSN 1423-0399.

von der Maase, H.; Hansen, S.W.; Roberts, J.T. et al. (2000). Gemcitabine and cisplatin versus methotrexate, vinblastine, doxorubicin and cisplatin in advanced or metastatic bladder cancer: results of a large, randomized, multinational, multicenter, phase III study. *Journal of Clinical Oncology*, Vol.18, No.17 (September 2000), pp. 3068-3077, ISSN 1527-7755.

Walz. J.; Shariat, S.F.; Suardi, N. et al. (2008). Adjuvant chemotherapy for bladder cancer does not alter cancer-specific survival after cystectomy in a matched case control study. *British Journal of Urology International*, Vol.101, No.11 (June 2008), pp. 1356-1361, ISSN 2042-2997.

Wiesner, C.; Pfitzenmaier, J.; Faldum, A. et al. (2005). Lymph node metastases in non-muscle invasive bladder cancer are correlated with the number of transurethral ressections and tumor upstaging at radical cystectomy. *British Journal of Urology International*, Vol.95, No. 3 (February 2005), pp. 301-305, ISSN 2042-2997.

Wigle, J.T. & Oliver, G. (1999). Prox1 function is required for the development of the murine lymphatic system. *Cell*, Vol.98, No.6 (September 1999), pp. 769-778, ISSN 0092-8674.

Wigle, J.T.; Harvey, N.; Detmar, M. et al. (2002). An essential role for Prox1 in the induction of the lymphatic endothelial cell phenotype. *The EMBO Journal*, Vol.21, No.7 (April 2002),pp. 1505-1513, ISSN 1460-2075.

Wiig, H.; Keskin, D. & Kalluri, R. (2010). Interaction between the extracellular matrix and lymphatics: consequences for lymphangiogenesis and lymphatic function. *Matrix Biology*, Vol.29, No.8 (August 2010), pp. 645-656, ISSN 0945-053X.

Williams, S.P.; Karnezis, T.; Achen, M.G. & Stacker SA. (2010). Targeting lymphatic vessel functions through tyrosine kinases. *Journal of Angiogenesis Research*, Vol.2 (August 2010), pp. 1-13, ISSN 2045-824X.

Wilting, J.; Hawighorst, T.; Hecht, M.; Christ, B. & Papoutsi, M. (2005). Development of lymphatic vessels: tumour lymphangiogenesis and lymphatic invasion. *Current Medicinal Chemistry*, Vol.12, No.26, pp. 3043-3053, ISSN 0929-8673.

Wright, J.L.; Lin, D.W. & Porter, M.P. (2008). The association between extent of lymphadenectomy and survival among patients with lymph node metastases undergoing radical cystectomy. *Cancer*, Vol.112, No.11 (June 2008), pp. 2401-2408, ISSN 1097-0142.

Yang, C.C.; Chu, K.C. & Yeh, W.M. (2004). The expression of vascular endothelial growth factor in transitional cell carcinoma of urinary bladder is correlated with cancer progression. *Urologic Oncology*, Vol.22, No.1 (January-February 2004), pp. 1-6, ISSN 1078-1439.

Yang, H.; Kim, C.; Kim, M.J. et al. (2011). Soluble vascular endothelial growth factor receptor-3 suppresses lymphangiogenesis and lymphatic metastasis in bladder cancer. *Molecular Cancer*, Vol.10 (April 2011), pp.36, ISSN 1476-4598.

Yoon, C.Y.; Lee, J.S.; Kim, B.S. et al. (2011). Sunitinib malate synergistically potentiates anti-tumor effect of gemcitabine in human bladder cancer cells. *Korean Journal of Urology*, Vol.52, No.1 (January 2011), pp. 55-63, ISSN 2005-6745.

Youssef, R.F. & Lotan, Y. (2011). Predictors of outcome of non-muscle-invasive and muscle-invasive bladder cancer. *Scientific World Journal*, Vol.11 (February 2011), pp. 369-381, ISSN 1537-744X.

Zhou, M.; He, L.; Zu, X. et al. (2011). Lymphatic vessel density as a predictor of lymph node metastasis and its relationship with prognosis in urothelial carcinoma of the bladder. *British Journal of Urology International*, Vol.107, No.12 (June 2011), 1930-1935, ISSN 2042-2997.

Zu, X.; Tang, Z.; Li, Y. et al. (2006). Vascular endothelial growth factor-C expression in bladder transitional cell cancer and its relationship to lymph node metastasis. *British Journal of Urology International*, Vol.98, No.5 (November 2006), pp. 1090-1093, ISSN 2042-2997.

7

Epidemiology and Polymorphisms Related to Bladder Cancer in Ecuadorian Individuals

César Paz-y-Miño and María José Muñoz
Instituto de Investigaciones Biomédicas, Facultad de Ciencias de la Salud,
Universidad de las Américas
Quito
Ecuador

1. Introduction

Bladder cancer (BC) is the fourth most common cancer in men and the eighth most common in women being the responsible for annual deaths of 150,000 and is the seventh most prevalent type of cancer worldwide (Parkin, et al., 2005; Jemal, et al., 2009; Altayli, et al., 2009; Covolo, et al., 2008; Marmot, et al., 2007). In Ecuador the incidence rates of BC are 5.4% in males and 1.6% in females taking into account all cases of cancer diagnosed (Cueva & Yepez, 2009). In Argentina, it was reported as the fourth and the fourteenth most commonly diagnosed malignancy in men and women, respectively, with age-standardized incidence rate per 100,000 people around 15.1 (men) and 2.6 (women) in the period 1998 - 2002 (Pou, et al., 2011). The estimated downward trend in bladder cancer mortality over the last decades has been previously reported in countries of the European Union (Bosetti, et al., 2008) as well as South and North America (Bosetti, et al., 2005).

Susceptibility to BC is considered to depend on interaction between genetic factors and environmental chemical carcinogens. Bladder cancer involves a heterogeneous cell population, and numerous factors are likely to be involved in tumorigenesis (Hirao, et al., 2009). These factors result in uncontrolled growth of the cell population, decreased cell death, invasion and metastasis, and may influence the patient's prognosis. Identification of the aggressive features of the cancer in patients with BC is very important for adequate management of this disease (Ha, et al., 2011).

Many studies have investigated the effects of gene polymorphism on the risk of cancer in humans (Paz-y-Miño, at al., 2010; Wacholder, et al., 2004; Marchini, et al., 2004). Single nucleotide polymorphisms (SNPs) are the most common type of gene polymorphism. Several millions of SNP variants have been identified. The risk of cancer associated with this type of polymorphism probably is not high, and the proportion of malignant tumors associated with a distinct polymorphism depends on the frequency of occurrence of this variant in the human population (Zaridze, 2008). Genetic polymorphisms that alter the activity of enzymes of biotransformation pathways have been reported to be associated with cancer development and progression (Franekova, et al., 2008).

In the other hand, molecular epidemiology of cancer studies, molecular markers of distribution of malignant tumors in the populations and their effects on individual are important to understand the risk of developing a disease. For an epidemiological study is very important not only the source of the biological material, but also the individual information, that could be the factors influencing the risk of developing cancer. Among these can mention lifestyle factors as smoking, alcohol consumption, nutrition/diet, physical activity, environmental factors as occupation and exposure to carcinogens at workplace, familial and individual medical history, and many other variables (Zaridze, 2008). Many epidemiological studies have been conducted to investigate the putative association between polymorphic genes for biometabolism, environmental carcinogens, and the development of urinary tract cancer (Souto Grando, et al., 2009).

The association between cigarette smoking and cancer of the urinary tract has been extensively investigated in epidemilogy (Zeegers, et al., 2000). Cigarette smoking is the main bladder cancer risk factor for both men (60%) and women (25%) (Paz-y-Miño, et al., 2010); approximately half of male urinary tract cancers and one third of female urinary tract cancers may be attributable to cigarette smoking (Hecht, 2003). Over 60 carcinogens have been identified in cigarette smoke. Among these are polycyclic aromatic hydrocarbons (PAHs) such as benzo[a]pyrene and aromatic amines, such as 2-naphtylamine and 4-aminobiphenyl, the organic benzene derivatives found in cigarettes and the reactive oxygen species (ROS) such molecular oxygen, hydrogen peroxide, and hydroxyl radicals (Ichimura, et al., 2004) increase the risk of developing this neoplasm by 25% (Paz-y-Miño, et al., 2010; Hecht, 2003; Luch, 2005). Molecular markers can be detected in tissues and biological liquids and characterize individual exposure to carcinogens, biological effect of the exposure, genetic susceptibility to the development of disease, and final result of carcinogenesis, i.e. tumor (Zaridze, 2008).

Many studies have indicated the relationship between different genetic polymorphisms and bladder cancer among the may appoint enzymes that perform a detoxifying function deactivate compounds and anions that are dangerous for the cell (Paz-y-Miño, et al., 2010). Cells are protected against metabolic ROS by several enzymatic and non-enzymatic defense systems, including superoxide dismutase (SOD), glutathione peroxidase (GPX) and reduced glutathione (Heistad, 2003). Three isoforms of SOD are present: Cu,Zn-SOD (SOD1 gene, cytosolic protein), Mn-SOD (SOD2 gene, mitochondrial protein) and EC-SOD (SOD3 gene, extracellular SOD) (Faraci & Didion, 2004). Manganese superoxide dismutase (MnSOD) has been the subject of particular interest as it is located in mitochondria and can be induced by several cytokines and by superoxide anion; it also appears to be involved in other processes, including tumor suppression and cellular differentiation (Charniot, et al., 2011).

In regards to GPX1, this is a major intracellular enzyme that catalyzes the degradation of peroxides by oxidizing glutathione with the formation of its conjugates, thereby preventing cellular injury (Deng, et al., 2008; Trošt, et al., 2010). Mutation in gene GPX1, which locates at chromosome 3p21, is one of the major factors regulating GPX1 activity. And among these, a genetic polymorphism at codon 198, resulting in either a proline (Pro) or leucine (Leu) at the corresponding position of the encoded peptide, have drawn increasing attention in the etiology of several cancers (Raaschou-Nielsen, et al., 2007; Ezzikouri, et al., 2010). In humans, the selenium-dependent activation of GPX 198Leu mutant enzyme is lower than for the GPX 198Pro wild-type enzyme (Hu, et al., 2010). And associations between low level of GPX1 activity in the circulation and increased risk of cancer were found in several cancer types including breast cancer (Arsova-Sarafinovska, et al., 2009; Hansen, et al., 2009); it is presumed that GPX1 Pro198Leu (C[T) polymorphism affecting GPX1 activity may be important for cancer development (Hu, et al., 2010).

The glutathione S-transferases (GSTs) are conjugation enzymes, which detoxify reactive chemical species, for example polycyclic aromatic hydrocarbons. Moreover these enzymes belong to a group of dimeric isozymes with various catalytic activities, which predominantly conjugate with electrophiles of glutathione conjugation and exert other noncatalytic functions. This isozyme is expressed in many tissues, including urinary bladder, and frequently overexpressed in carcinomas. The respiratory, urinary, and digestive tract epithelia express high levels of GSTP1 activity (Altayli, et al., 2009; Kopps, et al., 2008; Fishbain, et al., 2004)

There are five subclasses of the GST enzymes in humans: alpha, pi, mu, theta and zeta (Strange, et al., 2001). GSTM1, GSTT1, and GSTP1 are phase II enzymes (Rodriguez-Antona & Ingelman-Sundberg, 2006).

Altered substrate affinity has been shown in a polymorphism at exon 5 of the GSTP1 gene. Some studies have reported higher susceptibility to cancer in individuals carrying the variant GSTP1 allele, although contradictory results have also been obtained (Srivastava, et., 2005; Hu, et al., 1997).

A prevalent genetic polymorphism of the GSTP1 gene was reported differing only in a single A to G transition at nucleotide position 1578 corresponding to codon 105, resulting in an amino acid change from isoleucine to valine (Zimniak, et al., 1994; Harries, et al., 1997). The polymorphic forms were designated GSTP1a (Ile105, wild type) and b (Val105, mutant). Homozygosity for GSTP1 (Ile105Val) was found to be associated with a considerably higher risk for bladder cancer in patients in the United Kingdom (Harries, et al., 1997). In contrast, another study on Chinese benzidine workers diagnosed with bladder cancer indicated that GSTP1 Ile/Val and Val/Val polymorphism was a factor in disease occurrence (Ma, et al., 2003).

Association between oxidative stress and DNA damage has been well known and many studies have focused on the association between DNA damage and the development of certain diseases (Paz-y-Miño, et al., 2010; Padma, et al., 2011). DNA repair enzymes continuously monitor chromosomes to correct damaged nucleotide residues generated by exposure to cytotoxic compounds or carcinogens (Wood, et al., 2001). Recently, it has been hypothesized in many studies that polymorphisms in DNA repair genes reduce their capacity to repair DNA damage and thereby lead to enhanced cancer or other age-related disease susceptibility (Liu, et al., 2007; Povey, et al., 2007).

To date more than 100 DNA repair genes have been identified and their polymorphisms have been reported to be related with some diseases. Among them, polymorphisms of xeroderma pigmentosum complementation group D (XPD) and X-ray complementing group I (XRCC1) have been studied extensively (Clarkson & Wood, 2005; Paz-y-Miño, et al., 2011).

The human XRCC1 (X-ray repair cross-complementing group 1) gene is involved in single strand breaks and base excision repair (BER), it is located on chromosome 19q13.2, encodes for a 633 amino acids protein that plays an important role in BER and single-strand breaks repair (SSBR), following exposure to endogenous ROS or alkylating agents (Padma, et al., 2011; Vidal, et al., 2003; Marsin, et al., 2003). The XRCC1 is a scaffold protein that interacts with other many components of BER as DNA polymerase β, APE1, hOGG1, poly-(ADP-ribose) polymerase and DNA ligase III in the NH_2-terminal, central, and COOH-terminal regions, respectively (Sterpone & Cozzi, 2010). In 1998 Shen et al., described three polymorphisms of XRCC1 gene, which resulted in non-conservative aminoacid changes at evolutionary conserved regions: C → T substitution in codon 194 of exon 6 (Arg to Trp);

G → A substitution in codon 280 of exon 9 (Arg to His) and G → A substitution in codon 399 of exon 10 (Arg to Gln). All these single nucleotide polymorphisms (SNPs) could alter the XRCC1 function and impair DNA repair efficiency or accuracy (Shen, et al., 1998). Given the large number of polymorphic variants and due to the existence of substantial differences in bladder cancer incidence in different ethnic groups, it is very important determine the frequencies of polymorphisms of many genes in Ecuadorian population affected with bladder cancer. These analyses are of great interest since it allows determining the genetic constitution of the population.

2. Materials and methods

2.1 Biological samples and data collection

A total of 97 formalin-fixed, paraffin-embedded (FFPE) bladder cancer samples were obtained from males and females individuals affected with bladder cancer. These samples were collected from the Department of Urology of Carlos Andrade Marín Hospital in Quito and the Department of Pathology of the Solón Espinoza Ayala Oncologic Hospital of Ecuador (SOLCA). One hundred twenty peripheral blood samples from male and female individuals with a medical history without malignancy served as control. In both cases, all the individuals signed informed consent after receiving information about the study. The study protocol and consent forms were approved by the University Institutional Bioethics Committee.

The distribution of selected characteristics between cases and control groups is summarized in Table 1. As for gender, the group of healthy individuals consisted of 33% of women and 67% of men, while de group of affected individuals consisted of 43% of women and 57% of men. In regard to histological subtype, transitional cell carcinoma accounted for 89%, of total cancer cases; 1% cases consisted of adenocarcinoma, 6% presented urothelial papillary carcinoma and 4% affected individuals presented squamous cell carcinoma.

Characteristic	Cases Number	Control Number	Odds Ratio
Gender			5.3, 95% CI 2.9-9.5, p<0.001
Women	42	37	
Men	55	83	
Age	71 (>68)	41 (>66)	0.6, 95% CI 0.334-1.020, p<0.05
	26 (<68)	76 (<66)	
Age ($X \pm$ SD)	68 ± 5.5	66 ± 4.5	
Smoking status			23.95, 95% CI 1.28-4.07. p<0.05
Smoker	72	67	
Non-smoker	25	53	
Histotype	Male	Female	
Transitional cell carcinoma	47 (55%)	39 (45%)	
Adenocarcinoma	1 (100%)	0 (0%)	
Urothelial papillary carcinoma	4 (67%)	2 (33%)	
Squamus cell carcinoma	3 (75%)	1 (25%)	

$X \pm$ SD medium $\pm$ standard deviation
CI confidence interval

Table 1. Clinical-Pathological characteristic of bladder cancer and control individuals

Concerning cigarette consumption as a risk factor to develop bladder cancer, 74% and 56% of affected individuals and healthy individuals respectively used to smoke, whereas 26% of affected and 44% of controls never smoked.

2.2 Genotyping

The DNA of affected individuals was obtained using the Purelink Genomic DNA extraction kit (Invitrogen, Carlsbad, CA), while, DNA from peripheral venous blood samples was isolated by a "salting out" method (Sambrook, et al., 1989), stored in the nucleic acid data bank of the Biomedical Research Institute at the Universidad de las Américas. The mean concentration of the DNA samples was 80ng/mL measured in a Qubit® Fluorometer (Invitrogen, Carlsbad, CA). We proceeded to study single nucleotide polymorphisms (SNPs) in the GSTP1 (Ile105Val), GPX-1 (Pro198Leu), MnSOD (Ile58Thr) and XRCC1 (Arg399Gln) genes. Genotyping was performed through the polymerase chain reaction–restriction fragment length polymorphism technique (PCR-RFLP).

For GPX-1, MnSOD, GSTP-1 and XRCC1 genes amplification, a PCR final volume of 50µl was prepared, containing 4µl of DNA template, 34µl H_2O Milli-Q, 0,4µM of forward and reverse primers, (Table 2) 1.5mM MgCl 2,5µl 10 × buffer (200 mM Tris-HCl pH 8.4, 500 mM KCl), 0,2µm each deoxynucleotide triphosphate (dNTPs), and 2.5 U Taq DNA polymerase (Invitrogen). For a 191-bp fragment amplification and the analysis of the Pro198Leu polymorphism found in chromosome 3, we used the initial denaturation step lasted 10 min at 95ºC, then 35 cycles of 30 s at 56ºC, 30 s at 56ºC, 45 s at 72ºC and 3 min at 72ºC were needed. Digestion of PCR product was carried out during 2h at 37ºC with the ApaI (Promega, Madison, USA) restriction enzyme. The PCR-RFLP test revealed homozygous individuals (Pro/Pro), (Leu/Leu) or heterozygous (Pro/Leu) (Paz-y-Miño, et al., 2010; Ichimura, et al., 2004). For the amplification of the 145-bp fragment of the Ile58Thr found in chromosome 6, for the PCR reaction, samples were placed in a thermo cycler MJ Research PTC 200® (MJ-Research Inc., Watertown, MA) for the amplification. The initial denaturation step lasted 10 min at 95ºC, followed by 35 cycles of 30 s at 95ºC, 30 s at 55ºC, 1 min at 72ºC, and 10 min at 72ºC. For the 177-bp fragment amplification and the analysis of the Ile105Val polymorphism found in chromosome 11, codon 105, exon 5, once the PCR reaction was obtained, the samples were placed in the MultiGene Thermal Cycler TC9600-G for amplification (Labnet, Edison, NJ, USA). The initial denaturation lasted 5 min at 95ºC, followed by 35 cycles of 45 s at 94ºC, 30 s at 62ºC, 30 s at 72ºC, and 1 min at 72ºC. Digestion of the amplified fragment was performed during 2 h at 37ºC with 5 U of the Alw26I

Genes	Primers
GPX-1	Forward, 5'-AAGGTGTTCCTCCCTCGTAGGT-3'
	Reverse, 5'-CTACGCAGGTACAGCCGCCGCT-3'
MnSOD	Forward, 5'-ACTTCAGTGCAGGCTGAACAGC-3'
	Reverse, 5'-CTGGTCCCATTATCTAATAGCTT-3'
GSTP-1	Forward, 5'-ACCCCAGGGCTCTATGGGAA-3'
	Reverse, 5'-TGAGGGCACAAGAAGCCCCT-3'
XRCC1	Forward, 5'-CCCCAAGTACAGCCAGGTC-3'
	Reverse, 5'-TGCCCCGCTCCTCTCAGTAG-3'

Table 2. Sequences of the PCR primers

(Promega, Madison, WI, USA) restriction enzyme. Electrophoresis analysis revealed homozygous individuals (Ile/Ile), (Val/Val) or heterozygous (Ile/Val) (Paz-y-Miño, et al., 2011); whereas for a 242-bp fragment amplification and the analysis of the Arg399Gln polymorphism found in chromosome 19, codon 399, exon 10, the initial denaturation step lasted 5 min at 95°C, then 35 cycles of 45 s at 94°C, 1 min at 59°C, 30 s at 72°C and 3 min at 72°C. Digestion of amplicon was performed during 2 hours at 37°C with the MspI (Promega) restriction enzyme. The analysis revealed homozygote individuals (Arg/Arg), (Gln/Gln) or heterozygote individuals (Arg/Gln) (Wong, et al., 2008).

All the polymorphisms were genotyped using a PCR-RFLP assay. After amplification, PCR products were cleaved by 5U of the corresponding enzyme. After digestion, the fragments were separated by electrophoresis on a 3.0% agarose gel and visualized using ethidium bromide in a transilluminator under ultraviolet light.

2.3 Statistical analysis

All information obtained from the studied individuals was kept in a database and statistical analyses were performed using PASW Statistics 17 for Windows (SPSS, Chicago, IL). The allelic and genotypic frequencies of each single nucleotide polymorphism were calculated from the information provided by the genotypes; and the Hardy-Weinberg equilibrium was determined by using software available on the Internet (http://www.genes.org.uk/software/hardy-weinberg.shtml). Chi-square (X) analysis was performed to determine significant differences between the presence of Ile105Val, Pro198Leu, and Arg399Gln polymorphisms of the studied population. The risk of developing disease in the presence of the studied polymorphisms between affected and control groups was determined using the odds ratio test (OR). Data were analyzed using a 2x2 contingency table.

Table 3 shows the Hardy-Weinberg equilibrium and the genotypic and allelic frequency of the studied polymorphisms. For the GPX1 and MnSOD genes, the genotypic frequencies

Gene	Group	Genotype	Individual (%)	Genotypic Frequency	Allele Frequency
GPX-1	Affected (n = 97)	Pro/Pro	28 (29%)	0.29	0.39
		Pro/Leu	19 (19%)	0.19	
		Leu/Leu	50 (52%)	0.52	061
	Control (n = 120)	Pro/Pro	73 (61%)	0.61	0.79
		Pro/Leu	42 (35%)	0.35	
		Leu/Leu	5 (4%)	0.04	0.21
MnSOD	Affected (n = 97)	Ile/Ile	43 (44%)	0.44	0.68
		Ile/Thr	47 (49%)	0.48	
		Thr/Thr	7 (7%)	0.07	0.32
	Control (n = 120)	Ile/Ile	75 (62%)	0.63	0.82
		Ile/Thr	45 (38%)	0.37	
		Thr/Thr	0 (0%)	0.0	0.18

Table 3. Genotype Distribution and Allele Frequency of the pro198leu and ile58thr

bserved in both groups were in Hardy–Weinberg equilibrium (GPX1 cases, X = 0.36, ><0.05; controls, X = 0, p<0.05 and MnSOD; cases, X = 0.02; p<0.05; controls, X = 0.05; ><0.05), confirming that the study samples were obtained from a population in equilibrium. Regarding the GSTP1 Ile105Val polymorphism, we observed that the frequency of the Val allele in control individuals was 0.28 (Table 4). Concerning to the XRCC1 Arg399Gln polymorphism, we observed that the frequency of the Gln allele in control individuals was 0.98) (Table 4). The frequencies of both alleles for the individuals affected with bladder ancer are not shown but according to information reported in other studies could be orrelated with the results obtained from the Ecuadorian population.

Genes	Genotype	Genotypic frequency Control		Allele frequency Control	
GSTP1 Ile105Val	Ile/Ile	0.54		0.72	
	Ile/Val	0.36			
	Val/val		0.10		0.28
XRCC1 Arg399Gln	Arg/Arg	0.01		0.02	
	Arg/Gln		0.01		
	Gln/Gln		0.98	0.98	

Table 4. Genotypic distribution and allelic frequency of GSTP1 Ile105Val and XRCC1 Arg399Gln polymorphisms

3. Conclusion

Bladder cancer is an important cause of death worldwide, there are many known risk factors or this cancer including age, male sex, smoking habit, and exposure to carcinogens (Pou, et al., 2011). The results obtained from the analysis of four genes using PCR-RFLP technique to determine the presence of the polymorphisms pro198leu in the GPX-1 gene, ile58thr in the MnSOD gene, Ile105Val in the GSTP1 gene and Arg399Gln in the XRCC1 gene in Ecuadorian individuals affected with bladder cancer, although small, support other evidence that genetic polymorphisms of the detoxification enzymes can modify bladder cancer risk.

GSTP1 participates in the detoxification of polycyclic aromatic hydrocarbon in promoting the conjugation of carcinogenic electrophiles with glutathione, thus enhancing excretion in the urine. This gene has been reported to possess two variant alleles. A single base substitution at position 313 of exon 5, guanine for adenine, results in the presence of valine (Val), where originally isoleucine (Ile) was present (Cao, et al., 2005). The prevalence rates of these isoforms are entirely dependent on which ethnic group is being considered (Shimada, 2006). Some have suggested that GSTP1 genes have an increased risk for tobacco-related cancers, including bladder cancer (Souto Grando, et al., 2009). Regarding genetics, the GSTP1 gene encodes proteins that are believed to function in xenobiotic metabolism and play the role as regulator of apoptosis (Moyer, et al., 2008). We found an association between the polymorphism and bladder cancer (data not shown), these findings could be suggesting that the presence of the Val/Val variant could be associated with an increased risk of acquiring detoxification problems, whereas the combination of the Ile/Val and

Val/Val alleles could be associated with the risk of presenting a GSTP1 gene dysfunction. Those individuals presenting the GSTP1 Val/Val and GPX-1 Leu/Leu variables may have a higher risk of acquiring problems in the detoxification (Paz-y-Miño, et al., 2011; Cao, et al., 2005).

Altayli, et al., had reported that smokers with GSTP1 Val105Leu heterozygous genotype had a reduced risk of bladder cancer. Some other authors reported a statistically significant association between the Leu/Leu and Val/Leu genotypes and bladder cancer risk. There are other authors that reported no association between the Ile105Val polymorphism of the GSTP1 gene and laryngeal squamous cell cancer, gastric cancer, and colorectal cancer (Unal, et al., 2004; Cao, et al., 2005).

The GSTP1 Ile105Val polymorphisms appear to be associated with a modest increase in the risk of bladder cancer. Some studies conducted in Asiatic population shows higher risk of developing bladder cancer when GSTP1 Ile/Val and Val/Val versus genotype Ile/Ile were compared, whereas the Chinese population did not have a significant influence on the unadjusted summary odds ratio for GSTP1 Ile/Val and Val/Val compared with GSTP1 Ile/Ile (Ma, et al., 2003). In conclusion, the GSTP1 polymorphisms Ile/Val and Val/Val compared with Ile/Ile seem to be associated with a modest increase in the risk of bladder cancer (data not published).

Our results indicate that the Ile105 allele was associated with an increased risk of bladder cancer. In previous articles, several types of carcinoma have been studied, in which there appeared to be an approximately threefold increase in risk between those with the GSTP1 (Val/Val) allele and those with GSTP1 (Ile/Ile) variant for bladder carcinoma (Harries, et al., 1997).

Successful repair of damaged DNA relies on the coordinated action of many repair enzyme systems. Age dependent decline or imbalance of the activities of the DNA repair enzymes will result in the compromise of the overall capacity of repair for the damaged DNA molecules. Common polymorphisms in DNA repair enzymes have been hypothesized to result in reduced capability to repair DNA damage. XRCC1 is a DNA repair gene that is emerging as an essential element in the repair of both damaged bases and SSBs (Padma, et al., 2011). Additionally, XRCC1 is important in BER, the major repair pathway for nonbulky damaged bases, abasic sites, and DNA single-stranded breaks after treatment with ionizing radiation. Some reports in human populations suggested the 399Gln variant of XRCC1 was associated with greater DNA and chromosomal damage (Yoon, et al., 2011).

It has been suggested that changes in the XRCC1 protein, mainly in amino acid 399, increase the susceptibility for tumor development via genomic instability (Meza-Espinoza, et al., 2009). Nevertheless, another study did not find any effect of the Arg399Gln polymorphisms with regard to DNA damage (Pastorelli et al., 2002), even though it is not well known whether these polymorphisms produce a functional change in the protein. In any case, the risk of cancer depends on the involvement of several factors, and not only on the presence or combination of certain common genetic polymorphisms (Naccarati et al., 2007).

Earlier investigators reported that reduced DNA repair capacity resulting from genetic polymorphism was associated with increased risk for various cancers (Mittal, et al., 2008). In our study the Arg allele was found mainly in the population affected with bladder cancer. In our study, the results obtained show that the XRCC1 Arg399Gln polymorphism, the frequency of the Gln allele was higher in affected individuals when compared to the control group (data not show). Among the polymorphisms of the XRCC1 gene the Arg399Gln amino acid change alters the phenotype of XRCC1 protein and thereby result in deficient DNA repair. According to our data in case of codon 399 our study exhibited no risk for bladder cancer which was in accord with the Northern Italian population (Shen, et al., 2003). Kelsey et al., 2004 indicated a 40% reduction in risk for bladder cancer among patients with homozygous variant XRCC1 399 (AA) compared with those with wild-type allele carriers. However, Stern et al., 2001 observed contrasting results by showing low risk for AA genotype in bladder cancer patients (OR = 0.7), but with not significant p value. One of the most interesting findings was the obtained by Mittal, et al., 2008 in which XRCC1 codon 399 where AA genotype exhibited 5.27 folds increased recurrence risk (HR=5.27, p=0.04).

On the one hand, GPX1 is suggested to play an important role in moderating H_2O_2 under pathological conditions (Ardanaz, et al., 2010). Over-expression of GPX-1 is associated with a wide range of effects, including the prevention of apoptosis, the protection against toxicity and the reduction of DNA damage (Zhuo, et al., 2009). Given human epidemiological data indicating significant associations between polymorphisms in GPx-1 and the risk of several cancer types due to the important biological activities of the essential trace element selenium are mediated through the function of selenoenzymes (Ichimura, et al., 2004; Hu & Diamond, 2003; Mak, et al., 2006; Choi, et al., 2007; Peters, et al., 2008). In this article we show the relationship between the presence of the Pro198Leu variant of the GPX-1 gene and its association with the risk of developing bladder cancer.

Among the ninety-seven patients analyzed for the GPX1 gene, 28.87% harbored the P/P homozygous genotype, 19,58% were P/L heterozygous and 51.55% were L/L homozygous. Of the 120 controls analyzed for the GPX-1 gene, 60.83% were P/P homozygous, 35% were P/L heterozygous and 4.17% were L/L homozygous (Table 3). For the MnSOD gene in the affected population, 44.33% were I/I homozygous, 48.45% I/T heterozygous, and 7.22% T/T homozygous. For controls 62.5% I/I homozygous, 39.17% I/T heterozygous and 0% T/T homozygous. The allelic frequency of the (I/I) allele was 0.68 for the group of affected individuals and 0.32 for control group (Table 3). The frequencies of the GPX-1 and MnSOD null genotypes were, respectively 39 and 82% in the patients and 79 and 18% in the control group.

When comparing control subjects and those affected with bladder cancer, we found that the presence of the Pro198Leu polymorphism has a relationship with the risk of developing bladder cancer (OR = 3.8; 95% CI 2.1-6.8; p<0.001), therefore the presence of the allelic variant (L/L) decreases the unique redox characteristics of the glutathione peroxidase, which can reduce reactive oxygen species and thereby prevent damage of important biomolecules, including DNA, RNA, lipids, proteins, and membranes; reactive oxygen species–induced DNA damage is known to promote tumor progression (Peters, et al., 2008), thereby conferring risk of developing bladder cancer in the Ecuadorian population. Previous studies demonstrate that the carriers of the variant L/L have a four times greater risk of developing bladder cancer than the individuals with the P/P variant (Ichimura, et al., 2004; Hu & Diamond, 2003).

Table 5 shows the respective OR values of the GPX1 and MnSOD genotypes. We found an increased risk of bladder cancer associated with the genotypes for the GPX1 (P/L or L/L) OR = 3.8; 95% CI=2.1-6.8; p<0.001), while the MnSOD was not statistically significant (OR = 2.1; 95% CI=1.3-3.5; p>0.05). Possible modification of associations between genetic polymorphisms and bladder cancer risk was also achieved by stratifying cases based on old age (OR = 5.3; 95% CI 2.9-9.5; p<0.001), sex (OR = 0.6; 95% CI 0.33-1.02; p<0.05), and smoking history (OR = 2.3; 95% CI 1.28-4.07; p<0.05).

Pro198Leu	Pro/Pro	Pro/Leu	Leu/Leu	Chi-Square	Odds Ratio
Affected	29%	19%	52%	69.9, $p>$ 0.001	3.8, 95% CI 2.1-6.8, $p<0.001$
Control	61%	35%	4%		
Ile58Thr	Ile/Ile	Ile/Thr	Thr/Thr	Chi-square	Odds Ratio
Affected	44%	49%	7%	0.25, $p > 0.05$	2.1, 85% CI 1.3-3.5, $p>0.05$
Control	62%	38%	0%		

Table 5. Statistical Analysis

Several studies in different populations worldwide have reported, and an association between these variants with the risk of developing different types of cancer (Raaschou-Nielsen, et al., 2007; Ezzikouri, et al., 2010; Hu, et al., 2010; Arsova-Sarafinovska, et al., 2009; Hansen, et al., 2009). The incidence of these polymorphisms according to the population analyzed, for example: the allelic frequency of L/L in the Japanese population is 0.05, and in the Caucasian population it is 0.36 (Ichimura, et al., 2004; Hu & Diamond, 2003). Furthermore, it has been determined that variants in different populations increases 2.6 times of developing bladder cancer and 1.43 times of developing breast cancer (Ratnasinghe, et al., 2000).

About the age of individuals under study, it has been determined that the risk of acquire bladder cancer is increased in old aged individuals (OR = 0.6; 95% CI 0.334-1.020; p<0.05), and can be considered as a risk factor for developing this disease. Furthermore, it was determined that men are at five times more risk to develop this type of cancer than women (OR = 5.3; 95% CI 2.9-9.5; p<0.001).

Current scientific evidence considers tobacco as a carcinogenic in human, with a causal relationship also to urinary bladder cancer (Lagiou, et al., 2005), being one of the most important risk factors, responsible for almost one-third of bladder cancer deaths (Parkin, 2008). It has been determined that individuals who used to smoke are at two times more risk to develop bladder cancer than individuals that never smoke (OR = 2.3; 95% CI 1.28-4.07; p<0.05). These findings are supported because it has previously been reported that smoking results in lower GPX activity (Ravn-Haren, et al., 2006).

As a result of the ethnic differences, the distribution of the polymorphisms is affected; some studies have found that the risk of developing bladder cancer when a significant incidence of the L/L allelic variant exists, with the proportion of homozygous individuals for the L/L allele being low for the Asian population and high for the Caucasian population (Ichimura, et al., 2004; Hu & Diamond, 2003). These findings have been corroborated for the Ecuadorian population, due to the L/L genotype being present in a high proportion of individuals diagnosed with bladder cancer (n = 51; 51%).

Free radicals, which are produced naturally in the body, can cause oxidative damage of DNA, lipids, proteins and other cell constituents, contributing to the onset of cancer and other chronic diseases (Evans, et al., 2004). Several enzymes, including MnSOD, GSTP, are involved in the scavenging of free radicals and prevention of oxidative damage. MnSOD catalyzes the dismutation of superoxide radicals in mitochondria by converting anion superoxide into hydrogen peroxide and oxygen, being a primary source of defense against cellular oxidants, regulating mitochondrial transport. It plays a key role in protecting cells from oxidative stress, especially in people with a low intake of natural antioxidants (Vineis, et al., 2007) because low levels of MnSOD gene activity may cause oxidative stress, leading to the development of cancer, diabetes, and neurodegenerative diseases like Parkinson´s and Alzheimer´s (Paz-y-Miño, et al., 2010). Although low expression of MnSOD has often been suggested for different types of cancer, it has been demonstrated that overexpression of this protein inhibited cancerous growth implying it as a tumor suppressor gene (Tamimi, et al., 2004). In addition, MnSOD may exert its effect as a tumor suppressor, by altering pathways involving in cellular apoptosis and proliferation (Canan, et al., 2011).

It has been reported that the frequency of the ile58thr variant of the MnSOD gene does not have a high significance (Hu & Diamond 2003). However there are other reports that have found an association between genetic polymorphisms in MnSOD and myeloid leukemia (Vineis, et al., 2007) indicating that oxidative stress can play a role in cancer. When we compare the values reported with the values obtained in the study we performed, we confirmed that the incidence of the T/T allele maintains a low level within the Ecuadorian population. We have shown statistically that there is no significant difference between the bladder cancer group and the control group (Paz-y-Miño, et al., 2010).

In the same way when we calculate the related risk of this two polymorphism (Pro/Leu and Ile/Thr), a negative relationship between the tendency to develop bladder cancer was found (OR = 2.1; 95% CI 1.2-3.6; p>0.05), concluding that the individuals who present the pro198leu variant have an increased risk of developing bladder cancer; contrary to what we found for ile58thr polymorphism and being different from that reported by other authors (Clemente, et al., 2007). It is well known that the ile58thr polymorphism of the MnSOD gene varies within different populations, with an incidence of 11% in Japanese populations and 30% in Chinese populations, compared to the Caucasian populations, which has a 62% of incidence (Hori, et al., 2000; Ambrosone, et al. 1999).

Some authors have reported that the expression level of the manganese superoxide dismutase enzyme, varies within tissues and shows an increment in individuals with brain, skin, lung tumors, breast, bladder cancer and myeloid leukemia (Vineis, et al., 2007; Ichimura, et al., 2004; Clemente, et al., 2007; Ambrosone, et al., 1999), for this reason the present study is important because it allows a characterization of the Ecuadorian population with bladder cancer. Various ethnic groups exhibit significant differences in the distribution of alleles throughout the population, which may influence the interpretation of epidemiological and association studies, these region-specific epidemiological studies provide important information on the frequency of polymorphic allelic variants in various ethnic groups (Souto Grando, et al., 2009).

The very different findings in other populations might be caused by some confounding factors such as ethnicity, selection of control groups and characterization of cases, sample sizes, and gene–gene and gene–environment interactions. In conclusion, these results shown an association with increased risk of bladder cancer in the population studied. In addition, the results suggest that the genotypes of the polymorphisms may be associated with increased risk of bladder cancer.

4. References

Ambrosone, CB., Freudenheim, JL., Thompson, PA., Bowman, E., Vena, JE., Marshal, JR., Graham, S., Laughlin, R., Nemoto, T., & Shields, PG. (1999). Manganeso superoxide dismutase (MnSOD) genetic polymorphisms, dietary antioxidants and risk of breast cancer. *Cancer Research*; Vol.59, No.3, pp.602–606, ISSN 1538-7445.

Ardanaz, N., Yang, X.-P., Cifuentes, ME., Haurani, MJ., Jackson, KW., Liao, T-W., Carretero, OA., & Pagano, PJ. (2010). Lack of Glutathione Peroxidase 1 Accelerates Cardiac-Specific Hypertrophy and Dysfunction in Angiotensin II *Hypertension*, Vol. 55, No.1 pp.116-123, ISSN 0194911X.

Arsova-Sarafinovska, Z., Matevska, N., Eken, A., Petrovski, D., Banev, S., Dzikova, S., Georgiev, V., Sikole, A., Erdem, O., Sayal, A., Aydin, A., & Dimovski, AJ. (2009). Glutathione peroxidase 1 (GPX1) genetic polymorphism, erythrocyte GPX activity, and prostate cancer risk. *International Urology and Nephrology*, Vol.41, No.1, pp.63–70, ISSN 1573-2584.

Altayli, E., Gunes, S., Yilmaz, AF., Goktas, S., & Bek, Y. (2009). CYP1A2, CYP2D6, GSTM1, GSTP1, and GSTT1 gene polymorphisms in patients with bladder cancer in a Turkish population. *International Urology and Nephrology*, Vol.41, No.2, pp.259–266, ISSN: 1573-2584.

Bosetti, C., Malvezzi, M., Chatenoud, L., Negri, E., Levi, F., & La Vecchia, C. (2005). Trends in cancer mortality in the Americas, 1970–2000. *Annals of Oncology*, Vol.16, No.3, pp. 489–511, ISSN 1569-8041.

Bosetti, C., Bertuccio, P., Levi, F., Lucchini, F., Negri, E., & La Vecchia, C. (2008). Cancer mortality in the European Union, 1970–2003, with a joinpoint analysis. *Annals of Oncology*, Vol.19, No. 4, pp. 631–640, ISSN 1569-8041.

Canan Kucukgergin, C., Sanli, O., Tefik, T., Aydın, M., Ozcan, F., & Seckin, Ş. (2011). Increased risk of advanced prostate cancer associated with MnSOD Ala-9-Val gene polymorphism. *Molecular Biology Reports* (on-line). ISSN 1573-4978.

Cao. W., Cai, L., Rao, JY., Pantuck, A., Lu, ML., Dalbagni, G., Reuter, V., Scher, H., Cordon-Cardo, C., Figlin, RA., Belldegrun, A., & Zhang, EF. (2005). Tobacco smoking, GSTP1 polymorphism, and bladder carcinoma. *Cancer*, Vol.104, No.11, pp.2400–2408, ISSN 1097-0142.

Charniot, JC., Sutton, A., Bonnefont-Rousselot, D., Cosson, C., Khani-Bittar, R., Giral, P., Charnaux, N., & Albertini, JP. (2011). Manganese superoxide dismutase dimorphism relationship with severity and prognosis in cardiogenic shock due to dilated cardiomyopathy. *Free Radical Research*; Vol.45, No.4, pp.379-388, ISSN 1029-2470.

Choi, JY., Neuhouser, ML., Barnett, M., Hudson, M., Kristal, AR., Thornquist, M., King, IB., Goodman, GE., & Ambrosone, GB. (2007). Polymorphisms in Oxidative Stress–Related Genes Are Not Associated with Prostate Cancer Risk in Heavy Smokers. *Cancer Epidemiology Biomarkers & Prevention*, Vol.16, No.6, pp.1115-1120, ISSN 1538-7755.

Clarkson, SG., & Wood, RD. (2005). Polymorphisms in the human XPD (ERCC2) gene, DNA repair capacity and cancer susceptibility: an appraisal. *DNA Repair* Vol.4, No.10, pp.1068-74, ISSN 1568-7864.

Clemente, C., Elba, S., Buongiorno, G., Guerra, V., D'Attoma, B., Orlando, A., & Russo, F. (2007). Manganese superoxide dismutase activity and incidence of hepatocellular carcinoma in patients with Child-Pugh class. A liver cirrhosis: A 7-year follow-up study. *Liver International*, Vol.277, No.6, pp.791-797, ISSN 1478-3223.

Covolo, L., Placidi, D., Gelatti, U., Carta, A., Scotto Di Carlo, A., Lodetti, P., Piccichè, A., Orizio, G., Campagna, M., Arici, C., & Porru, S. (2008). Bladder cancer, GSTs, NAT1, NAT2, SULT1A1, XRCC1, XRCC3, XPD genetic polymorphisms and coffee consumption: a case-control study. *European Journal of Epidemiology*, Vol.23, No.5, pp.355-362, ISSN 1573-7284.

Cueva, P., & Yépez, J. (2009). *Cancer Epidemiology in Quito 2003-2005*. Quito, AH, Editorial: National Cancer Registry (NCR), SOLCA. ISBN 9942-9958. Quito-Ecuador.

Deng, FY., Liu, YZ., Li, LM., Jiang, C., Wu, S., Chen, Y., Jiang, H., Yang, F., Xiong, JX., Xiao, P., Xiao, SM., Tan, LJ., Sun, X., Zhu, XZ., Liu, MY., Lei, SF., Chen, XD., Xie, JY., Xiao, GG., Lian, SP., & Deng, HW. (2008). Proteomic analysis of circulating monocytes in Chinese premenopausal females with extremely discordant bone mineral density. *Proteomics* Vol.8, No.20, pp. 4259-4272, ISSN, 1615-9861.

Evans, MD., Dizdaroglu, M., & Cooke, MS. (2004). Oxidative DNA damage and disease: induction, repair and significance. *Mutation Research*, Vol.567, No. 1, pp.1-61, ISSN 0027-5107.

Ezzikouri, S., El-Feydi, AE., Afifi, R., Benazzouz, M., Hassar, M., Pineau, P., & Benjelloun, S. (2010). Polymorphisms in antioxidant defence genes and susceptibility to hepatocellular carcinoma in a Moroccan population. *Free Radical Research;* Vol.44, No.2, pp.208-216, ISSN 1029-2470.

Faraci, FM., & Didion, SP. (2004). Vascular protection: superoxide dismutase isoforms in the vessel wall. *Arteriosclerosis, Thrombosis, and Vascular Biology*, Vol.24, No.8, pp.1367-1373 ISSN 10795642.

Franekova, M., Halasova, E., Bukovska, E., Luptak, J., & Dobrota, D. (2008). Gene polymorphisms in bladder cancer. *Urologic Oncology*, Vol.26, No.1, pp.1-8, ISSN, 1078-1439.

Fishbain, DA., Fishbain, D., Lewis, J., Cutler, RB., Cole, B., Rosomoff, HL., & Rosomofff, RS. (2004). Genetic testing for enzymes of drug metabolism: does it have clinical utility for pain medicine at the present time? *Pain Medicine*, Vol.5, No.1, pp.81-93, ISSN, 1526-4637.

Ha, Y-S., Yan, C., Jeong, P., Kim, W., Yun, S-J., Kim, I., Moon, S-K., & Kim, W-J. (2011). GSTM1 Tissue Genotype as a Recurrence Predictor in Nonmuscle Invasive Bladder Cancer. *Journal of Korean Medical Science*, Vol. 26, No.2, pp. 231-236, ISSN 1598-6357.

Hansen, RD., Krath, BN., Frederiksen, K., Tjønneland, A., Overvad, K., Roswall, N., Loft, S., Dragsted, LO., Vogel, U., & Raaschou-Nielsen, O. (2009). GPX1 Pro(198)Leu polymorphism, erythrocyte GPX activity, interaction with alcohol consumption and smoking, and risk of colorectal cancer. *Mutation Research*, Vol.664, No. 1-2, pp.13-19, ISSN 0027-5107.

Harries, LW., Stubbins, MJ., Forman, D., Howard, GC., & Wolf, CR. (1997). Identification of genetic polymorphisms at the glutathione S-transferase Pi locus and association with susceptibility to bladder, testicular and prostate cancer. *Carcinogenesis* Vol.18, No.4, pp.641-644, ISSN 1460-2180.

Hecht, EM. (2003). Tobacco carcinogens, their biomarkers and tobacco induced cancer. *Nature Reviews Cancer*, Vol.3, No.10, pp.733-744, ISSN 1474-175X.

Heistad, DD. (2003). Oxidative stress and vascular disease. *Arteriosclerosis, Thrombosis, and Vascular Biology*, Vol.26, No.4, pp.689 - 695, ISSN 10795642.

Hirao, Y., Kim, W., & Fujimoto, K. (2009). Environmental factors promoting bladder cancer. *Current Opinion in Urology*, Vol.19, No.5, pp. 494-499, ISSN 1473-6586.

Hori, H., Ohmori, O., Shinkai, T., Kojima, H., Okano, C., Suzuki, T., & Nakamura, J. (2000). Manganese superoxide dismutase gene polymorphism and achizophrenia: Relation to tardive dyskinesia. *Neuropsychopharmacology*, Vol.23, No.2, pp.170-177. ISSN 0893-133X.

Hu, X., Ji, X., Srivastava, SK., Xia, H., Awasthi, S., Nanduri, B., Awasthi, YC., Zimniak, P., & Singh, SV. (1997). Mechanism of differential catalytic efficiency of the two polymorphic forms of the human glutathione Stransferase P1-1 in the glutathione conjugation of carcinogenic diol epoxide of chrysene. *Archives of Biochemestry and Biophysics* Vol.345, No.1, pp.32–38, ISSN 0003-9861.

Hu, YJ., & Diamond, AM. (2003). Role of glutathione peroxidase 1 in breast cancer: Loss of heterozygosity and allelic differences in response to selenium. *Cancer Research* Vol.63, No.12, pp.3347–3351, ISSN 1538-7445.

Hu, J., Zhou, GH., Wang, N., & Wang, YJ. (2010). GPX1 Pro198Leu polymorphism and breast cancer risk: a meta-analysis. *Breast Cancer Research and Treatment*, Vol.124, No.2, pp. 425-431, ISSN 1573-7217.

Ichimura, Y., Habuchi, T., Tsuchiya, N., Wang, L., Oyama, C., Sato, K., Nishiyama, H., Owag, O., & Kato, T. (2004). Increased risk of bladder cancer associated with a glutathione peroxidase 1 codon 198 variant. *The Journal of Urology*, Vol. 172, No.2, pp.728-32, ISSN 0022-5347.

Jemal, A., Siegel, R., Ward, E., Hao, Y., Xu, J., & Thun, M. (2009). Cancer statistics, 2009. *CA A Cancer Journal for Clinicians*, Vol.59, No.4, pp. 225-249, ISSN 1542-4863.

Kelsey, KT., Park, S., Nelson, HH., & Karagas, MR. (2004). A population-based case-control study of the XRCC1 Arg399Gln polymorphism and susceptibility to bladder cancer. *Cancer Epidemiology Biomarkers & Prevention*, Vol.13, pp.1337-1341, ISSN 1538-7755

Kopps, S., Angeli-Greaves, M., Blaszkewicz, M., Prager, HM., Roemer, HC., Löhlein, D., Weistenhöfer, W., Bolt, HM., & Golga, K. (2008). *Glutathione S-Transferase P1 Ile105Val* Polymorphism in Occupationally Exposed Bladder Cancer Cases. *Journal of Toxicology and Environmental Health, Part A*, Vol.71, No.13-14, pp.898–901, ISSN 1087-2620.

Lagiou, P., Adami, HO., & Trichopoulos, D. (2005). Causality in cancer epidemiology. *European Jounal of Epidemiology*, Vol.20, No.7, pp.565–574, ISSN 1573-7284.

Liu, G., Zhou, W., Yeap, BY., Su, L., Wain, JC., Poneros, JM., Nishioka, NS., Lynch, TJ., & Christiani, DC. (2007). XRCC1 and XPD polymorphisms and esophageal adenocarcinoma risk. *Carcinogenesis*, Vol.28, No.6, pp.1254-8, ISSN 1460-2180.

Luch, A. (2005). Nature and nurture—lessons from chemical carcinogenesis. *Nature Reviews Cancer*, Vol.5, No.2, pp.113–125, ISSN 1474-175X.

Ma, Q., Lin, G., Qin, Y., Lu, D., Golka, K., Geller, F., Chen JG., & Shen JH. (2003). GSTP1 A1578G (Ile105Val) polymorphism in benzidine-exposed workers: An association with cytological grading of exfoliated urothelial cells. *Pharmacogenetics*, Vol.13, No.7, pp.409–415, ISSN 0960-314X.

Marchini, J., Cardon, L., Phillips, M., & Donnelly, P. (2004). The effects of human population structure on large genetic association studies *Nature Genetics*, Vol.36, No.5, pp.512-517, ISSN 1061-4036.

Mak, JC., Leung, HC., Ho, SP., Kow, FW., Cheung, AH., & Chang-Yeung, MM. (2006). Polymorphisms in manganese superoxide dismutase and catalase genes: Functional study in Hong Kong Chinese asthma patients. *Clinical and Experimental Allergy*, Vol.36, No.4, pp.440-447, ISSN 1365-2222.

Marsin, S., Vidal, AE., Sossou, M., Ménissier-de Murcia, J., Le Page, F., Boiteux, S., De Murcia, G., & Radicella, JP. (2003). Role of XRCC1 in the coordination and stimulation of oxidative DNA damage repair initiated by the DNA glycosylase hOGG1," *The Journal of Biological Chemistry;* Vol.278, No.45, pp.44068–44074, ISSN 1083-351X.

Marmot, M., Atinmo, T., Byers, T., Chen, J., & Hirohata, T. (2007). *Food, nutrition, physical activity, and the prevention of cancer: a global perspective,* World Cancer Research Fund / American Institute for Cancer Research, ISBN, 13-9780972252225, AICR, Washington DC.

Meza-Espinoza, JP., Peralta-Leal, V., Gutierrez-Angulo, M., Macias-Gomez, N., Ayala-Madrigal, ML., Barros-Nuñez, P., Duran-Gonzalez, J., Leal-Ugarte, E. (2009). *XRCC1* polymorphisms and haplotypes in Mexican patients with acute lymphoblastic leukemia. *Genetics and Molecular Research;* Vol.8, No.4, pp.1451-1458, ISSN 1676-5680.

Mittal, RD., Singh, R., Manchanda, PK., Ahirwar, D., Gangwar, R., Kesarwani, P., Mandhani, A. (2008). XRCC1 codon 399 mutant allele. A risk factor for recurrence of urothelial bladder carcinoma in patients on BCG immunotherapy. *Cancer Biology & Therapy,* Vol.7, No.5, pp.647-652. ISSN 1555-8576.

Moyer, A., Salavaggione, O., Wu, T., Moon, I., Eckloff, B., Hildebrandt, MA., Schaid, DJ., Wieben, ED., & Weinshilboum, RM. (2008). Glutathione S-transferase P1: gene sequence variation and functional genomic studies. *Cancer Research;* Vol.68, No.18, pp.4791-4801, ISSN 1538-7445.

Naccarati, A., Pardini, B., Hemminki, K. & Vodicka, P. (2007). Sporadic colorectal cancer and individual susceptibility: a review of the association studies investigating the role of DNA repair genetic polymorphisms. *Mutation Research* Vol.635, No.2–3, pp.118–145, ISSN 0027-5107.

Padma, G., Mamata, M., Ravi Kumar, K., & Padma, T. (2011). Polymorphisms in two DNA repair genes (*XPD* and *XRCC1*) – association with age related cataracts. *Molecular Vision;* Vol.12, No.17, pp.127-133, ISSN 1090-0535.

Pastorelli, R., Cerri, A., Mezzetti, M., Consonni, E., & Airoldi, L. (2002). Effect of DNA repair gene polymorphisms on BPDE-DNA adducts in human lymphocytes. *International Journal of Cancer.* Vol.100, No.1, pp.9-1, 1097-0215.

Parkin, DM. (2008). The global burden of urinary bladder cancer. *Scandinavian Journal of Urology and Nephrology. Supplementum.* Vol.218, pp.12–20, ISSN 03008886.

Parkin, D., Bray, F., Ferlay, J., & Pisani, P. (2005). Global cancer statistics, 2002. *CA A Cancer Journal for Clinicians,* Vol.55, No.2, pp. 74-108, ISSN 1542-4863.

Paz-y-Miño, C., Muñoz, MJ., López-Cortés, A., Cabrera, A., Palacios, A., Castro, B., Paz-y-Miño, N., & Sánchez, ME. (2010). Frequency of Polymorphisms pro198leu in *GPX-1* Gene and ile58thr in *MnSOD* Gene in the Altitude Ecuadorian Population With Bladder Cancer. *Oncology Research,* Vol.18, No.8, pp.395–400, ISSN 0965-0407.

Paz-y-Miño, C., Muñoz, MJ., Maldonado, A., Valladares, C., Cumbal, N., Herrera, C., Robles, P., Sánchez, ME., & López-Cortés, A. (2011). Baseline determination in social, health, and genetic areas in communities affected by glyphosate aerial spraying on the northeastern Ecuadorian border. *Reviews on Environmental Health,* Vol.26, No.1, pp.45-51, ISSN 2191-0308.

Peters, U., Chatterjee, N., Hayes, RB., Schoen, RE., Wang, Y., Chanock, SJ., & Foster, CB. (2008). Variation in the Selenoenzyme Genes and Risk of Advanced Distal Colorectal Adenoma. *Cancer Epidemiology Biomarkers & Prevention*, Vol.17, No.5, pp.1144-1154, ISSN 1538-7755.

Pou, S., Osella, A., & Diaz, M. (2011). Bladder cancer mortality trends and patterns in Córdoba, Argentina (1986–2006). *Cancer Causes Control*; Vol.22, No.3, pp. 407–415, ISSN 1573-7225

Povey, JE., Darakhshan, F., Robertson, K., Bisset, Y., Mekky, M., Rees, J., Doherty, V., Kavanagh, G., Anderson, N., Campbell, H., Mackie, RM., & Melton, DW. (2007). DNA repair gene polymorphisms and genetic predisposition to cutaneous melanoma. *Carcinogenesis*, Vol.28, No.5, pp.1087-93, ISSN 1460-2180.

Raaschou-Nielsen, O., Sørensen, M., Hansen, RD., Frederiksen, K., Tjønneland, A., Overvad, K., & Vogel, U. (2007). GPX1 Pro198Leu polymorphism, interactions with smoking and alcohol consumption, and risk for lung cancer. *Cancer Letters*, Vol.247, No.2, pp. 293–300, ISSN 0304-3835.

Ratnasinghe, D., Tangrea, JA., Andersen, MR.,Barrett, MJ., Virtamo, J., Taylor, PR., & Albanes, D. (2000). Glutathione peroxidase codon 198 polymorphism variant increases lung cancer risk. *Cancer Research* Vol.60, No.22, pp.6381–6383, ISSN 1538-7445.

Ravn-Haren, G., Olsen, A., Tjønneland, A., Dragsted, LO., Nexø, BA., Wallin, H., Overvad, K., Raaschou-Nielsen, O., & Vogel, U. (2006). Associations between GPX1 Pro198Leu polymorphism, erythrocyte GPX activity, alcohol consumption and breast cancer risk in a prospective cohort study. *Carcinogenesis*, Vol.27, No.4, pp.820 – 825, ISSN 0143-3334.

Rodriguez-Antona, C., & Ingelman-Sundberg, M. (2006). Cytochrome P450 pharmacogenetics and cancer. *Oncogene*, Vol.25, No.11, pp.1679–1691, ISSN, 0950-9232.

Sambrook, J., Fritsch, E.F., & Maniatis, T. (1989). *Molecular Cloning: A Laboratory Manual*. Cold Spring Harbor Laboratory Press, ISBN, 0-87969-577-3, New York, USA.

Shen, M., Hung, RJ., Brennan, P., Malaveille, C., Donato, F., Placidi, D., Carta, A., Hautefeuille, A., Boffetta, P., & Porru, S. (2003). Polymorphisms of the DNA Repair Genes XRCC1, XRCC3, XPD, Interaction with Environmental Exposures, and Bladder Cancer Risk in a Case-Control Study in Northern Italy. *Cancer Epidemiology Biomarkers & Prevention*, Vol.12, pp.1234-1240, ISSN 1538-7755

Shen, MR., Jones IM., & Mohrenweiser, H. (1998). Nonconservative amino acid substitution variants exist at polymorphic frequency in DNA repair genes in healthy humans," *Cancer Research*; Vol.58, No.4, pp.604–608, ISSN 1538-7445.

Shimada, T. (2006). Xenobiotic-metabolizing enzymes involved in activation and detoxification of carcinogenic polycyclic aromatic hydrocarbons. *Drug Metabolism and Pharmacokinetics*. Vol.21, No.4, pp.257-276, ISSN 1880-0920.

Souto Grando, J., Kuasne, H., Losi-Guembarovski, R., Rodrigues, I., Mitsu-Matsuda, H., Fuganti, PE., Pereira, E., Libos, F., Paes de Menezez, R., de Freitas, MA., & de Syllos, IM. (2009). Association between polymorphisms in the biometabolism genes CYP1A1, GSTM1, GSTT1 and GSTP1 in bladder cancer. *Clinical and Experimental Medicine*, Vol.9, No.1, pp.21–28, ISSN 1591-9528.

Srivastava, DSL., Mishra, DK., Mandhani, A., Mittal, B., Kumar, A., & Mittal, RD. (2005). Association of genetic polymorphism of glutathione S-transferase M1, T1, P1 and susceptibility to bladder cancer. *European Urology*, Vol.48, No2, pp.339–344, ISSN 1569-9056.

Stern. MC., Umbach, DM., van Gils, CH., Lunn, RM., & Taylor, JA. (2001). DNA Repair Gene *XRCC1* Polymorphisms, Smoking, and Bladder Cancer Risk. *Cancer Epidemiology Biomarkers & Prevention*, Vol.10, pp.125-131, ISSN 1538-7755.

Sterpone, S., & Cozzi, R. (2010). Influence of XRCC1 Genetic Polymorphisms on Ionizing Radiation-Induced DNA Damage and Repair. *Journal of Nucleic Acids*, pp.1-6 ISSN 2090-0201.

Strange, RC., Spiteri, MA., Ramachandran, S., & Fryer, AA. (2001). Glutathione-S-transferase family of enzymes. *Mutation Research* Vol.482, No.1–2, pp.21–26, ISSN 0027-5107.

Tamimi, RM., Hankinson, SE., Spiegelman, D., Colditz, GA., & Hunter, DJ. (2004). Manganese superoxide dismutase polymorphism, plasma antioxidants, cigarette smoking, and risk of breast cancer. *Cancer Epidemiology, Biomarkers & Prevention*, Vol.13, No.6, pp.989-996. ISSN 1538-7755.

Trošt, Z., Trebše, R., Preželj, J., Komadina, R., Bitenc-Logar, D., & Marc, J. (2010). A microarray based identification of osteoporosis related genes in primary culture of human osteoblasts, *Bone*, Vol. 46, No.1, pp.72–80, ISSN 8756-3282.

Unal, M., Tamer, L., Ateş, NA., Akbas, Y., Pata, YS., Vayisoğlu, Y., Ercan, B., Görür, K., & Atik, U. (2004). Glutathione S-transferase M1, T1, and P1 gene polymorphism in laryngeal squamous cell carcinoma. *American Journal of Otolaryngology*, Vol.25, No.5, pp.317–322 ISSN 1532-818X

Vidal, AE., Boiteux, S., Hickson, ID., & Radicella, JP. (2003). XRCC1 coordinates the initial and late stages of DNA abasic site repair through protein-protein interactions," *The EMBO Journal*, Vol.20, No.22, pp. 6530–6539, ISSN 0261-4189.

Vineis, P., Veglia, F., Garte, S., Malaveille, C., Matullo, G., Dunning, A., Peluso, M., Airoldi, L., Overvad, K., Raaschou-Nielsen, O., Clavel-Chapelon, F., Linseisen, JP., Kaaks, R., Boeing, H., Trichopoulou, A., Palli, D., Crosignani, P., Tumino, R., Panico, S., Bueno-De-Mesquita, HB., Peeters, PH., Lund, E., Gonzalez, CA., Martinez, C., Dorronsoro, M., Barricarte, A., Navarro, C., Quiros, JR., Berglund, G., Jarvholm, B., Day, NE., Key, TJ., Saracci, R., Riboli, E., & Autrup, H. (2007). Genetic susceptibility according to three metabolic pathways in cancers of the lung and bladder and in myeloid leukemias in nonsmokers. *Annals of Oncology*, Vo.18, pp. 1230–1242. ISSN 1569-8041.

Wacholder, S., Chanock, S., Garcia_Closas, M., El Ghormli, L., & Rottiman, N. (2004). Assessing the Probability That a Positive Report is False: An Approach for Molecular Epidemiology Studies *Journal of the National Cancer Institute*, Vol.96, No.6, pp.434-442, ISSN 1460-2105.

Wong, RH., Chang, SY., Ho, SW., Huang, PL., Liu, YJ., Chen, YC., Yeh, YH., & Lee, HS. (2008). Polymorphisms in metabolic GSTP1 and DNA – repair XRCC1 genes with an increased risk of DNA damage in pesticide exposed fruit growers. *Mutation Research*, Vol.654, No. 2, pp.168 – 75, ISSN 1383-5718.

Wood, RD., Mitchell, M., Sgouros, J., & Lindahl, T. (2001). Human DNA repair genes. *Science*, Vol.291, No.5507, pp.1284-1289, ISSN 1095-9203.

Yoon, HH., Catalano, PJ., Murphy, KM., Skaar, TC., Philips, S., Powell, M., Montgomery, EA., Hafez, MJ., Offer, SM., Liu, G., Meltzer SJ., Wu, X., Forastiere, AA., Benson, AB., Kleinberg, LR., & Gibson, MK. (2011). Genetic variation in DNA-repair pathways and response to radiochemotherapy in esophageal adenocarcinoma: a retrospective cohort study of the Eastern Cooperative Oncology Group. *Bio Med Central Cancer*, Vol.17, No.11, pp.176. ISSN 1471-2407.

Zaridze, D. (2008). Molecular Epidemiology of Cancer. *Biochemistry (Moscow)*, Vol. 73, No.5, pp. 532-542, ISSN 0006-2979.

Zeegers, MPA., Tan, FES., Dorant, E., & Van den Brandt, P. (2000). The impact of characteristics of cigarette smoking on urinary tract cancer risk. A meta-analysis of epidemiologic studies. *Cancer*, Vol.89, No.3, pp.630–639, ISSN 1097-0142.

Zimniak, P., Nanduri, B., Pikula, S., Bandorowicz-Pikula, J., Singhal, SS., Srivastava, SK., Awasthi, S., & Awasthi, YC. (1994). Naturally occurring human glutathione S-transferase GSTP1-1 isoforms with isoleucine and valine in position 104 differ in enzymic properties. *European Journal of Biochemistry*, Vol.224, No.3, pp.893–899, ISSN 1742-4658.

Part 3

Clinical Presentation and Diagnosis

8

Clinical Presentation

Samer Katmawi-Sabbagh
Kettering General Hospital NHS Trust
United Kingdom

1. Introduction

Bladder cancer can occur at any age. However, it is known to be a disease of the middle-aged or elderly patient. The incidence is variable in different countries and the risk factors includes male sex, increasing age, smoking, occupational exposure to carcinogens, chronic inflammation, drugs such as phenacitin and cyclophosphamide, and pelvic radiation. In this chapter, we will discuss the different symptoms and signs that the bladder cancer patient could present with, keeping in mind that non of these presenting features are unique for bladder cancer.

2. Haematuria

Haematuria is the presenting symptom in up to 80% of patients with bladder cancer(Cummings et al., 1992). It could be Visible (previously called gross or frank haematuria), or Non Visible (previously called Dipstick or Microscopic haematuria). It is usually intermittent rather than constant, therefore, if a second urine specimen is free of any haematuria after a previous positive sample, investigations are still warranted in a bladder cancer age range patient. It may be initial or terminal if the lesion is at the bladder neck or in the prostatic urethra. The history of smoking or occupational exposure to certain chemicals is relevant. The Renal Association and British Association of Urological Surgeons joint consensus statement uses the abbreviations VH and NVH to refer to visible and non visible haematuria respectively (Kelly et al., 2009). They also define significant haematuria as the one that is visible (VH), Symptomatic non visible (sNVH)ie: associated with lower urinary tract symptoms, and persistent asymptomatic (aNVH)ie: without association with any urinary tract symptoms. Persistence was defined as 2 out of 3 positive urine samples. Microscopic or non visible haematuria (NVH) is defined as more than 3 Red blood cells (RBCs) per high-powered field(HPF) on a spun specimen by the American Urological Association. However, Campbell-Walsh definition is more than 5 RBCs per HPF for spun urine and more than 2 RBCs per HPF for unspun urine. The degree of haematuria does not correlate with the stage or the grade of the bladder cancer but cancer pick up rate is different. Cancer diagnosis is about 20-25% for the VH and 5-10% for the NVH (Khadra et al.,2000; Edwards et al.,2006). Majority of cancers discovered when investigating haematuria are bladder ones and the rarity relate to the upper urinary tract. Haematuria is an alarming presentation especially when asymptomatic. It requires extensive examination and investigations to rule out underlying pathologies and in particular bladder or upper urinary tract cancers. The role of purposely designed one-stop haematuria clinic has been developed

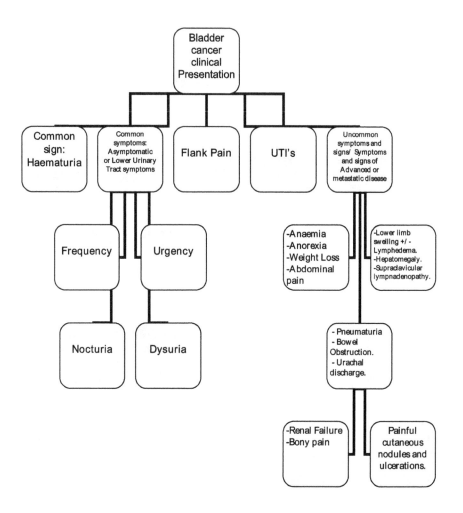

Fig. 1. Diagram showing the common and uncommon presenting symptoms and signs of bladder cancer.

and some evidence is existent that it could well reduce the time to cancer diagnosis and treatment (Katmawi-Sabbagh et al., 2010). Patients will require full history and examination including detailed information abouthaematuria, its duration and any associated symptoms. Smoking, occupation and exposure to chemicals and drugs should be documented. Abdominal, genital, and rectal examinations will be required in men. Vaginal examination is also important as vaginal bleeding is sometimes mistaken as haematuria in women. Details of required investigations will be discussed at different chapter of this book. Common causes of haematuria are listed below in Table 1:

	Infective	Neoplasic	Others
Kidney	-Pylonephritis -Tuberculosis(TB)	-Renal cell carcinoma -Transitional cell carcinoma (TCC). - Squamous cell carcinoma (SCC).	-Trauma -Stones. -Nephrological: IgA nephropathy, diabetes, Alport's syndrome, interstitial nephritis, papillary necrosis.
Ureter	-Ureteritis -Tuberculosis	-TCC -Adenocarcinoma. -SCC	-Trauma. -Stones.
Bladder	-Bacterial cystitis. -TB cystitis. -Schistosomiasis	-TCC -Adenocarcinoma -SCC	-Trauma -Stones -Foreign bodies.
Prostate	-Bacterial prostatitis -Granulomatous prostatitis.	-Prostate cancer. -Benign prostatic hypertrophy.	-Trauma - Iatrogenic: Post biopsy.
Urethra and penis	-Urethritis.	-SCC. -TCC.	-Trauma. -Stricture. -Iatrogenic: catheterization.

Table 1. Common causes of Haematuria based on the anatomical location and the causative factors.

3. Lower urinary tract symptoms

Frequency, nocturia, urgency, and urge incontinence are symptoms of vesical irritability. These could be seen in association with haematuria in bladder cancer patients (with or without the presence of dysuria or suprapubic pain). These symptoms were previously named as irritative symptoms and they have association with diffuse carcinoma in situ (CIS) as well as invasive cancer (Farrow et al., 1977).

4. Flank pain

Flank pain can be a symptom of advanced bladder cancer representing ureteric obstruction due to invasion of bladder muscular wall or the ureter. Tumours cause hydronephrosis as they become invasive (Figure 2). This is usually seen with high grade TCC rather than low grade (Table 2).
Alternatively hydronephrosis with or without pain could happen when there is involvement of the ureteric orifice (Leibovitch et al., 1993).

1973 World Health Organisation (WHO) grading
Grade 1: Well differentiated Grade 2: Moderately differentiated Grade 3: Poorly differentiated
2004 WHO grading – Flat lesions:
Hyperplasia (flat lesion without atypia or papillary) Reactive Atypia (flat lesion with atypia) Atypia of unknown significance Urothelial dysplasia Urothelial Carcinoma in situ (CIS)
2004 WHO grading – Papillary lesions:
Urothelial Papilloma (wich is a completely benign lesion) Papillary urothelial neoplasm of low malignant potential Low-grade papillary urothelial carcinoma High-grade papillary urothelial carcinoma

Table 2. WHO grading in 1973 and in 2004 (Sauter el al.,2004)

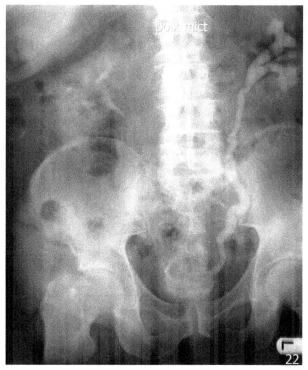

Fig. 2. An Intravenous urography (I.V.U) of a 76 year old man presented with haematuria and left sided loin pain. It shows left sided hydroureteronephrosis and large filling defect in the bladder. Cystoscopy confirmed a bladder tumour and histology revealed invasive G3 pT2 transitional cell carcinoma of the bladder.

'yelonephritis may result if obstruction is complicated with infection. Flank pain and hydronephrosis could also be seen in cases of retroperitoneal metastasis. Flank pain caused by a bladder tumour is rarely encountered as the obstruction arises gradually. It should be distinguished from the one caused by a urinary stone which could also be associated with a degree of haematuria, but the colicky pain caused by a stone is normally of sudden onset and of higher intensity than that caused by a gradually occurring obstruction. Another differential diagnosis is the flank pain caused by a clot colic related to a bleeding from upper urinary tract transitional cell carcinoma or renal cell carcinoma.

5. Recurrent urinary tract infections (UTI's)

Recurrent urinary tract infections (UTI's) can be the first presentation of patients with necrotic infected bladder tumours. Therefore, it is always recommended to investigate recurrent UTI's with cystoscopic examination to rule out associated bladder tumour. It is also believed that bladder stones, long term catheters, and ova of Schistosoma haematobium (bilharziasis) are all implicated in the development of squamous cell carcinoma of the bladder via the mechanism of chronic inflammation of bladder mucosa.

6. Rare presentation symptoms and signs / symptoms and signs of advanced or complicated disease

The natural history of bladder cancer can be classified as follows:
- No further recurrence following initial presentation, diagnosis and treatment.
- Local recurrence, which can occur on a single occasion or on multiple occasions. The recurrent tumours are usually of the same stage and grade as the primary tumour. Clinically patient may be asymptomatic or represent with haematuria or any other local symptoms.
- Local Progresssion, which represent an increase in the local staging with time, the appearance of distant metastases and subsequent death. It is rare to encounter the symptoms and signs of advanced disease in the first presentation but patients with local recurrence and progression do represent with some of these symptoms and signs that are discussed below.

6.1 Anaemia, Anorexia, weight loss and abdominal mass:
Patients with large volume disease, muscle invasive tumours, or metastatic disease do sometimes present with these symptoms. The mass is properly assessed during bimanual examination under general anaesthesia and if it is immobile, this suggests that it is fixed to adjacent structures. Palpable masses that remain after local resection are likely to be extensive (non organ confined or T3 disease). The Tumour, Node, Metastasis(TNM) classification approved by the Union Internationale Contre le Cancer, which was updated in 2009 is shown in the table 3 (Sobin et al 2009):

T Primary tumour.
TX primary tumour cannot be assessed.
T0 No evidence of primary tumour.
Ta Noninvasive papillary carcinoma.
Tis carcinoma in situ:`Flat tumour`
T1 Tumour invades subepithelial connective tissue.
T2 Tumour invades muscle

T2a Tumour invades superficial muscle (inner half)
T2b Tumour invades Deep muscle (outer half)
T3 Tumour invades perivesical tissue:
T3a Microscopically
T3b Macroscopically (extravesical mass)
T4 Tumour invades any of the following: Prostate, Uterus, Vagina, Pelvic Wall, abdominal wall.
    T4a Tumour invades prostate, uterus, or vagina.
    T4b Tumour invades pelvic wall or abdominal wall.

N Lymph Nodes Nx Regional lymph nodes cannot be assessed. N0 No regional lymph node metastasis N1 Metastasis in a single lymph node in the true pelvis (hypogastric, Obturator, external iliac, or presacral). N2 Metastasis in multiple lymph nodes in the true pelvis (hypogastric, Obturator, external iliac , or presacral). N3 Metastasis in a common iliac lymph node(s).
M Distant metastasis Mx Distant metastasis cannot be assessed. M0 No distant metastasis. M1 Distant metastasis.

Table 3. 2009 TNM classification of urinary bladder cancer

6.2 Lower limb swelling and lymphedema:
This is normally caused by occlusive pelvic lymphadenopathy or venous obstruction in the context of advanced disease.

6.3 Hepatomegaly and supraclavicular lymphadenopathy:
both are signs of metastatic disease.

6.4 Pneumaturia:
uncommon presentation of bladder cancer after enterovesical fistula formation. These type of fistulas are commoner with benign causes such as diverticular and crohn's disease. (Dawam et al.,2004). Nevertheless, pneumaturia warrants further investigations with urine cytology and cystoscopy with bladder biopsy if any neoplastic lesions could be seen.

6.5 Small bowel obstruction:
uncommon and unusual presentation caused by large and advanced disease (Aigen et al.,1983).

6.6 Renal failure:
caused be blocked ureters due to extensive muscle invasive disease or unilateral blockage in case of malfunctioning or absent contralateral kidney. This could also be related to retroperitoneal metastasis.

6.7 Painful cutaneous nodules and ulcerations:
very unusual and rare site of metastasis (Fujita et al., 1994;Block et al.,2006).

6.8 Urachal discharge (mucus or bloody):
a very rare presentation of adenocarcinoma, which is a rare histological subtype of bladder cancer. The tumour could be in the urachus itself or at the dome of the urinary bladder. It could also present with mucosuria.

6.9 Bony pain: a rare symptom that could be seen in cases of bony metastasis (Figure 3).

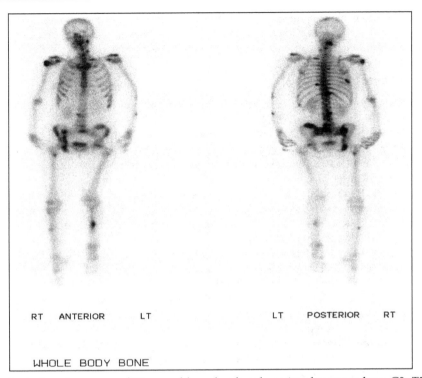

RT ANTERIOR LT   LT POSTERIOR RT

WHOLE BODY BONE

Fig. 3. An isotope bone scan of 38 year-old smoker female patient known to have G3pT2a bladder transitional cell carcinoma. She presented 2 years after radical radiation therapy with left sided hip pain. The bone scan shows wide spread metastasis (Spine, Pelvis, left forearm, left tibia, right femur and tibia).

7. Clinical conditions that could predispose to delayed presentation

7.1 Spina bifida patients

Patients with spinal bifida and bladder cancer present at a young age with variable tumour histology and advanced stage and they also have poor survival. These patients have neuropathic bladder dysfunction in addition to the fact that bladder augmentation is a significant risk factor for developing bladder cancer. Presenting symptoms are often atypical.

Although there has been suggestion of a role for annual serial bladder biopsies (Game et al., 1999) but it is not clear yet if screening would be beneficial for earlier detection and improved outcome. However, bladder cancer should be a consideration in this patient population, even in young adults (Austin et al. 2007).

7.2 Blind and colour blind patients

In a study of 200 bladder cancer patients, we found that those who had colour blindness (21 patients) did present with higher grade and stage disease compared to non colour blind population. The hypothesis is that these patients do not promptly notice the red colour of their urine at earlier stage, However, this is not proven. There is not sufficient evidence for screening of colour blind patients for bladder cancer. However, it is advisable to keep these findings in mind when assessing colour blind patients as they may help in case finding and early diagnosis of bladder cancer in this group of patients (Katmawi-Sabbagh et al., 2009).

8. References

Aigen AB, Schapira HE, Metastatic carcinoma of prostate and bladder. Causing intestinal obstruction. Urology 1983;21: 464-466.

Austin JC, Elliott S, Cooper CS. Patients with Spina bifida and bladder   cancer: Atypical presentation, advanced stage and poor survival. J Urol 2007; 178(3): 798-801

Block CA, Dahmoush L, Konety BR. Cutaneous metastases from transitional cell carcinoma of the bladder. Urology 2006.67:846.

Cummings KB, Barone JG, Ward WS. Diagnosis and staging of bladder cancer. Urologic Clinic of N Am 1992;3: 455-465.

Dawam D, Patel S, Kouriefs C, Masood S, Khan O, Sheriff MK. A "Urological" enterovesical fistula. J Urol 2004;172:943-944.

Edwards TJ,Dickson AJ,Natale S,Gosling J,Mcgrath J. A prospective analysis of the diagnostic yield resulting from attendance of 4020 patients at a protocol-driven haematuria clinic.BJU 2006;97:301-305.

Farrow GM, Utz DC, Rife CC, Greene LF. Clinical observations in 69 cases of in situ carcinoma of the urinary bladder. Cancer Res 1977; 37: 2794.

Fujita K, Sakamoto Y, Fujime M, Kitagawa R. Two cases of inflammatory skin metastasis from transitional cell carcinoma of the urinary bladder. Urol Int 1994;53:114-116.

Game X, Villers A, Malavaud B, Sarramon J. Bladder cancer arising in a Spina bifida patient. Urology 1999;54:923.

Katmawi-Sabbagh S, Haq A, Jane S, Subhas G, Turnham H. Impact of colour blindness on recognition of Haematuria in bladder cancer. Urol Int 2009; 83(3): 289-290

Katmawi-Sabbagh S, Hussain T, Al-Sudani M, England R, Khan Z. The role of the one-stop haematuria clinic in reducing time to diagnsis and treatment of Urological cancers. Italian Journal of Urology and Nephrology 2010;62(3):331-332.

Kelly JD,Fawcett D, Goldberg L. Assessment and investigation of non- visible haematuria in the primary care setting. BMJ 2009; 338:a3021

Khadra MH, Pickard RS, Charlton M. A prospective analysis of 1930 patients with hematuria to evaluate current diagnostic practice. J Urol 2000;163:524-527

Leibovitch I, Ben-Chaim J, Ramon J, Madjar I, Engelberg IS, Goldwasser B. The significance of ureteral obstruction in invasive transitional cell Carcinoma of the urinary bladder. J Surg Oncol 1993; 52: 31-35.

Sauter G, Algaba F, Amin M. Tumours of the urinary system: Non - Invasive urothelial neoplasias. In: Eble JN, Sauter G, Epstein JI, Sesterhenn I. WHO classification of tumours of the urinary system And male genital organs. Lyon, France: IARCC Press; 2004.

Sobin LH, Gospodarowicz MK, wittekind C. TNM classification of Malignant tumours (UICC International Union Against Cancer). Ed 7. New York, NY:Wiley-Blackwell;2009. p.262-265.

Part 4

Infectious Agents and Bladder Cancer

9

Bladder Cancer and Schistosomiasis: Is There a Difference for the Association?

Mohamed S. Zaghloul and Iman Gouda
Radiation Oncology and Pathology Departments,
Children's Cancer Hospital and National Cancer Institute,
Cairo University, Cairo,
Egypt

1. Introduction

Bladder cancer represents a significant worldwide health problem with an estimated 386,300 new cases and 150,200 deaths in 2008 worldwide. The majority of bladder cancer occurs in males and there is a 14-fold variation in incidence internationally. The highest incidence rates are found in the countries of Europe, North America, and Northern Africa (Jemal et al.2011). Smoking and occupational exposures are the major risk factors in Western countries, whereas chronic infection with Schistosoma hematobium (SH) in developing countries, particularly in Africa and the Middle East, accounts for about 50% of the total burden. The majority of bladder cancers associated with schistosomiasis are squamous cell carcinoma **(Figure 1)**.

Although the majority of bladder cancers, present with disease confined to the superficial layer of the bladder wall, approximately 20-40% of the patients will present with or subsequently develop invasive cancer. Bladder cancer is morphologically heterogeneous; more than 90 % of bladder cancer cases are urothelial (UC, transitional cell, TCC) carcinoma, whereas primary squamous cell carcinoma (SCC), adenocarcinoma, small cell carcinoma and other rare tumors are less common (Lopez-Beltran and Cheng, 2006). Urothelial cell carcinoma can present mixed with other malignant components **(figure 2)**. These mixed forms of bladder histologies include squamous differentiation (present in 20 - 60% of bladder cancer cases), adenocarcinoma or glandular differentiation (10%), sarcomatoid (7%), micropapillary (3.7%) and lymphoepitelioma-like carcinoma. About 1 in 25 Western men and 1 in 80 women will be diagnosed with bladder cancer (BC) sometime in their life. In many developing countries, life expectancy is much lower than Westerns, which is one of the reasons why overall BC incidence (not age-specific incidence) is lower in these developing countries (Albertson and Pinkel, 2003). It is associated with substantial morbidity and mortality. History of Tobacco smoking not only increases the incidence of BC, but also it can increase the tumor grade, its size and the number of tumor lesions (Muscheck et al, 2000). Chronic schistosomal cystitis was related for a long period to the development of BC in areas endemic for schistosomiasis like Egypt. In these areas, risk factors are many, including exposure to schistosomiasis, increased smoking rate and exposure to carcinogenic chemicals (Kallioniemi et al, 1992).

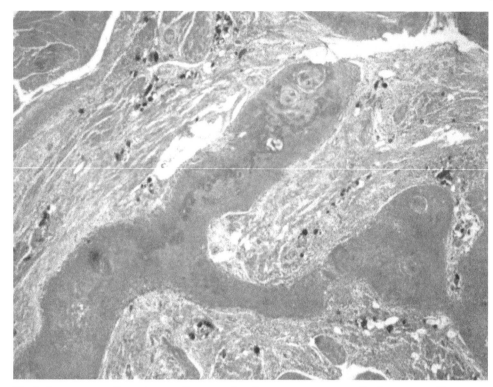

Fig. 1. Squamous cell carcinoma. Groups of malignant squamous cells show central keratin nests formation. Aggregates of calcified bilharzias eggs are seen between groups of malignant cells.

Although smoking is still recognized as a major risk factor of cancers including bladder cancer, the increasing incidence of bladder cancer, despite the reduction in smoking in the United States, suggests that other environmental factors may be playing an increasing role in the development of bladder cancer. Unlike the common belief, risk factors such as positive family history, parent's consanguinity, exposure to pesticides and chronic cystitis seem to play now more important roles than bilharziasis and smoking in the development of this disease in Egypt, yet reports on larger numbers of patients are needed to support this conclusion (Zarzour et al, 2008).

2. Bladder cancer formation

Urothelial tumor is characterized by its multifocality. There have been two theories proposed to explain the frequency of this Urothelial tumor multifocality. One theory, the monoclonal theory, suggests that multiple tumors arise from a single transformed cell that proliferates and spreads throughout the urothelium. The second theory, the field-effect theory, explains tumor multifocality as a development secondary to the field cancerization effect. In the last scenario, carcinogens cause independent transforming genetic alterations at different sites in the urothelial lining leading to multiple genetically defective tumors

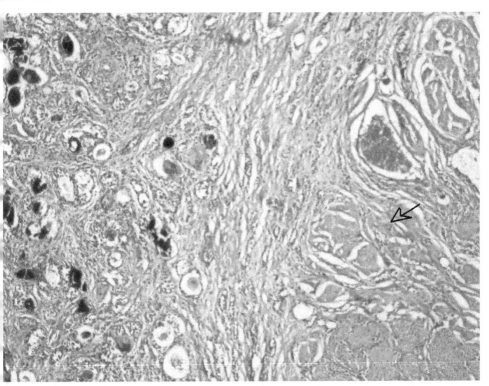

Fig. 2. Invasive urothelial cell carcinoma. Small groups of cells with glandular differentiation on the right are seen infiltrating muscle layer (arrow). Bilharzial granulomas are seen on the left.

(Cheng et al, 2010). That may highlight the existence of different histopathologies in the same specimen. A recent study suggests that both field cancerization and monoclonal tumor spread may coexist in the same patient (Jones et al, 2005). In this study, molecular evidence supported an oligoclonal origin for multifocal Urothelial carcinoma. Field cancerization, which is an important cause of multicenteric squamous cell carcinoma (SCC) of head and neck postulates that multifocal Urothelial carcinoma arises in the same way. The independent transformations are a consequence of external cancer-causing influences. Premalignant changes, such as dysplasia or carcinoma in situ (CIS) are often found in Urothelial mucosa distant from an invasive bladder cancer. Furthermore, various theories have been proposed to combine the two mechanisms. Early or preneoplastic lesions may arise independently with specific clone and pseudomonoclonality (Hafner et al, 2002). The modern carcinogenesis model suggests that malignancy represents clonal expansion of one or a few cancer stem cells that proliferate through asymmetric differentiation and can diversify into heterogeneous cancer cell lineages. Asymmetric differentiation means that following cell division, one daughter cell retains the capacity to divide again and the other daughter cell possesses genetic plasticity, allowing phenotypic variation in the offspring. When tumors arise from Chromosomal Somatic Changes (CSC) of progenitor cells, a specific set of genomics, epigenomic and/ or microenvironment niche alterations is essential for continued clonal expansion. Therefore, each CSC and its pro/zaxgency possess a unique set of genetic, epigenetic and phenotypic features. Genetic alterations of stromal somatic cells assist CSCs in the niche to promote cancer development and progression (Cheng and Zhang, 2008). Since the sixties of the last century, meaningful chromosomal changes were subsequently reported in human cancer. With the establishment of different new methods, detection of these changes became more apparent and allowed better understanding of the process of evolving of different kinds of cancer. Each new method widened the recognition of karyotypic changes, increasing the resolution of cytogenetic details until the limit of microscopic visualization were almost reached. The evolution of cytogenetics encompasses also molecular approaches such as fluorescent in situ hybridization (FISH) and comparative genomic hybridization (CGH) whether metaphasic or array. These techniques have revealed novel and otherwise cryptic rearrangements, as well as providing chromosomal information for cases in which conventional cytogenetic analysis is not possible (Sendberg and Meloni-Ehrg, 2010).

A meta-analysis examining urine markers for surveillance showed that Fluorescence In Situ Hybridization (FISH) test had a median sensitivity of 79% and median specificity of 70% in detecting genetic abnormalities in cells present in urine using FISH (Van Rhijin et al, 2005). The main disadvantages of FISH are the lack of standardization of the criterion for a positive test, the low sensitivity of detecting low-grade tumors, its expense, and the need for specially trained laboratory personnel to perform the test (Degtyar et al, 2004 & Lokeshwar et al, 2005). Combined testing with other assays may improve the effectiveness of this biomarker. Several markers have shown promise as noninvasive biomarkers of bladder cancer, and some may be useful as therapeutic targets. To date, however, none have found a strong niche in clinical care because of the lack of evidence demonstrating that outcomes are altered on a practical basis. In addition, at this time, none of these markers can supplant cystoscopy, and most add little advantage to the combination of cystoscopy and cytology.

3. Schistosomiasis

Schistosomiasis infect 200 million people according to the World Health Organization and is endemic in as much as 76 tropical developing countries. S. hematobium (SH) is associated with bladder cancer. Schistosomes are dioecious parasitic blood flukes, which have a mammalian host and an intermediate invertebrate host: fresh water snails (Kuper et al, 2000). There are four human schistosomes :S. haematobium, S. mansoni, S. japonicum, S. mekonji. The S. haematobium, like other schistosomes is dioecious and the adult female lives in-copulo in the gynecophoral canal of the male; this species of schistosome lives in the venules of the human urinary bladder. Eggs laid in the urinary bladder produce irritation and eventual fibrosis, contributing to the events that lead to human carcinogenicity (Fried et al, 2011).

All schistosoma infections follow direct contact with fresh water that harbors free-swimming larval forms of the parasite known as cercariae. Cercariae penetrate the skin. The cercariae shed their bifurcated tails, and the resulting schistosomula enter capillaries and lymphatic vessels en route to the lungs. After several days, the worms migrate to the portal venous system, where they mature and unite. Pairs of worms then migrate to the vesical plexus and veins draining the ureters. Egg production commences four to six weeks after infection and continues for the life of the worm, usually three to five years. Eggs pass from the lumen of blood vessels into adjacent tissues, and many then pass through the bladder mucosa and are shed in the urine. The life cycle is completed when the eggs hatch, releasing miracidia that, in turn, infect specific freshwater snails (Bulinus species).After two generations - primary and then daughter sporocysts — within the snail, cercariae are released (Ross et al, 2002).

4. Schistosoma-Associated Bladder Cancer (SA-BC)

Schistosomiasis was first linked to urinary bladder cancer in Egypt in 1911 (Ferguson et al, 1911). The incidence of urinary bladder cancer in the Middle East and Africa is greater in areas with high rather than low SH prevalence; the aforementioned study noted that 60% of the Egyptian population was at risk of infection with SH, with rural school children at particular risk because of their proximity to contaminated water. The overall prevalence of SH infection in Egypt was 37–48% that decreased due to the antibilharzial campaign to 3 % (Ministry of Health and Population, 2004). The urinary bladder cancer accounted for about 31% of the total incidence of cancers in Egypt that subsequently decreased to 12% in recent years. However still, it is the most common type of cancer in males and the second most prevalent, after breast cancer, in females (Gouda et al, 2007). In Egypt, Iraq, Zambia, Zimbabwe, Malawi and Sudan, the incidence of SA-BC peaks at 40–49 years of age; the male to female ratio for bladder cancer is 5:1 in endemic and 3:1 in non-endemic areas. This relates to the fact that it is agricultural workers, mainly men, who have daily exposure to water infected with SH cercariae. (Makhyoun et al, 1971). Mechanicaly, there are several factors that may contribute to the oncological potential of schistosomia infection. Schistosoma ova deposited in the bladder provoke an intense inflammatory reaction, associated with the production of oxygen-derived free radicals, which may induce genetic mutations or promote the production of carcinogenic compounds (such as N-nitrosamines and polycyclic aromatic hydrocarbons) (Marletta 1988 & Rosin et al, 1994) ,leading to malignant transformation. Shokeir (2004) showed that schistosomiasis is often accompanied by chronic bacterial super-infection, which may in itself predispose to squamous cell (SC) neoplasia. Bacteria found to accompany schistosomiasis can promote the formation of N-nitrosation of amines, adding to those from other sources such as the diet. A 54–81% incidence of SCC was found in all cases of bladder cancers in endemic areas, opposed to 3–10% in Western countries. The higher incidence of SCC is probably due to exposure to carcinogens such as N-nitroso compounds that are abundantly present in the urine of patients with SH (Tricker et al,1989). International Agency for Research on Cancer (IARC) found that the intensity of infection was determined by urinary egg counts and confounded by smoking, a recognized cause of bladder cancer in non-endemic countries, and the combination was strongly considered. Positive association between bladder cancer and SH infection was detected, with odd ratios ranging from 2 to 14. The more heavily infected individuals were with this schistosome, the more likely they were to develop bladder cancer, and at a younger age (IARC, 1994).

Most of the pathological findings of schistosomiasis are due to an inflammatory and immunological response to egg deposition. Granulomatous areas form around the eggs and induce an exudative cellular response consisting of lymphocytes, polymorphonuclear leukocytes and eosinophil. The early stage of SH infection is characterized by egg deposition in the lower ureters and urinary bladder. Resultant perioval granulomas, fibrosis and muscular hypertrophy are seen histologically. In the ureter, lesions can cause stenosis, leading to hydronephrosis. In the urinary bladder, masses of large granulomatous inflammatory polyps containing eggs are found at the bladder apex, dome, trigone and posterior wall. Polyps may ulcerate and slough, producing haematuria. Hyperplasia of the urothelium occurred in 38% of the autopsied SH cases as opposed to 21% in non-infected cases; also, metaplasia in 31.6% versus 11.5% and dysplasia in 27.2% versus 8.5% cases were found. Late-stage infections were characterized by schistosomal bladder ulcers and sandy patches, and irregularly thickened or atrophic mucosa in the posterior bladder or trigone area. Histologically, fibrosis with some round cell infiltration was seen; old granulomas containing calcified or disintegrating eggs were also seen (Smith and Christie, 1986). The inflammatory and fibrotic response to egg deposition could lead to calcification of the urinary bladder, infection and stone disease and these changes are frequently associated with urinary bladder cancer (EL-Bolkainy et al, 1981). These lesions may be at least partially responsible to the reported clinical picture of SA-BC. Furthermore, the following sequence of events in SH-induced carcinogenesis has been suggested: chronic infection leads to schistosoma eggs being trapped in the bladder wall. Proliferation of cells in the bladder mucosa results from constant irritation and inflammation. Clones of neoplastic cells develop, stimulated by N-nitrosamines and other environmental carcinogens such as cigarette smoke and pesticides (Abdel et al, 2000). The importance of urinary retention, whether from fibrosis and obstruction of the urinary bladder neck or from voluntary causes such as pain on urination, in prolonging the exposure of the bladder mucosa to various exogenous and endogenous carcinogens was documented. Schistosome-induced urinary stasis allows increased absorption of carcinogens and therefore plays an integral role in carcinogenesis. Recurrent bacterial urinary tract infections are associated with squamous cell carcinoma of the urinary bladder, even in the absence of SH infection (Genile et al, 1985). Carcinogenesis of SH involving an initiating and promoting effect has been described. First, the damage occurs to the DNA template which, unless repaired, leads to irreversible changes in the complementary strand of DNA produced during the S-phase of the cell cycle. Somatic mutation results when the altered strand is used as a template. The promotion phase followed by stimulation of cell proliferation. Different cancer-associated genes, notably protoncogenes/oncogenes and tumor suppressor genes, were known to be associated with numerous human cancers; recent efforts have been made to study the specific genes involved in the induction of SA-BC. Cell exposed to SH cell total antigen (warm exttract) was found to divide faster than those not exposed to the parasite and died much less. This was probably due to increased level of bcl2, a protein involved in cancer apoptosis that may lead to SH carcinogenic ability in bladder urothelium (Botelho et al, 2009). The urothelium of mice exposed to SH total antigen showed dysplasia, low grade intra-urothelial neoplasm, non-invasive malignant flat lesions in 70 % of the tested mice after 40 weeks of exposure. Carcinoma of the bladder frequently harbors gene mutations that constitutively activate the receptors tyrosine kinase Ras pathway (Wu, 2005). The Ras gene product is a monometric membrane-localized G protein of 21 Kd that functions as a molecular switch linking receptors and non-receptors tyrosine kinase activation to downstream cytoplasmic or nuclear events. Each mammalian cell contains at least three distinct Ras proto-oncogenes encoding closely related but distinct protein, Kras, Hras and Nras. Activating mutation in these Ras protein, result in constitutive signaling. Thereby stimulating cell proliferation and inhibiting apoptosis. Oncogenic mutations in the Ras gene are present in approximately 30% of all human cancer (Adjer, 2001). Botelho et al (2010) used the dysplastic bladders induced by SH in mice and screened them by sequencing for mutations in Kras codon hotspots gene. They concluded that the parasite abstract has carcinogenic ability possibly through oncogenic mutation of Kras gene.

5. Genetic changes in SA-BC

Among the most common genetic changes in bladder cancer is the loss of heterozygosity (LOH) on chromosomes 9p and 9q, which is found regardless of tumor grade and stage (Jacobs et al,2010 & McConkey et al, 2010). A prospective study stated that there was no evident line of demarcation between schistosomiasis-associated and non schistosomiasis-associated bladder cancer in terms of LOH of microsatellite markers on chromosome 9. This suggests that data obtained from schistosoma-associated bladder cancer can be extrapolated to bladder cancer induced by a schistosomiasis independent mechanism (Abdel Wahab et al, 2005). DNA microsatellites are highly polymorphic repeats found throughout the genome, and microsatellite markers can detect cancer-associated alterations in genetic material, including microsatellite instability and LOH (Nielsen et al, 2006). A more recent analytical tool that has been developed to detect genomic instability in urinary DNA uses small nucleotide polymorphisms (SNPs). SNP chips have a potential advantage over microsatellite analysis in that they can screen more than 300 genetic loci at once compared with 13-20 loci, which leads to a greater sensitivity of the detection of molecular changes (Hoque et al, 2003).

6. Cytogenetics for understanding carcinogenesis

Carcinogenesis is a complex process in which normal cell growth is modified as a result of the interaction of multiple factors, including xenobiotics and endogenous constituents. Carcinogenic process results from the accumulation of both genetic and epigenetic changes that are driven by instability of cellular genome and alterations in inter- or intra-cellular communication, which disrupt the cell proliferation regulation process (Loeb and loeb, 2000). Cytogenetics is concerned with the task of finding recurrent (repeated) or specific abnormalities associated with cancer, and continues to provide crucial diagnostic and prognostic information. In current practice, cytogenetic data often serve as a guide in other studies, ranging from the exploration of cytogenetic findings with various methodologies, singly or in combination, including fluorescence in situ hybridization (FISH), polymerase chain reaction (PCR), or microarray-based technologies such as comparative genomic hybridization (CGH), both metaphasic (mCGH) and array (aCGH), to the use of immunohistochemical techniques by the pathologist. Cytogenetic data also provide key background information for the recognition and identification of genes (and their networks) involved in cancer. Progress in understanding the cytogenetic and molecular basis of neoplastic transformation has strengthened the conception of cancer as a genetic disease. Thus, the finding of apparently normal karyotypes in abnormal cells presents an enigma. It can be assumed that cryptic genetic changes are involved in such cases. Newer technologies highlight the more complicated and perplexing aspects of cancer that have eluded more traditional cytogenetic studies. For example, molecular studies have demonstrated fusion genes associated with many tumors like prostate and lung cancers that are not discernible cytogenetically. These findings raise the strong possibility that more epithelial carcinomas, which are usually associated with numerous or complex karyotypic alterations, will be shown to have cryptic primary genetic alterations (Sandberg et al,2010)

7. Requirements and limitations of cancer cytogenetic studies

Cytogenetic techniques require the presence of dividing cells (preferably in the metaphase stage) for the visualization of chromosomes. Thus, fresh specimens are necessary for establishing either short-term or long-term cultures (Sandberg, 1990, Brigge and Sandberg, 2000, Sandberg and Chen, 2001& Gersen and Keagle, 2005). Nevertheless, useful genetic information can be obtained from fixed specimens with appropriate FISH or other molecular techniques (Gersen and Keagle, 2005). Cytogenetic changes represent genetic mechanisms that are thought to be responsible for the biology of the respective clinical conditions, and have become important components of diagnostic and prognostic criteria. There are two different classes of genetic alterations associated with cancer: activation of oncogenes and inactivation of tumor suppressor genes. Rearrangements are a common source of activating mutations. Another scenario is exemplified by chromosome translocations, inversions, or insertions that lead to formation of fusion oncogenes. The oncogene fusion mechanism has received increased attention, because many of these fusions lead to activation of protein tyrosine kinases (PTKs) in various types of cancer. Most of the cytogenetic changes involve activation of receptor proteins, especially PTKs. Receptor PTKs are a highly regulated family of proteins in normal cells, but may undergo activating mutations or structural alterations to become oncoproteins in human malignancies. As already noted, oncogenic activation of PTKs can result from genetic lesions such as point mutations, deletions, or overexpression by gene amplification. Alternatively, chromosomal rearrangements such as translocations, inversions, and insertions that lead to formation of an oncogenic gene fusion can involve receptor PTK or other PTK encoding genes as fusion partners. Another type of gene rearrangement involves tumor suppressor genes, whose products normally serve as brakes on cell growth and runaway cell proliferation. Inactivation of tumor suppressor genes leads to uncontrolled cell proliferation and downregulation of apoptosis (programmed cell death)(Jones and Baylin, 2002 & Feinberg and Tycko, 2004). The activation of oncogenes sometimes results from complex genetic rearrangements. In each of the fusion genes the kinase domain of the neural-associated receptor tyrosine kinase gene is fused to an activating domain of another gene. The same genes may be altered in a number of different tumors, but apparently at varying chronologies in tumor development and associated with different genetic changes. In many tumors, a specific translocation may be the only alteration present. Many cases, however, display additional structural or numeric karyotypic changes that may be responsible for, or at least are associated with, disease progression(Sandberg, 1990). The relevance of additional abnormalities is also reflected by alterations in the expression of a number of genes apart from those involved in the translocations. The exact cause or causes of these additional alterations is unknown, and it remains uncertain whether the primary translocation per se is responsible for the basic genetic process underlying the tumor genesis. These additional changes usually vary from tumor to tumor, even among tumors with the same diagnosis. Tumors with specific translocations may exhibit a variety of anomalies, with or without additional chromosome changes, at the molecular level. Carcinomas being diagnosed relatively late in their development, thus allow for the genesis of chromosomal rearrangements in addition to the primary genetic event. Although some of the chromosomal changes have been related to prognosis and tumor biology yet, few recurrent or repeated chromosomal anomalies have been identified as characterizing these tumors (Teixeira et al, 2006).

MicroRNAs (miRNAs) constitute a rapidly developing field of study at many levels. The miRNAs are short segments of RNA (~22 bases in length) that affect mRNA functions, most often by suppressing translation of the protein product or by promoting degradation of them. An important value of miRNAs is that they can be detected and quantified in a variety of samples, including plasma and formalin-fixed, paraffin-embedded tissues. This makes them a valuable testing tool, particularly in the clinical arena(Wijnhoven et al, 2007, Grady and Tewari, 2010 & Ferracin et al, 2010)

In cancer, the combination of cytogenetic and molecular studies (FISH, SKY, PCR, CGH, and related methodologies) can more clearly define pathogenetic pathways and the biologic functions of molecular markers than either approach alone. Such a dual approach should lead to less empiric and more biologically oriented approaches to tumor classification and, ultimately, to more efficient clinical use of biomarkers (Wang,2002 & Balsara et al, 2002). Findings based on the combination of cytogenetic and molecular approaches have improved the criteria for diagnosis of cancer. The hypothesis that specific clones of spontaneously evolving aneuploidies or karyotypes, rather than specific mutations, generate the individuality of cancers (Fabarius et al, 2008), may apply to at least some of, if not all, the conditions .Cancer development not only depends on genetic alterations but also on epigenetic changes (Jones and Baylin, 2007). These changes modify gene expression through DNA methylation, histone modifications, chromatin remodeling, and/or the expression of noncoding RNA(Esteller, 2007 & Zaratiegui et al, 2007).

Epigenetic gene silencing in cancer was thought to be restricted to focal events that silenced isolated genes (Smith and Costello, 2006). However, recent findings have indicated that epigenetic silencing can extend to a whole chromosomal region and has been reported to involve DNA methylation and/or histone modification in various cancers (bladder, breast, colorectal, and prostate cancer) (Coolen et al, 2010).

The development of cancer is often a multistage process where the disruption of specific subsets of genes can result in cells expressing a malignant phenotype. However, the series of mutations leading to malignancy has only been elucidated for a small number of human cancers (e.g., polyposis of the colon, retinoblastoma). There has been no entirely specific cytogenetic aberration identified for bladder cancer, but various nonrandom deletions, gains of chromosomes, polyploidisation, and formation of isochromosomes have been observed (Gibas and Gibas, 1997).

8. Bladder cancer cytogenetics and epigenetics

Chromosome 1 has been reported as being the most frequently involved chromosome in rearrangements; other chromosomes commonly reported in bladder cancer include chromosomes 3,5,7, and 9 (Heim and Mitelman, 1995). Yunis and Soreng (1984) suggested that there was a relationship between chromosomal fragile sites and oncogenesis. It is believed that fragile sites provide regions of the genome that are more susceptible to damage and that this contributes to the carcinogenic process because of subsequent changes to gene function or dosage. Bladder cancer is a very heterogenous disease cytogenetically, which suggests that the pathogenesis of the disease may not be consistent for every case. A possible scenario of pathogenesis could be the disruption of a nonconsistent set of cell regulatory genes compounded with disruption to genes that have a phenotypic effect on the bladder. Sustained disruptions to fragile regions as a result of prolonged exposure to clastogens in vivo are likely to lead to enduring chromosomal rearrangements and associated gene alterations. The heterogeneity of cytogenetic findings in bladder cancer hints that there might be different "fingerprints" or accumulations of genetic changes that individually lead to bladder cancer and that fragile sites may be providing a gateway for oncogenesis for some cases. Different combinations of these damaged sites could result in varying cancer phenotypes, depending upon which particular genes were located at the sites susceptible to the mutagens.

Protoncogenes encode proteins that ultimately enhance cell proliferation. Events that convert protoncogenes to oncogenes can lead to uncontrolled cell proliferation and carcinogenesis (Badawi et al, 1995). The RAS oncogene and its potential association with urinary bladder cancer was studied, though still not totally clear. The RAS oncogene encodes a 21-kDa protein that affects signal transmission between the nucleus and tyrosine kinase receptors. H-RAS activation was estimated in bladder cancer to range between 7% and 17%, with its expression being similar with or without concurrent schistosomal infection. The TP53 tumor suppressor gene, located on the short arm of chromosome 17, encodes a protein that regulates DNA damage repair and controls aspects of the cell cycle involving cellular apoptosis and senescence. TP53 mutation results in a reduction of DNA damage surveillance leading to instability of the genome and malignant transformation (Strohmeyer and Slamon, 1994). The overexpression of the BCL-2 gene in SA-BC patients was found to be up-regulated in squamous but not transitional cell cancers of the urinary bladder. Therefore, this BCL-2 overexpression is consistent with the predominance of SCC in SA-BC. Upregulation of this gene overrides programmed cell apoptosis increasing the risk of genomic instability and may interact with various proto-oncogenes facilitating tumorigenesis. Mutations of TP53 were found in 73% of tumors, BCL-2 expression in 32% and abnormalities of both TP53 and BCL-2 in 13%. Loss of the normal reciprocal control mechanism for apoptosis was suggested in the subset of patients with overexpression of both TP53 and BCL-2 (Chaudhary et al, 1997).

Furthermore, cyclooxygenase-2 is overexpressed in SA-BC. The quantitative relationship between cyclooxygenase-2 expression and tumor grade was statistically significant. The cyclooxygenase-2 role in the complex multi-stage process of SA-BC carcinogenesis was proposed: pro-inflammatory cytokines such as interleukin-1, tumor growth factor-β and tumor necrosis factor-alpha, are generated by activated macrophages in the inflammatory lesions. These cytokines and growth factors are potent inducers of cyclooxygenase-2 production. By-products of uncontrolled cyclooxygenase activity together with endogenous genotoxins produce oxidative and nitrosative stress creating lipid peroxidation by-products. Additional mutations are induced: TP53, H-RAS, deletion of p16 and p15, increased epidermal growth factor receptor, c-erb-2 and tumor necrosis factor-alpha. Increased prostaglandin production up-regulates cyclooxygenase-2, decreases killer T-cell activity, increases BCL-2 and glutathione-S-transferase. These changes increase tumorgenicity by decreasing cell apoptosis, creating immunosupression. Prostaglandin products of cyclooxygenase-2 cause tumor progression and eventual metastasis by down-regulating adhesion molecules, increasing the degradation of extracellular matrix and increasing angiogenesis (El-Sheikh et al, 2001).

9. Natural history of SA-BC

The association between SA-BC and SH was established through case-controlled studies and through the close correlation of the incidence of bladder cancer with the prevalence of SH within different geographic areas. Moreover, the association was based on the frequent association of tumors with the presence of parasitic eggs and egg-induced granulomatous pathology involving bladder tissues *(Figure 2)*. Despite that linkage between SH and bladder cancer, only limited data are available on cytopathologic findings in SA-BC. The cellular mechanisms linking SH infestation with bladder cancer formation are not yet defined. In some cases, severe metaplasia in bladder urothelium may represent a precancerous transformation, whereas in others it may merely serve as a marker of prolonged inflammation, which is associated with high cancer risk (Hodder et al, 2000). Keratinizing or adenomatous metaplasia per se has a strong association with cancer formation in patients with chronic irritation due to bladder stones, chronic infection, or prolonged catheterization.

SA-BC was defined by characteristic pathology (i.e., squamous carcinoma, transitional cell carcinoma, or adenocarcinoma, rather than mainly transitional) and cellular and molecular biology that differ from non-Schistosoma-associated bladder cancer (NSA-BC). Few studies have analysed the cytogenetic and molecular genetic abnormalities in SA-BC and some compared DNA copy number changes in SA-BC and NSA-BC (Kallioniemi et al, 1992,Tsutumi et al, 1998, Muscheck et al,2000, Fadl-Elmula et al, 2002 & Albertson and Pinkel, 2003). Further future studies are needed to characterize the genetic alterations in schistosomal bladder tumors and their role in bladder cancer induction.

These studies used metaphase CGH to obtain overview of chromosomal alterations in SA-BC. The value of pooled DNA in aCGH was shown to be advantageous in detecting recurrent changes associated with specific histopathologic or clinical features (Kendziorski et al, 2005). Two more recent studies used aCGH, rather than metaphase CGH (Armengol et al, 2007 & Vauhkonen et al, 2007). Array CGH provides higher density region-specific coverage and direct mapping of aberrations to the genome sequence, as well as higher throughput (Albertson and Pinkel, 2003). This ensures greater accuracy in comparing two groups of tumors (e.g., SA-BC and NSA-BC). Muscheck et al. (2000) demonstrated deletion similarities in Schistosoma-associated transitional cell carcinoma (SA-TCC) and Schistosoma-associated squamous cell carcinoma (SA-SCC), compared to what has been previously reported by Kallioniemi et al. (1992) on NSA-TCC and Tsutsumi et al. (1998) on NSA-SCC. The previous investigators (Kallioniemi et al,1992,Tsutsumi et al,1998, Muscheck et al, 2000, Fadl-Elmula et al, 2002 & Albertson and Pinkel, 2003) used the technique of CGH on individual tumor tissues, not pooled tissues of similar pathologies. Armengol et al. (2007) used an excellent technique of combining similar pathological types into pools of tissue arising from patients having similar pathological subtypes. These pooled DNAs revealed recurrent primary changes covering secondary changes that vary from case to case. The pooled specimens of SA-BC tumors showed no schistosomiasis specific changes, compared with pools of NSA tumors. The comparison between SA-TCC and NSA-TCC and that between SA-SCC and NSA-SCC gave similar results. DNA copy number profiles of urinary bladder SA adenocarcinoma revealed similarities to that of SA-TCC and SA-SCC reported by Vauhkonen et al. (2007). The results in these two publications showed that the detailed analysis of individual genes revealed a set of genes with the same copy number changes in all bladder carcinomas, including both SA and NSA tumors. Armengol et al. (2007) concluded that there are no major cytogenetic differences among different urinary bladder epithelial tumors, regardless of the suspected carcinogen. All the detected imbalances in SA-BC have been repeatedly reported in NSA-BC that suggested that cytogenetic profiles of chemical- and Schistosoma-induced carcinoma are largely similar in the reports of Muscheck et al. (2000) and Fadl-Elmula et al. (2002). Patients having SA-BC usually present late with more advanced stage, due to the repeated SH infestations having similar symptoms. The decreased intensity of schistosomal infestation in Egypt led to a changing pattern of the clinicoepidemiologic features of SA-BC. A decreased SCC/TCC ratio (increase in the percentage of TCC and decrease in that of SCC), lowering of the tumor stage and increase in the mean age incidence and percentage of pelvic nodal involvement have been reported. The reported clinicoepidemiologic differences between SA-BC and SNA-BC are now continuously decreasing and the features of SA-BC is slowly approaching that of NSA-BC as reported by Koraitim et al. (1995) and Zaghloul et al. (2008). These changing features were attributed to the decreased intensity of schistosomal infestation in the urinary bladder, as a higher degree of schistosomal infestation and egg deposition was found more frequently with SCC and a lower with TCC (Zaghloul et al, 2008 & Zaghloul, 2010). Furthermore, these changes are repeatedly evident with the predominance of TCC over the SCC type, and a decrease of male predominance. If these changes continue with the same rate, bladder cancer in Egypt is expected to become identical in features to that of Western countries in the near future (Gouda et al, 2007).

10. Clinical presentation

Clinical presentations in SA-BC and SNA-BC are similar with few minor differences. Hematuria, dysuria and necroturia are the main symptoms in both situations. However, SA-BC patients usually had experienced these symptoms beforehand as a result of simple schistosomal cystitis. This may be the reason of their relatively late presentation. Table (1) showed the postcystectomy pathological staging in SA-BC and SNA-BC large studies. The early stages (Pa, Pis, P1) were fewer in SA-BC than that in SNA-BC in both the Urothelial and non-urothelial pathology. The pelvic nodal involvement was nearly similar in SA-BC (range: 16.7% - 25.5%) , Urothelial SNA-BC (range: 16.3% - 45%) and non-urothelial SNA-BC (21.8% - 23%). The clincopathologic differences between SA-BC and SNA-BC were previously summarized as late presentation, with younger median age and a higher percentage of squamous cell carcinoma category (Zaghloul, 1994).

11. Treatment of non-muscle invasive (superficial) bladder cancer

Treatment of superficial bladder cancer remains to be transurethral resection and bladder biopsy (TURBT) with and without intravesical BCG or chemotherapy instillation. Although this treatment type is very popular in Urothelial cancer, it is less popular in non-urothelial SNA-BC and SA-BC, probably due to the rarity of the non-invasive stages and the presence of many lesions either precancerous or cancerous in the bladder mucosa.

12. Treatment of muscle-invasive bladder cancer

Radical cystectomy

Muscle-invasive bladder cancer is mostly treated with radical cystectomy in many parts of the world. Radical cystectomy procedure includes removal of the bladder, seminal vesicles and prostate together with perivesical fat and peritoneal coverage, in addition to bilateral

Author	Number of Patients	PTa,is,1 %	PT2 %	PT3 %	PT4 %	Nodal involvement
Pure Urothelial Carcinoma (SNA-BC)						
Bassi et al (1999)	338	32.8	19.8	42.0	19.8	NM
Stein et al, (2001)	1057	39.9	23.5	23.5	13	23.3
Cheng et al, (2003)	303	36.1	28.6	25.5	9.9	16.3
Shariat et al, (2006)	958	22	35	31	12	23
Urothelial & Non-urothelial (SNA-BC)						
Rogers et al, (2006)	955	21	33	32	14	23
Lughezzani et al, (2010)	12003	13.4	38.9	28.1	19.6	21.8
Scosyrev et al,(2009)	1422	14.8	29	29.3	26.8	
Urothelial & Non-urothelial (SA-BC)						
El Said et al, (1997)	420	1	3.8	70.7	24.5	16.7
Zaghloul, (1996)	357	0	33.3	47.9	18.8	24.4
El Makresh et al,(1998)	185	7	25	64	7	16
Zaghloul et al, (2006)	192	3.6	28.1	51.6	16.7	25.5
Ghoneim et, (2008)	2720	10.5	63.9	16.6	9.0	20.4
Zaghloul et al, (2008)	5071	1.9	30.1	54.9	13.1	21.9
Khaled et al, (2005)	180	1.2	5.8	14.1	11.5	16.6
Ali-El-Dein, (2009)	180	10.0	62.8	25.0	2.2	18.3

Table 1. Postcystectomy pathological stages and nodal involvement in pure Urothelial and mixed Urothelial and non-urothelial schistosoma-non associated and schistosoma associated bladder cancer in large series.

endopelvic lymphadenectomy (with varying level of dissection) in male patients. In females, it includes removal of the bladder, its perivesical fat and peritoneal coverage, urethra, uterus, ovary and anterior wall of the vagina (anterior pelvic excentration) (Ghoneim et al, 1997 & Stein et al, 2001). A review of recent literature of treatment results of different types of bladder cancer showed that applying the same treatment yielded nearly the same level of results if comparing the same pathological stage (Zaghloul, 2006 & Zaghloul et al, 2006). Similar 5-year overall survival rates were found in SA-BC, pure Urothelial and combined

Urothelial and non-urothelial SNA-BC types (Table 2). The results were slightly higher in Stein et al. (2001) (NSA-BC) and Zaghloul et al.(2006) (SA-BC) as both studies reported neoadjuvant or adjuvant radiotherapy and /or chemotherapy as a part of treatment in more than one third of their patients. Furthermore, this conclusion applies for comparison of disease-free survival, overall survival, or local control rates for radical cystectomy or even in adjuvant and neoadjuvant radiotherapy types of treatment for SA-BC and NSA-BC (Zaghloul, 2006 & 2010). The treatment end-results of radical cystectomy was not affected by

Author	Patients #	PT1	PT2	PT3	PT4	Nodal involvement
Pure Urothelial Carcinoma (SNA-BC)						
Cheng et al, (2003)	218	---	50	28	17	11
Stein et al, (2001)	1054	74	81/68*	47	44	35
Medersbacher et al, (2003)	507	76	62	40	49	26
Takahashi et al, (2004)	466	81	74	47	38	50
Dhar et al, (2006)	385	---	63	19	NM	9
Ho et al, (2009)	148	77	68	65	11	37
Manoharan et al, (2009)	432	79	60	43	17	22
Urothelial & Non-urothelial (SNA-BC)						
Nishiyama et al, (2004)	1113	82	84/69*	59	43	35
Niu et al, (2008)	356	---	73/44*	22	0	8
Gupta et al, (2008)	502	90	78	70/58*	46	NM
Urothelial & Non-urothelial (SA-BC)						
Ghoneim et al, (1997)	1026	73	66	47/31*	19	23
El Mekresh et al, (1985)	185	83		41		21
Khaled et al, (2005)	180	55		12		6
Zaghloul et al, (2006)	192	100	100/47	40	44	31
Zaghloul et al, (2007)	216	100	51	40	30	31
Ghoneim et al, (2008)	2720	82	75/53	40	30	27

*= a/b, NM = not mentioned

Table 2. The 5-y survival of each pathological stage in Schistosoma-non associated and schistosoma associated bladder cancer patients in large radical cystectomy patients.

the association with schistosomiasis, nor tumor cell type (Urothelial or non-urothelial) in most of the recently published literatures (Ghoneim et al, 1997, Stein et al, 2001, Zaghloul et al, 2006) (Table 2). Favorable end-results were reported for patients with pathologically organ confined disease. These results were constant for both SA-BC (ranged from 47% to 83%), and SNA-BC (ranged from 50% to84%). However, the results were significantly worse when reporting upon locally advanced tumors (PT3N0M0, PT4aN0M0 or Any N). Again, these worse results were experienced by both SA-BC and SNA-BC patients (Ghoneim et al, 1997 & 2008,Stein et al, 2001,Gschwend et al, 2002, Chang et al, 2003, Medersbacher et al, 2003, Nishiyama et al, 2004, Takahashi et al, 2004, Rogers et al, 2006 & Lughezzani et al, 2010). Regardless of the old belief that aberrant differentiation leads to worse results, yet many authors reported similar results of these aberrant variants to UC when comparing stage to stage. Rogers et al (2006) reported a 5-year progression-free survival rate of 60±2% after radical cystectomy for UC and 55±11% for SCC. This difference was statistically insignificant. Patients with UC or SCC had statistically significant higher progression-free survival rates than non-UC non-SCC patients including those having adenocarcinoma. Another study containing considerable number of adenocarcinoma patients was conducted using 17 Surveillance, Epidemiology and End Results (SEER) and it showed a difference of statistical significance in adenocarcinoma patients who underwent RC at a more advanced disease stage than their UC counterparts. Another recent study using a similar SEER database demonstrated that SCC was more aggressive than Urothelial cancer after adjusting for common prognostic factors, such as stage and grade (Scosyrev et al, 2009). Scosyrev et al (2009) concluded that SCC was an independent predictor of mortality among patients with stage III and IV disease, and among patients with stage I and II disease who did not undergo cystectomy as part of their treatment. Therefore, squamous histology was not associated with increased mortality among patients with stage I and II disease when treated with cystectomy. Moreover, Ploeg et al (2010) studied all invasive bladder cancer cases treated in The Netherlands during a 12 year period of (1995-2006). They concluded that the relative survival of muscle-invasive adenocarcinoma patients were equal to that of UC patients. For stage II and III disease, adenocarcinoma patients had even better outcome. Muscle-invasive SCC patients showed worse survival regardless of stage. In SA-BC, Ghoneim et al (2008) demonstrated that SCC (1345 patients) had 10 year overall survival rate (OS) of 53.05% (95% CI: 51-57) compared to 48.49% (44-53 for pure UC (705 patients) and 51.18 % (CI: 45-58) for adenocarcinoma (262 patients). Those patients who had UC with squamous or adenomatous metaplasia (286 patients) showed a lower 10-year OS of 42.78% (CI: 36-49). The lowest 10-year OS was experienced by those patients who had undifferentiated pathology (122 patients) having 10-year OS of 34.23 (CI: 24-45). It is clear from this large-number single institution study that the OS of SCC, UC and adenocarcinoma were similar and having the same profile. They demonstrated that although the univariate analysis was significant (Undifferentiated carcinoma had much lower OS), the multivariate analysis proved that tumor cell type is not an independent working factor determining the OS. The only significant prognostic factors were stage, grade and pelvic nodal involvement. Many authors cautiously concluded that RC treatment end-results were not affected by tumor histology or etiology but affected by other prognostic factors like stage, grade, nodal involvement, lymphovascular invasion, angiogenesis, P53, P21, Retinoblastoma genes (Rb) and other biological factors. These prognostic and predictor factors were shown in many SA-BC and SNA-BC studies to have varying weight effect (Ghoneim et al, 2008,Scosyrev et al, 2009,Ploeg et al, 2010 & Zaghloul, 2010).

13. Preoperative and postoperative radiotherapy

The rationale of preoperative radiotherapy is to prevent intraoperative seeding of tumor cells in the operative field and to sterilize microscopic extensions in the perivesical tissues. In the English literature, there are 6 randomized trials addressing the issue of adding preoperative radiotherapy to RC. Two of these 6 studies were on SABC (Awwad et al, 1979 & Ghoneim et al, 1985). Only one (Awwad et al, 1979) showed the benefit of adding preoperative radiotherapy. Most of the other 5 studies showed this effect on high stage and high grade tumors. On the other hand, there were no differences in statistical values in earlier cases. Meta-analysis of these randomized studies showed a corrected odd ratio of 0.94 (95% CI: 0.57-1.55), indicating no benefit for adding preoperative radiotherapy in BC (Huncharek et al,1998).

Postoperative radiotherapy (PORT) has the advantage of dealing with microscopic cells that are easier to sterilize. It allows better identification of the group of patients that may benefit from this adjuvant therapy. One large prospective randomized trial proved the benefit of PORT in locally advanced SA-BC. The 5-year disease-free survival (DFS) rate was 49 and 44 % for hyperfractionated (HF) and conventional fractionation (CF) PORT, respectively compared with 25% for cystectomy alone patients (Zaghloul et al,1992). This effect was constant across all tumor cell type, all muscle-invasive stages and grades in SA-BC. These results were replicated in a non-randomized prospective controlled Radiation Therapy Oncology Group (RTOG) trial on SNA-BC (Reisinger et al,1992). The results ot the 2 studies were nearly identical when compared stage by stage (Zaghloul, 1994). The only difference was the high GIT late complication rate reported by Reisinger et al study. They reported 37% (15 out of 40 patients) developed intestinal obstruction after PORT. Nine out of these 15 patients required surgery and 3 died. On the contrary, Zaghloul et al (1992) reported 5% and 18% all grades of late GIT complications for the HF and CF respectively. Only 4% and 5% out of the HF and CF group respectively necessitated surgical interference. Similar low levels of late GIT complications were experienced by other retrospective studies reported on SA-BC and SNA-BC (Cozzarini et al,1999, Zaghloul et al,2002, Zaghloul et al, 2006).

Abdel Moneim et al (2011) compared, in a prospective randomized trial, preoperative and postoperative radiotherapy in SA-BC. They administered the same dose of 50 Gy in 5 weeks to both groups. The study reported both similar treatment end-results and late complication rates for the two randomized pre- and postoperative groups.

14. Neoadjuvant and adjuvant chemotherapy

Neoadjuvant and adjuvant chemotherapy have been utilized in bladder cancer, in an attempt to improve the outcome for patients with high risk muscle-invasive disease. At least 50% of these patients developed distant metastasis after radical cystectomy. Several meta-analysis of prospective, randomized trials indicated that patients undergoing neoadjuvant chemotherapy with methotrexate, vinblastine, doxorubicin and cisplatin (MVAC) prior to cystectomy have an approximate 5.0 - 6.5 % survival advantage over those who underwent surgery alone (Winquist et al, 2004 & Vaughn et al, 2005). However, some investigators still argue that this neoadjuvant advantage is small and chemotherapy might be better targeted to those at highest risk of relapse after surgery. Furthermore, many elderly patients or who have comorbidities will not tolerate MVAC chemotherapy. Therefore, many investigators tried adjuvant chemotherapy in a supposed more favorable situation. In reality, adjuvant

chemotherapy yielded a modest, statistically significant improvement in survival over cystectomy alone (Vale, 2006 & Ruggeri et al, 2006).
The Egyptian bladder cancer cooperative group compared Neoadjuvant chemotherapy using gemcitabine-cisplatin regimen to cystectomy alone in 109 SA-BC patients, in a prospective controlled randomized study. The one-year survival rate was 54% for the cystectomy alone patients compared to 69% for the neoadjuvant chemotherapy patients (Khaled et al, 2003).

15. Bladder preservation trimodality treatment

Since the late 1980s, many centers investigated the bladder preservation strategy as an alternative to radical cystectomy. The rationale of this strategy depends on 3 goals: first, eradication of the local disease, second, elimination of potential micrometastasis and third, maintenance of the best possible quality of life (QoL) through organ preservation (Rodel, 2004). Several treatment protocols were carried out by different investigators. However, they all characterized 3 main and essential procedures with varying timing and varying minute details. The first main procedure is maximal TURBT. This is to be followed by neoadjuvant chemotherapy or radiochemotherapy (second procedure) and then after cystoscopic assessment, followed by either radical radiotherapy or consolidation radiochemotherapy for the complete responders (third procedure). There was another group treated with radiochemotherapy after TURBT. Cystoscopic assessment will segregate the complete responder (CR) for bladder-conserving management and those showing less than CR to undergo salvage cystectomy (Zaghloul and Mousa,2010). The 5-year OS rates ranged between 39% and 58% and the 5-year survival with native bladder preservation ranged from 36% to 43% (Tester et al, 1993,Kachnic et al, 1997, Shipley et al, 1998, Sauer et al, 1998 & Arias et al, 2000). Saba et al (2010) reported similar results for UC (SA-BC and SNA-BC) in Egypt using a trimodality treatment. Complete remission was achieved in 79% of cases after initial radiochemotherapy using gemcitabine- cisplatin regimen. The 5-year OS rate for patients with initial CR was 68% which is comparable to the results in SNA-BC in the western countries treated with trimodality therapy. Moreover, Sabba et al (2010) found that the association with schistosomiasis had no significant impact on the results of therapy for their patients.

16. References

Abdel MM, Hassan A, El-Sewedy S. Human bladder cancer, schistosomiasis, N-nitroso compounds and their precursors,International Journal of Cancer 2000; 88: 682–683.

Abdel Wahab AH, Abo-Zeid HI, El-Husseini MI, Ismail M, El-Khor AM. Role of loss of heterozygosity on chromosomes 8 and 9 in the development and progression of cancer bladder. J Egypt Natl Canc Inst. 2005; 17(4):260-9.

Adjei AA. Blocking oncogenic Ras signaling for cancer therapy. J Natl Cancer Inst 2001; 93: 1062-1074.

Albertson DG, Pinkel D. Genomic microarrays in human genetic disease and cancer. Hum Mol Genet 2003;12: 145-152.

Ali-El-Dein B. Oncological outcome after radical cystectomy and orthotopic bladder substitution in women. Eur J Surg Oncol. 2009 ;35(3):320-5.

Arias F, Domínguez MA, Martínez E, et al. Chemoradiotherapy for muscle invading bladder carcinoma. Final report of a single institutional organ-sparing program. Int J Radiat Oncol Biol Phys. 2000 ;47(2):373-8

Armengol G, Eissa S, Lozano JJ, Shoman S, Sumoy L, Caballı´n MR, Knuutila S. Genomic imbalances in Schistosoma-associated and non Schistosoma-associated bladder carcinoma: an array comparative genomic hybridization analysis. Cancer Genet Cytogenet 2007;177: 16-19.

Awwad HK, Baki HA, El Bolkainy *et al.*: Preoperative irradiation of T3 carcinoma in Bilharzial bladder. *Int. J. Radiat. Oncol. Biol.Phys.* 1979; 5: 787–794.

Badawi AF, Mostafa MH, Prober tA,. O'ConnorPJ. Role of schistosomiasis in human bladder cancer: evidence of association, aetiological factors, and basic mechanisms of carcinogenesis, European Journal of Cancer Prevention 1995;4: 45–49.

Balsara BR, Pei J, -Testa JR. Comparative genomic hybridization analysis. Methods Mol Med 2002;68:45-57.

Bassi P, Ferrante GD, Piazza N *et al.* Prognostic factors of outcome after radical cystectomy for bladder cancer, a retrospective study of homogenous patient cohort. *J. Urol.* 1999; 161, 1494–1497

Botelho M, FerreiaAC, Olivieira MJ, Domingues A, Machado JC, de Costa JM. Schistosoma haematobium total antigen and decreased apoptosis of normal epithelial cells. Int. J Parasitol 2009;39: 1083-1091.

Botelho MC, Machado JC, deCosta JM. Schistosoma hematobium and bladder cancer. Virulence 2010; 1: 2, 84-87.

Bridge JA, Sandberg AA. Cytogenetic and molecular genetic techniques as adjunctive approaches in the diagnosis of bone and soft tissue tumors. Skeletal Radiol 2000;29: 249-58.

Chaudhary KS, Lu KS, Abel PD, et al. Expression of bcl-2 and p53 oncoproteins in schistosomiasis-associated transitional and squamous cell carcinoma of the urinary bladder, British Journal of Urology 1997;79: 78–84.

Cheng L, Weaver AL, Leibovich BC et al. Predicting the survival of bladder carcinoma patients treated with radical cystectomy. Cancer 2000;88: 2326-2332.

Cheng L , Zhang D. Molecular genetic pathology. Humana Press/Sprnger, NY, USA 2008.

Cheng L, Davidson D, Mac Lennan GT, et al. The origin of Urothelial cancer. Exp Review Anticancer Ther 2010; 10 (6): 865-880.

Coolen MW, Stirzaker C, Song JZ, et al. Consolidation of the cancer genome into domains of repressive chromatin by long-range epigenetic silencing (LRES) reduces transcriptional plasticity. Nat Cell Biol 2010;12(3):235–246.

Cozzarini C, Pelegrini D, Fallini M *et al.*: Reappraisal of the role of adjuvant radiotherapy in muscle-invasive transitional cell carcinoma of the bladder.Int. J. Radiat. Oncol. Biol. Phys.*1999;* 45:221.

Degtyar P, Neulander E, Zirkin H, et al. Fluorescence in situ hybridization performed on exfoliated urothelial cells in patients with transitional cell carcinoma of the bladder. Urology. 2004;63:398-401.

Dhar NB, Campbell SC, Zippe CD *et al.* Outcomes in patients with Urothelial carcinoma of the bladder with limited pelvic lymph node dissection. BJU Int. 2006; 98(6), 1172–1175.

El-Bolkainy MN, Mokhtar NM,. Ghonim MA, HusseinMH. The impact of schistosomiasis on the pathology of bladder carcinoma, Cancer; 1981;48: 2643–2648.

El-Mekresh MM, el-Baz MA, Abol-Enein H, Ghoneim MA. Primary adenocarcinoma of the urinary bladder: a report of 185 cases. Br J Urol. 1998 ;82(2):206-12.

El-Moneim HA, El-Baradie MM, Younis A, Ragab Y, Labib A, El-Attar I. A prospective randomized trial for postoperative vs. preoperative adjuvant radiotherapy for muscle-invasive bladder cancer. Urol Oncol 2011 Feb 24 [Epub ahead of print]

El-Said A, Omar S, Ibrahim AS. et al. Bilharzial bladder cancer in Egypt. A review of 420 cases of radical cystectomy. Jap J Clin Oncol 1979; 9: 117-122.

El-Sheikh SS, Madaan S, Alhasso A, Abel P, Stamp G, Lalani EN. Cyclooxygenase-2: a possible target in Schistosomaassociated bladder cancer, British Journal of Urology 2001;88:921–927.

Esteller M. Cancer epigenomics: DNA methylomes and histone-modification maps. *Nat Rev Genet.* 2007;8(4):286–298.

Fabarius A, Li R, Yerganian G, Hehlmann R, Duesberg P. Specific clones of spontaneously evolving karyotypes generate the individuality of cancer. Cancer Genet Cytogenet 2008;180: 89-99.

Fadl-Elmula I, Kytola S, Leithy ME, et al. Chromosomal aberrations in benign and malignant bilharzia-associated bladder lesions analyzed by comparative genomic hybridization. BMC Cancer 2002; 2:5.

Feinberg AP, Tycko B. The history of cancer epigenetics. Nat Rev Cancer 2004;4:143-53.

Ferguson A.R., Associated bilharziasis and primary malignant disease of the urinary bladder with observations on a series of forty cases, Journal of Pathology and Bacteriology 1911; 16:76–94.

Ferracin M, Veronese A, Negrini M. Micromarkers: miRNAs in cancer diagnosis and prognosis. Expert Rev Mol Diagn 2010;10:297-308.

Fried B, Reddy A, Mayer D. Helminths in human carcinogenesis. Cancer letters 2011; 305 (2): 239-249.

Gentile JM. Schistosome related cancers: a possible role for genotoxins, Environmental Mutagenesis 1985;7: 775–785.

Gersen SL, Keagle MB. Editors. The principles of clinical cytogenetics. 2nd ed. Totowa. NJ; Humama Press. 2005: 42-43.

Ghoneim MA, Ashamalla AG, Awwad HK, Whitmore WF Jr: Randomized trial of cystectomy with or without preoperative radiotherapy for carcinoma of the bilharzial bladder. J. Urol.1985; 134, 266–268.

Ghoneim MA, El-Mekresh MM, El-Baz MA, El-Attar IA, Ashamallah A. Radical cystectomy for carcinoma of the bladder: critical evaluation of the results in 1,026 cases. J Urol 1997;158:393-399.

Ghoneim MA, Abdel-Latif M, el-Mekresh M *et al.*: Radical cystectomy for carcinoma of the bladder: 2,720 consecutive cases 5 year later. *J. Urol.2008;* 180(1), 121–127.

Gibas Z, Gibas L. Cytogenetics of bladder cancer. Cancer Genetics Cytogenetics 1997;95:108-15.

Gouda I, Mokhtar N, Bilal D, El-Bolkainy T, El-Bolkainy NM. Bilharziasis and bladder cancer: a time trend analysis of 9843 patients. J Egypt Natl Canc Inst. 2007; 19(2):158-62.

Grady WM, Tewari M. The next thing in prognostic molecular markers: microRNA signatures of cancer. Gut 2010; 59:706-8.

Gschwend JE, Dahm P, Fair WR. Disease specific survival as endpoint of outcome for bladder cancer patients following radical cystectomy.Eur Urol. 2002 ; 41(4):440-8.

Gupta NP, Kolla SB, Seth A et al. Radical cystectomy for bladder cancer: A single center experience. Indian J Urol 2008; 24 (1): 54-59.

Hafner C, Knuechel R, Hartmann A, Clonality and multifocal Urothelial carcinoma: 10 years of molecular genetic studies. Int J Cancer 2002; 101: 1-5.

Heim S, Mitelman F. Cancer cytogenetics. 2nd edition. New York: Wiley-Liss Inc., 1995.

Ho CH, Huang CY, Lin WC *et al.*: Radical cystectomy in the treatment of bladder cancer: oncological outcome and survival predictors. J. Formos. Med. Assoc. 2009; 108(11), 872–878.

Hodder SL, Mahmoud AA, Sorenson K, et al. Predisposition to urinary tract epithelial metaplasia in Schistosoma haematobium infection. Am J Trop Med Hyg 2000;63:133-138.

Hoque MO, Lee CC, Cairns P, Schoenberg M, Sidransky D. Genome-wide geneticcharacterization of bladder cancer: a comparison of high-density single-nucleotide polymorphism arrays and PCR-based microsatellite analysis. *Cancer Res.* 2003;63:2216-2222.

Huncharek M, Muscat J, Geschwind JF: Planned preoperative radiation therapy in muscle invasive bladder cancer. Results of metaanalysis. Anticancer Res.1998: 18: 1931–1934.

IARC, Monograph on the evaluation of carcinogenic risks to humans: schistosomes, liver flukes and Helicobacter pylori, WHO: International Agency for Research on Cancer 1994; 61: 9-175.

Jacobs BL, Lee CT, Montie JE. Bladder cancer in 2010: how far have we come? CA Cancer J Clin. 2010;60(4):244-72.

Jemal A, Bray F, Center MM, Ferlay J, Ward E, Forman D. Global cancer statistics. CA Cancer J Clin 2011; 61: 69-90.

Jones PA, Baylin SB. The fundamental role of epigenetic events in cancer. Nat Rev Genet 2002;3:415-28.

Jones PA, Baylin SB. The epigenomics of cancer. *Cell.* 2007;128(4):683–692.

Jones TD, Wang M, Eble JN, et al Molecular evidence supporting field effect in urothelial carcinogenesis. Clin Cancer Res. 2005; 11(18):6512-9.

Kallioniemi A, Kallioniemi OP, Sudar D, Rutovitz D, Gray JW, Waldman F, Pinkel D. Comparative genomic hybridization for molecular cytogenetic analysis of solid tumors. Science 1992;258: 818-821.

Kachnic LA, Kaufman DS, Heney NM, et al. Bladder preservation by combined modality therapy for invasive bladder cancer.J Clin Oncol. 1997 ; 15(3):1022-9.

Kendziorski C, Irizarry RA, Chen KS, Haag JD, Gould MN. On the utility of pooling biological samples in microarray experiments.Proc Natl Acad Sci U S A. 2005;102(12):4252-4257.

Khaled H, Zaghloul M, Ghoneim M, et al: Gemcitabine and cisplatin as neoadjuvant chemotherapy for invasive bladder cancer: Effect on bladder preservation and survival. Proc Am Soc Clin Oncol 2003; 22:411, (abstr 1652).

Khaled H, El-Hattab O, Moneim DA, Kassem HA, Morsi A, Sherif G: A prognostic index (bladder prognostic index) for bilharzial-related invasive bladder cancer. Urol. Oncol. 2005; 23, 254–260.

Koraitim MM, Metwalli NE, Atta MA, El-Sadr. Changing age incidence and pathological types of schistosoma-associated bladder carcinoma. J Urol 1995;154: 1714-1716.

Kuper H, Adami HO, Trichopoulos D. Infections as a major preventable cause of human cancer. J Intern Med 2000; 248: 171-83

Loeb K and Loeb I. The significance of multiple mutation in tumor. Carcinogenesis. 2000;21: 379-385.

Lokeshwar VB, Habuchi T, Grossman HB, et al. Bladder tumor markers beyond cytology: International Consensus Panel on bladder tumor markers. Urology. 2005; 66:35-63.

Lopez-Beltran A, Cheng L. Histologic variants of Urothelial carcinoma: differential diagnosis and clinical implications. Hum Paththol 2006; 37: 1371-1388.

Lughezzani G, Sun M, Jeldres C et al.: Adenocarcinoma versus urothelial carcinoma of the urinary bladder: comparison between pathologic stage at radical cystectomy and cancer-specific mortality. Urology 2010; 75(2):376–381.

Madersbacher S, Hochreiter W, Burkhard F, et al. Radical cystectomy for bladder cancer today: a homogeneous series without neoadjuvant therapy. J Clin Oncol 2003;21:690-696.

Makhyoun NA., El-Kashlan KM, Al-Ghorab MM, Mokhles AS. Aetiological factors in bilharzial bladder cancer, Journal of Tropical Medicine and Hygiene 1971; 74: 73-78.

Manoharan M, Ayyathurai R, Soloway MS: Radical cystectomy for urothelial carcinoma of the bladder: an analysis of perioperative and survival outcome. BJU Int. 2009; 104(9), 1227–1232.

Marletta MA. Mammalian synthesis of nitrite, nitrate, nitric oxide, and nnitrosating agents. Chem Res Toxicol 1988; 1: 249–57.

McConkey DJ, Lee S, Choi W, et al. Molecular genetics of bladder cancer: Emerging mechanisms of tumor initiation and progression. Urol Oncol. 2010; 28(4):429-40.

Ministry of Health and Population, Egypt, Department of Endemic Diseases, Prevalence of schistosomiasis in Egypt over time, 2004.

Muscheck M, Abol-Enein H, Chew K, Moore D 2nd, Bhargava V, Ghoneim MA, Carroll PR, Waldman FM. Comparison of genetic changes in schistosome-related transitional and squamous bladdercancers using comparative genomic hybridization. Carcinogenesis 2000; 21:1721-1726.

Nielsen ME, Gonzalgo ML, Schoenberg MP, Getzenberg RH. Toward critical evaluation of the role(s) of molecular biomarkers in the management of bladder cancer. World J Urol. 2006; 24:499-508.

Nishiyama H, Habuchi T, Watanabe J, Teramukai S, Tada H, Ono Y, Ohshima S, Fujimoto K, Hirao Y, Fukushima M, Ogawa O. Clinical outcome of a large-scale multi-institutional retrospective study for locally advanced bladder cancer: a survey including 1131 patients treated during 1990-2000 in Japan. Eur Urol 2004;45: 176-181.

Niu HT, Xu T, Zhang YB et al.: Outcomes for a large series of radical cystectomies for bladder cancer. Eur. J. Surg. Oncol. 2008; 34(8), 911–915.

Ploeg M, Aben KK, Hulsbergen-van de Kaa CA *et al.*: Clinical epidemiology of nonurothelial bladder cancer: analysis of The Netherlands Cancer Registry. *J. Urol.*2010; 183(3), 915-920.

Reisinger S, Mohiuddin M, Mulholland S: Combined pre- and post-operative adjuvant radiation therapy for bladder cancer – a ten year experience. Int. J. Radiat. Oncol. Biol.Phys. 1992; 24: 463-468.

Rödel C. Current status of radiation therapy and combined-modality treatment for bladder cancer. Strahlenther Onkol. 2004 ;180(11):701-9.

Rogers CG, Palapattu GS, Shariat SF *et al.*: Clinical outcomes following radical cystectomy for primary nontransitional cell carcinoma for the bladder compared with transitional cell carcinoma of the bladder. *J. Urol.*2006; 175: 2048-2053

Rosin MP, Saad el Din Zaki S, Ward AJ, Anwar WA. Involvement of inflammatory reactions and elevated cell proliferation in the development of bladder cancer in schistosomiasis patients. *Mutat Res* 1994; 305 : 83– 92.

Ross AGP, BartlyPB, Sleigh AC, et al. Schistosomiasis. N Engl J Med, 2002; 346(16): 1212-1220.

Ruggeri EM, Giannarelli D, Bria E et al. Adjuvant chemotherapy in muscle-invasive bladder cancer: a pooled analysis from phase III studies. Cancer 2006; 106:783-788.

Sabaa MA, El-Gamal OM, Abo-Elenen M, Khanam A. Combined modality treatment with bladder preservation for muscle invasive bladder cancer. Urol. Oncol. 2010; 28, 14-20.

Sandberg AA. The chromosomes in human cancer and leukemia. 2nd ed. New York. Elsevier, 1990.

Sandberg AA, Chen Z. Cytogenetic analysis. Methods Mol Med 2001; 55: 3-41

Sandberg AA, Meloni-Ehrig AM. Cytogenetics and genetics of human cancer: methods and accomplishments.Cancer Genet Cytogenet. 2010;203(2):102-26.

Sauer R, Birkenhake S, Kühn R, Wittekind C, Schrott KM, Martus P. Efficacy of radiochemotherapy with platin derivatives compared to radiotherapy alone in organ-sparing treatment of bladder cancer. Int J Radiat Oncol Biol Phys. 1998 ;40(1):121-7

Scosyrev E, Yao J, Messing E: Urothelial carcinoma versus squamous cell carcinoma of bladder: is survival different with stage adjustment? *Urology 2009*; 73: 822-827.

Shokeir AA. Squamous cell carcinoma of the bladder: pathology, diagnosis and treatment. *BJU Int* 2004; 93: 216-20.

Shariat SF, Karakiewicz PI, Palapattu GS. Outcomes of radical cystectomy for transitional cell carcinoma of the bladder: a contemporary series from the Bladder Cancer Research Consortium. J Urol. 2006 ;176(6):2414-22;

Shipley WU, Winter KA, Kaufman DS, et al. Phase III trial of neoadjuvant chemotherapy in patients with invasive bladder cancer treated with selective bladder preservation by combined radiation therapy and chemotherapy: initial results of Radiation Therapy Oncology Group 89-03. J Clin Oncol. 1998 ;16(11):3576-83

Smith JH, Christie JD. The pathobiology of Schistosoma haematobium infection in humans, Human Pathology 1986; 17: 333-345.

Smith JS, Costello JF. A broad band of silence. *Nat Genet*. 2006; 38(5):504-506.

Stein JP, Lieskovsky G, Cote R, et al. Radical cystectomy in treatment of invasive bladder cancer: long-term results in 1,054 patients. J Clin Oncol 2001; 19: 666-675.

Strohmeyer TG, Slamon DJ. Proto-oncogenes and tumor suppressor genes in human urological malignancies, Journal of Urology 1994;151: 479–1497.

Takahashi A, Tsukamoto T, Tobisu K et al.:Radical cystectomy for invasive bladdercancer, results of multi-institutional pooled analysis. Jpn. J. Clin. Oncol. 2004; 34: 14–19.

Teixeira MR. Recurrent fusion oncogenes in carcinomas. Crit Rev Oncogenesis 2006;12:257-71.

Tsutsumi M, Tsai YC, Gonzalgo ML, Nichols PW, Jones PA. Early acquisition of homozygous deletions of p16/p19 during squamous cell carcinogenesis and genetic mosaicism in bladder cancer. Oncogene 1998;17:3021-3027.

Tricker AR, Mostafa MH, Spiegelhalder B, Preussmann R. Urinary excretion of nitrate, nitrite and N-nitroso compounds in schistosomiasis and bilharzial bladder cancer patients, Carcinogenesis1989; 10 : 547–552.

Tester W, Porter A, Asbell S et al. Combined modality program with possible organ preservation for invasive bladder carcinoma: results of RTOG protocol 85–12. Int. J. Radiat. Oncol. Biol. Phys.1993; 25(5), 783–790.

Vale CL. Advanced Bladder Cancer Meta-analysis Collaboration. Adjuvant chemotherapy for invasive bladder cancer. Cochrane Database Syst Rev2006:CD006018.

van Rhijn BW, van der Poel HG, van der Kwast TH. Urine markers for bladder cancer surveillance: a systematic review. Eur Urol. 2005;47:736-748.

Vaughn DJ, Malkowicz SB. Neoadjuvant chemotherapy in patients with invasive bladder caner. Urol Clin North Am. 2005; 32: 231-237.

Vauhkonen H, Bohling T, Eissa S, Shoman S, Knuutila S. Can bladder adenocarcinomas be distinguished from schistosomiasisassociated bladder cancer by using comparative genomic hybridization analysis? Cancer Genet Cytogenet 2007;177:153-157.

Wang N. Methodologies in cancer cytogenetics and molecular cytogenetics. Am J Med Genet 2002;115:118-24.

Wijnhoven BPL, Michael MZ, Watson DI. MicroRNAs and cancer.Br J Surg 2007;94:23-30Winquist E, Kichner TS, Segal R et al. Neoadjuvant chemotherapy for transitional cell carcinoma of the bladder: a systematic review and meta-analysis. J Urol 2004; 171: 561-569.

Wu XR. Urothelial tumorigenesis: a tale of divergent pathway. Nat Rev Cancer 2005;5: 713-725.

Yunis JJ, Soreng AL. Constitutive fragile sites and cancer. Science 1984;226:1199–204.

Zaratiegui M, Irvine DV, Martienssen RA. Noncoding RNAs and gene silencing. Cell. 2007;128(4):763–776.

Zarzour AH, Selim M, Abd-Elsayed AA, Hameed DA, Abdelaziz MA. Muscle invasive bladder cancer in Upper Egypt: the shift in risk factors and tumor characteristics. BMC Cancer 2008; 8: 250-255.

Zaghloul MS: Radiation as adjunctive therapy to cystectomy for bladder cancer.Is there a difference for bilharzial association? Int. J. Radiat. Oncol. Biol. Phys.1994; 28: 783.

Zaghloul, M.S.,: Distant metastasis from bilharzial bladder cancer. Cancer 77: 743-749, 1996.

Zaghloul MS : Adjuvant radiation therapy for locally advanced bladder cancer. Touchbriefings, US oncological disease 2006 issue 2, 86-9.

Zaghloul MS. Adjuvant and neoadjuvant radiotherapy for bladder cancer: revisited. Future Oncol. 2010; 6(7):1177-1191.

Zaghloul MS, Mousa AG. Trimodality treatment for bladder cancer: does modern radiotherapy improve the end results? Expert Rev Anticancer Ther. 2010 ;10(12):1933-44

Zaghloul MS, Awwad HK, Omar S et al.: Postoperative radiotherapy of carcinoma in bilharzial bladder. Improved disease-free survival through improving local control. Int.J. Radiat. Oncol. Biol. Phys.1992; 22: 511–517.

Zaghloul MS, Mohran TZ, Saber RA, Agha N: Postoperative radiotherapy in bladder cancer. J. Egypt. Nat. Cancer Inst.2002; 14: 161–168.

Zaghloul MS, Nouh A, Nazmy M, Ramzy S, Zaghloul A, Sedira MA, Khalil E. Long-term results of primary adenocarcinoma of the urinary bladder: a report on 192 patients. Urol Oncol 2006; 24:13-20.

Zaghloul MS, El Baradie Nouh MA, Abdel-Fatah S, Taher A and Shalaan M. Prognostic index for primary adenocarcinoma of the urinary bladder. Gulf J Oncol 2007. 1 (2), 47- 54.

Zaghloul MS, Nouh A, Moneer M, El-Baradie M, Nazmy M, Younis A. Time-trend in epidemiological and pathological features of schistosoma-associated bladder cancer. J Egypt Natl Canc Inst. 2008 ;20(2):168-74..

10

Role of HPV in Urothelial Carcinogenesis: Current State of the Problem

G.M. Volgareva, V.B. Matveev and D.A. Golovina
N.N. Blokhin Cancer Research Center of the Russian Academy of Medical Sciences,
Russia

1. Introduction

Human papillomaviruses (HPV) of the so-called high risk types (HR-HPV) cause cervical cancer (CC). Carcinomas in other organs such as vagina, vulva, penis, oropharynx and rectum are known to be aetiologically heterogeneous with respect to HPV (zur Hauzen, 2000, 2008; Gillison & Shah, 2003; International Agency for Research on Cancer [IARC], 2008). HPV-positive cancer in those organs including cervix uteri differs from HPV-negative one in molecular-genetic profile, morphology as well as in clinical peculiarities (Morrison et al., 2001; Gillison & Shah, 2003).

Carcinogenicity of the HR-HPV is determined by two viral genes, E6 and E7. Their expression is recognized as a necessary condition for conversion of virus-infected cell from normal to malignant state. Viral oncoproteins E6 and E7 can interact with various cellular proteins and thus preclude their normal functioning. Among numerous activities of viral oncoproteins the following two are usually regarded as principal ones. E7 is capable of binding to retinoblastoma protein pRb, and E6 can interact with p53. Therefore both above mentioned tumor suppressors become inactivated and then degraded. Cellular functions such as proliferation, apoptosis, DNA repair etc., controlled by pRb and p53, become disturbed (zur Hauzen, 2000, 2008; IARC, 2008).

Since CC is a frequent female malignancy many research groups were occupied in search of early diagnostic markers for this cancer type. Experience thus obtained extends usually to HPV-associated carcinomas of other organs after necessary validation. Attempts to detect HR-HPV DNA by PCR did not leads in those studies to designing of a reliable diagnostic test because cancer *in situ* and invasive CC developed in a small proportion of women with HR-HPV-positive dysplasia (zur Hauzen, 2000). So specificity of the given approach turned out to be low despite the known very high PCR sensitivity. Current attempts to improve early diagnostics of CC and some other HPV-associated cancers are mostly focused on search of genes in virus-infected host cell whose expression becomes unconvertably altered under the influence of viral oncoproteins (Santin et al., 2005).

One of these genes is *INK4a* encoding p16^{INK4a} protein, an inhibitor of cyclin D-dependent kinases Cdk 4/6 (Serrano et al., 1993). *INK4a* transcription in displastic and cancer cells becomes much more active in comparison with its level in normal epithelium being triggered by HR-HPV oncoprotein E7; the content of p16^{INK4a} in a cell increases correspondingly (Li et al., 1994; Khleif et al., 1996; Sano et al., 1998; Kaneko et al., 1999; Klaes et al., 2001). This phenomenon formed experimental grounds for the immunohistochemical test which is currently widely applied in early CC diagnostics (Klaes et al., 2001, 2002; Milde-Langosch et al., 2001; Volgareva et al., 2002, 2004, 2006). This test is becoming popular in diagnostics of HR-HPV-associated carcinomas of other localizations (Begum et al., 2007; Kim et al., 2007).

Bladder cancer (BC) takes 7-th place in the global cancer incidence making up ~ 2-5% of all neoplasms. BC is 2.5-6 times more frequent in men than in women: 260000 new BC cases are registered annually among men and only 76000 among women. Bladder tumors are rare in people under 35 years old; however BC has become younger recently (Parkin et al., 2003). It seems reasonable to mention in this connection the data of Scandinavian investigators (Litlekalsoy et al., 2007) concerning dynamics of the BC molecular markers. They reported that significant shift in the BC molecular profile occurred during 70 years. This shift possibly reflects some alterations in the set of BC causative factors which might have taken place during these years.

In Russia BC makes up ~ 3 % of all malignant tumors; the trend has been registered for the steady elevation of new cases number (Chissov et al., 2010). Mortality among male BC patients in Russia is higher (> 7 in many regions) than the highest indices for countries from the WHO mortality list; as to female BC patiens, mortality figures do not differ in this group from those in other European countries (Zaridze, 2009).

BC development is a multistage process with unpredictable course. Several risk factors for BC are known (Zaridze et al., 1992; Dinney et al., 2004). Among these factors are: geographic region (BC morbidity may vary worldwide up to tenfold); professional occupation (there are about 40 professions at high risk); smoking; nutritional habits and drinking water quality; use of certain medicines; parasitic diseases caused by some Trematoda (Schistosomas). Possible significance of some other factors is still under discussion including irradiation, hereditary predisposition, some other.

Association of some biological agents with BC development might be suggested from results of one study in ~ 6000 patients cohort (Adami et al., 2003). Various organs had been transplanted to those patients with consequent immunosuppressor treatment. BC incidence in this group turned out to be 2-4 times higher as compared with corresponding index for the population as a whole. Carcinomas with proven causative role of HPV occurred in this group of patients even more frequently. Thus prevalence of vulvar and vaginal cancer was 20 times higher than expected one, and that for rectal and oropharyngeal cancer – 10 and 5 times higher, respectively.

The problem of HPV involvement in urinary bladder carcinogenesis is not novel. Historically one of the first indications to the possible linkage between these viruses and BC was the fact that secondary BC occurrence in women with primary CC was significantly higher (five to six-fold) than its occurrence in general population (Bailar, 1963; Newell et al., 1974, 1975). The interpretation of that data in favor of real HPV involvement in urothelial carcinogenesis became possible later after the discovery of HR-HPV carcinogenicity for cervical epithelium by H. zur Hausen and co-authors (Durst et al., 1983, zur Hauzen, 2000, 2008). However definitive commentary on those results as proving HPV carcinogenicity for urinary bladder is still difficult due to the known fact that both CC and BC are more frequent among smoking women.

One more evidence in favour of HPV involvement into BC development was obtained in observations carried out on immunodeficient patients with benign or malignant bladder

neoplasms where HPV DNA was found (Del Mistro et al., 1988; Kitamura et al, 1988; Querci della Rovere et al., 1988; Maloney et al., 1994).
The International Expert Group on HPV selected over twenty studies dedicated to HPV role in BC which had been published in 1991-2001 worldwide. The authors had detected HPV DNA in BC specimens by PCR, *in situ* hybridization and/or Southern blot hybridization. Percentage of HPV-positive cases in these communications varied from 0 up to 82.6 %. Therefore the experts included BC into the category of cancers for which aetiological role of HPV remains unclear – "inadequate evidence" (IARC, 2008).

2. The recent data warn against HPV underestimation as a risk factor in urinary bladder carcinogenesis

Several researchers have published recently some data proving topicality of the HPV problem in BC aetiology (Barghi et al., 2005; Yang et al., 2005; Helal Tel et al., 2006; Moonen et al., 2007; Badawi et al., 2008).
Thus ~ 36 % of transitional-cell BC specimens from Iran (21 out of 59 studied) harboured HPV DNA (Barghi et al., 2005). HPV 18 predominated over other types of the viruses (it was found in 17 patients out of 21, - 81 %); - viruses of the given type are second most frequent causative agents for CC (the first place belongs to HPV16). Urinary bladder tissues from 20 non-oncological patients were taken for control in this study and HPV18 DNA was detected in 1 patient with heavy cystitis. Possibility of precancerous alterations in the latter case could not be ruled out. The authors concluded that HPV may play role of a causative BC factor.
Similar was the opinion by the researchers from the Netherlands who carried out study of BC specimens from 107 patients and found DNA of various HPV types in ~ 15 %; HR-HPV DNA was detected in ~ 8 % (Moonen et al., 2007). Percentage of HR-HPV DNA-positive specimens increased with progression of clinical stage of BC (Ta, T1 and T2-T4), making 0, 12.5 and 18.2 % respectively
Group of investigators from Egypt and USA presented data on HPV-positivity of 27 Schistosoma-associated BC cases (Yang et al., 2005). All of them harboured HPV16. Highly sensitive variety of PCR was used in the study. The results reported by another group from Egypt (Helal Tel et al., 2006) differ dramatically from the data of H. Yang et al. These authors found HPV 16/18 DNA in a single Schistosoma-associated BC specimen (squamous cancer *in situ*) out of 64 studied. Much lower sensitivity of *in situ* hybridization used in the last study for HPV DNA detection in comparison with the method used by H. Yang et al. may be responsible for such a sharp data discrepancy. The total sum of BC specimens examined by A. Helal Tel et al. was 114 including 67 transitional-cell, 32 squamous and 15 other. The above mentioned case was the only HPV-positive BC in this study. The results obtained enabled the authors to conclude that HPV do not play any significant role in pathogenesis of urinary bladder in Egypt.
The data reported by these two research groups, H. Yang et al. and A. Helal Tel et al. and mutually exclusive inferences made by the investigators warn against underestimation of HPV as a risk factor in BC genesis. Essential in this connection is the fact that results reported by H. Yang et al. were confirmed recently by another research group from Egypt (Badawi et al., 2008). The authors using PCR detected HR-HPV DNA (belonging to types 16,18 and 52) more frequently in BC specimens than in urothelial biopsies from cystitis patients. The PCR data were compared with the data on antibody to HPV16 protein L1

detection in blood serum of the HPV16-positive BC patients; perfect coincidence of these results took place. The association was observed in this study between HPV-positivity of BC and its propensity for relapse. The authors concluded that HPV participates in BC genesis in combination with other risk factors, including Schistosomas which were commonly found in the group of patients examined. The authors recommend detection of antibodies to HPV L1 to optimize the treatment of BC patients and their further follow-up .

3. Aspects of the problem to be addressed

Thus a glimpse into the problem of HPV role in BC gives idea of its complexity. Therefore we rise the following questions:

1. What reasons may be the for conflicting data communicated by different research groups? Are there any ways to optimize the methodology of the study and get uniform data?
2. What is the incidence of HPV-positivity among urothelial dysplasia and BC specimens obtained from Russian patients keeping in mind ethno-geographic BC heterogeneity?
3. Have there been any attempts to investigate the role of papillomaviruses in urothelial carcinogenesis in experimental models?
4. What benefits may it bring to practical oncourology provided that a certain role of HPV in BC is accepted by medical community?

4. What reasons may be for conflicting data communicated by different research groups? Are there any ways to optimize the methodology of the study and get uniform data?

The authors usually explain the conflicting data character by different research groups by either of the following factors:

1. objective ethno-geographic heterogeneity of BC and
2. technical peculiarities of studies.

Concerning the first factor, a relationship seems to be evident between the state of the excretory organ lining, on the one hand, and environmental factors such as drinking water quality, regional and ethnic specificity of food, endemic urinary bladder parasitic diseases, etc., on the other hand. Each of these factors may influence the HPV-BC association rate. This statement could be verified by comparison of HPV-positivity in BC from different regions worldwide done by the same research group with unified technical approaches. Such studies have never been carried out as far as we know .

The second group of factors includes small numbers of specimens tested in some works; application of a single test for viral DNA detection (most commonly PCR or *in situ* hybridization, wherein both techniques have benefits and limitations); detection of only one or two HPV types, usually HPV16 and HPV18, which are most frequent in CC, while other HPV types might be involved in carcinogenesis in urinary bladder. The data by C. De Gaetani et al. prove the latter point (De Gaetani et al., 1999). Using *in situ* hybridization with probe to 31/33/35 viral types the authors detected HPV DNA positivity in 60 % of BC specimens, while the index turned out to be 24 % with probe to the types 16/18 .

In addition, a predominant majority of groups which publish data on high incidence of HR-HPV DNA in BC made no attempts to confirm viral genome expression and in particular *E6/E7* expression.

Contamination should be mentioned also besides the above-listed factors. It may be either laboratory (admixing of products of viral genome amplification to the samples under study) or patient related. The former is a well-known source of false-positivity of PCR data. Possibility of the latter is to be kept in mind in studies of BC specimens particularly. If any adjacent organ (vulva, penis, urethra) is HPV-infected, casual bladder contamination with HPV-harbouring cell(s) might occur through blood during surgical operation or by endoscope during cystoscopy. False HPV-positivity data may occur both in PCR done to screen materials for viral DNA presence and in reverse-transcription PCR (RT-PCR) study of viral genome expression as well.

Thereby complex approach seems to be reasonable to study possible HPV role in urothelial carcinogenesis. Techniques are reasonable which enable to detect DNA not only of HPV16 and HPV18 but of other types of viruses as well. To check up whether viral oncogenes *E6* and *E7* are expressed in DNA-HPV-positive specimens methods seem to be appropriate of both viral mRNA *E6/E7* detection (by RT-PCR) and viral oncoproteins E6 and E7 revelation (by immunohistochemistry). In female BC cases it may be reasonable to examine patient's cervical epithelium for HPV infection.

5. What is the incidence of HPV-positivity among urothelial dysplasia and BC specimens obtained from Russian patients?

The given section presents data of two independent studies of Russian patients with urinary bladder oncological conditions including results of our own complex approach to HPV detection in BC specimens.

5.1 Attempts to determine occurrence of HPV-positivity in bladder urothelium

DNA of HPV16 and HPV18 was found in ~ 50 % of urinary bladder dysplasia and carcinoma in situ specimens by in situ hybridization; an attempt to detect HPV of other types (6, 11, 31, 33 and 51) gave negative results (Frank et al., 2002).

We have screened 130 transitional BC specimens (1-3 grade) obtained by transurethral resections for HPV DNA using several PCR versions with primers to *L1*, *E6* and *E7* genes of the viral genome (Volgareva et al., 2007, 2008, 2009; Trofimova et al., 2009). Our tests included application of literary primers My09/11 and GP5-GP6 to *L1* enabling one to detect HPV of various types; these primer sets are commonly used in similar studies (Resnik et al., 1990; van den Brule et al., 1990). HPV16 genetic material was found in ~ 40% of the specimens tested, DNA of other HPV types was not found. Viral genome expression was confirmed at the level of mRNA by RT-PCR in some of the specimens (Volgareva et al., 2009; Trofimova et al., 2009). Viral oncoprotein E7 was spotted by immunohistochemistry in ~30% of DNA HPV16-positive cases (Cheng et al., 2009; Volgareva et al., 2009 a,b). BC specimens stained positively with polyclonal anti-E7 HPV16 serum (done by Fiedler et al., 2004) turned out to be positive also when stained by monoclonal antibodies to HPV16 E6 and E7 from Neodiagnostic (Cheng et al., 2009). Five examples of BC specimens' screening for HPV are presented in Table 1 and Figure 1.

The fact that HPV16 oncoprotein E7 is detected in ~30% of BC specimens means that HPV16 plays some role in urothelial carcinogenesis in Russian patients. However in case of urothelial malignization some deviations there seem to exist from the known role of these viruses in cervical carcinogenesis. Signs testifying to the truth of the given assumption are as follows.

Case No	DNA*	RNA**	Protein E7*** (type of staining)
1	-	not studied	-
2	+	+	+ (diffuse)
3	+	+	+ (diffuse)
4	+	-	+ (focal)
5	+	-	+ (focal)

* HPV DNA was detected by PCR, viral typing carried out either by PCR with type-specific primers or by restriction fragment length polymorphism test (Astori et al.,1997). Specimens 2-5 appeared to harbour DNA of HPV16.
** reverse-transcription PCR was carried out with primers to E6/E7 HPV16.
*** immunohistochemical staining was performed with polyclonal serum to HPV16 oncoprotein E7 (Fiedler et al., 2004). The type of staining was either diffuse (over 25% of stained cells in a cancer tissue) or focal (less than 25% of stained cancer cells).

Table 1. Data of the complex approach to HPV detection in five BC specimens. Case 1: Transitional BC relapse, focuses of squamous metaplasia, 3-d grade, muscle-invasive. Case 2: Transitional BC, 3-d grade, muscle-invasive. Case 3: Transitional BC, 2-d grade, submucosal invasion, no muscle cells on the slide. Case 4: Transitional BC, focuses of squamous metaplasia, 2-3-d grade, growth within mucous layer, no invasion into muscle. Case 5. Transitional BC, 3-d grade, submucosal invasion, no muscle cells on the slide.

Firstly, along with BC specimens expressing viral oncoprotein E7 in a predominant majority of cancer cells throughout cancer tissue (as was usually the case with CC in our previous studies, - the so-called "diffuse staining"; - Volgareva et al., 2006) we observed some BC cases in which E7 was registered only in certain groups of cancer cells or in separate cells, - the so-called "focal staining" (Table 1, cases 4 and 5; Fig. 1d,e). It should be underlined in this connection that we confirmed HPV16 genome expression at the level of mRNA by RT-PCR for some of such BC specimens. However it was not in every BC specimen studied that the results of RT-PCR and immunohistochemistry coincided: cases 4 and 5 in Table 1 serve as examples of the lack of the data homogeneity. Focal character of HPV16 genome expression registered immunohistochemically may perhaps be responsible for this discrepancy: HPV16-harbouring cells detected by staining in a certain section of a BC specimen might not occur in another section of the same specimen from which mRNA was obtained. It is also important that in all such specimens HPV16 E7-expressing cells were found in the internal layers of cancer tissue but not at its brims (Fig. 1d,e). This observation enables one to rule out the above-mentioned possibility of the urinary bladder intrapatient contamination with cells of some adjacent HPV-infected organ. Focal HPV16 E7 expression in some BC specimens in our study is in a good agreement with the data by C. De Gaetani et al. on HPV DNA detection in BC by in situ hybridization (De Gaetani et al., 1999). These investigators had at their disposal several biopsy samples for each of ten patients under study. It was from only one out of ten patients that the test results were permanently positive in all biopsies, while in the rest nine cases only a quota of samples was DNA HPV-positive.

Secondly, in some cases of focal E7 expression BC cells contain this viral oncoprotein only in a cytoplasm (Fig 1e). Its ability to get bound to the nuclear pRb remains under question in such cases.

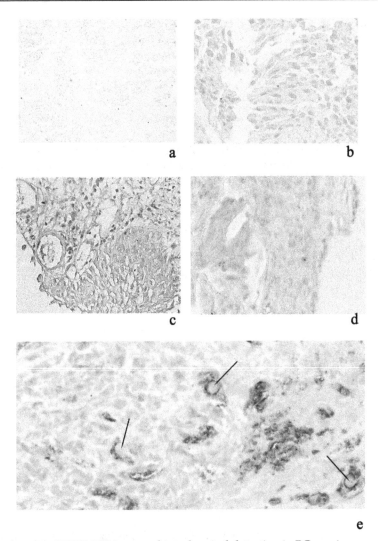

Fig. 1. Results of the HPV16 E7 immunohistochemical detection in BC specimens. Specimens' numbers match to those in Table 1. a Negative reaction with E7-specific serum in specimen N1. b, c Diffuse staining of specimens NN 2 and 3, respectively. d, e Focal staining of specimens NN 4 and 5, respectively. Uncoloured nuclei of three cells expressing E7 in a cytoplasm are indicated with arrows in "e".

Thirdly, the results of our repeated examination of the female patient with relapsing BC turned out to be quite unexpected. In her original tumor removed surgically in 2004 we detected HPV16 DNA, *E7* mRNA as well as protein E7 (the latter spotted independently in two laboratories with different antibodies) (Volgareva et al., 2009 b; Cheng et al., 2009). The patient is a hard smoker. For more than 20 years she had worked at a chemical factory and had been exposed with solvents and aniline dyes. Three BC relapses took place in 2005-2008.

During this period the patient undervent surgery, chemotherapy and BCG treatment. At the next relapse in 2009 we performed repeated study. Neither HPV DNA nor protein E7 were found in BC cells. Colposcopy study was also performed and HPV DNA tested in cervical cells by PCR; the results of both analyses proved absence of HPV in cervical epithelium of the patient (Volgareva et al., 2010a). Could there occur a total clearance from virus-harbouring cells due to surgical and other treatments in this patient? Further observations on similar cases are desirable to answer in the affirmative.

5.2. Study of *INK4a* expression in DNA HPV16-positive bladder cancer specimens
To verify the fact of HPV16 genome expression in 50 DNA HPV16-positive BC specimens we studied cellular *INK4a* expression at the levels of mRNA (Fig. 2) and respective protein p16^{INK4a} (Fig. 3) (Volgareva et al., 2010b). The above mentioned phenomenon of the *INK4a* overexpression indicating to HR-HPV E7 activity in cervical cells served as a rationale. In 12 BC specimens under study the HPV16 *E7* expression had been detected at the mRNA and/or protein level. Five conditionally normal urothelial specimens obtained from the same BC patients were studied as well. In some BC cases associated with HPV16 DNA we detected *INK4a* overexpression at the both levels (Fig. 2, patients A,B and E; Fig. 3c).

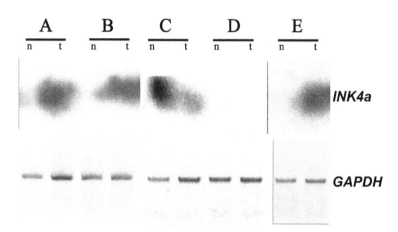

Fig. 2. Analysis of expression of *INK4a* by RT-PCR in BC specimens obtained from five patients (A, B, C, D and E); t - urinary bladder carcinoma, n – morphologically normal tissue adjacent to tumour.
The top-panel electrophoregram developed after Southern blot hybridization with the *INK4a*-specific radio-active probe according to Nguyen and co-authors (Nguyen et al., 2000).
The bottom panel: results with *GAPDH*-specific primers as a control for stability and concentration of RNA; amplification products visualized by staining with ethidium bromide.

Incidence of p16^{INK4a}- overexpressing BC specimens was ~ 10% (Fig. 3c), however as opposed to CC in BC it did not correlate with HPV16 E7 expression in any case (Figures 2c and 3d present lack of such correlation for one and the same BC specimen).

We don't regard this result as evidence disproving the role of HPV in urinary bladder carcinogenesis. The point is, according to literature data, that factors determining *INK4a* expression in HPV-associated BC may differ in essence from those in HPV-positive CC. Thus in BC, in contrast to CC, *INK4a* undergoes frequent deletions, point mutations or promoter methylations (Ruas, Peters, 1998; Aveyard, Knowles, 2004; Gallucci et al., 2007). Due to any of these events its expression at the level of protein $p16^{INK4a}$ may become partly or fully lost. For example, homozygous *INK4a* deletions depriving cell of $p16^{INK4a}$ synthesis were found in ~ 30-50 % of BC specimens (Aveyard, Knowles, 2004; Gallucci et al., 2007). Thus our data might prove unsuitability of $p16^{INK4a}$ for role of the HPV-associated BC marker.

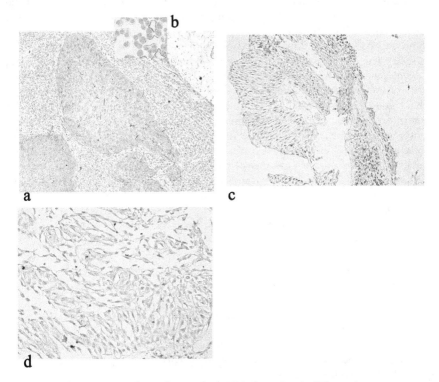

Fig. 3. Results of the immunohistochemical $p16^{INK4a}$ detection in BC specimens.
a. Positive control: HPV16 – harbouring cervical cancer, diffuse staining.
b. Negative control: cells of HCT line (smear), negative reaction with $p16^{INK4a}$-specific antibodies.
c. BC, diffuse staining.
d. BC specimen represented as N3 in Table 1 and "c" in Fig. 1, negative reaction with $p16^{INK4a}$-specific antibodies.

5.3 Summary
The results obtained in two independent samplings of urothelial dysplasia and BC from Russian patients show as a whole that HR-HPV DNA-positivity reaches up to ~ 40-50 %.

Presence of viral DNA in cancer cells is frequently accompanied by expression of viral oncogenes. These results are in agreement with the notion that HR-HPV may take part in BC initiation either solely or in combination with other factors, in particular chemical carcinogens. There are certain reasons still to assume some difference in the action of these viruses in urothelium in comparison with their manifestation in cervical epithelium.

6. Have there been any attempts to investigate the role of papillomaviruses in urothelial carcinogenesis in experimental models?

Urinary bladder similarly to other parts of urinary system (renal pelvis, ureter, etc.) is lined with epithelium of a special kind, the so-called transitional epithelium (Henle epithelium). The question is of particular interest in this connection whether HPV can cause oncogenesis in urinary bladder lining.

M. Campo and co-authors addressed this problem in vivo in cattle (Campo et al., 1992; Campo, 2002). The investigators demonstrated that bovine papillomavirus BPV-2 takes part in BC development under both spontaneous and experimental infection. An important peculiarity of their model is that BPV-associated BC develops commonly in animals being fed with a certain kind of plant, namely bracken fern. Besides BC these animals are affected often with carcinomas in various segments of gastrointestinal tract. When studied particularly bracken fern appeared to contain a number of ingredients which possess mutagenic, carcinogenic and immunosuppressive activities.

The thesis of a species-specific character of papillomavirus infection is well-known (IARC, 2008). In view of this point an exact extrapolation of the data by M. Campo et al. to human papillomaviruses and their possible role in human urothelial oncogenesis seems not quite correct. There are yet some indirect evidences that such extrapolation is not fully groundless. They are as follows. First of all, these researchers found among various histological BC types substantial quota of transitional carcinomas, the type of BC predominating among human patients in many countries including Russia. Secondly, bracken fern similarly to cattle promotes in a human organism carcinogenesis just in gastrointestinal tract. In the regions where it is consumed as food (Brazil in particular) HPV16 is commonly found in dysplasia and carcinoma specimens of esophagus (Campo et al., 1999, as cited in Campo, 2002). Thirdly, transactivation of HPV16 promoter was achieved in experimental model by quercetine, one of the mutagenic ingredients of bracken fern; in such a way it was demonstrated that some types of human cancer in which HPV are being regularly detected may be aetiologically similar to corresponding cancer types of cattle (Campo et al., 1999, as cited in Campo, 2002).

C. Reznikoff and co-authors carried out study on HPV oncogenicity in human urothelial cells in vitro (Reznikoff et al., 1994). The authors transformed isogenic mucosal cells of ureteral uroepithelium obtained from a healthy donor by HPV16 E6 and/or E7 gene(s). Cellular immortalization occurred after the integration of either of these viral oncogenes into host chromosomes. Simultaneous integration of both of them led to similar effect. Phenotypic and genotypic alterations were more prominent in cells immortalized by E6 alone or in combination with E7 than in cells harbouring sole E7. Neither of the transformed cell clones formed tumors when inoculated into nude mice. Some chromosomal alterations found in the transformed cells were identical to karyotype abnormalities found by other researchers in clinical specimens from BC patients. The authors inferred that the phenomena taking place in vitro may correspond to initial stages of urothelial oncogenesis in vivo.

Thus the results obtained in experimental models show that there is no good cause to eliminate papillomaviruses from the list of potential carcinogens in urinary bladder urothelium of Homo sapiens.

7. What benefits may it bring to practical oncourology provided that a certain role of HPV in BC is accepted by medical community?

If this notion is accepted new prospects for BC prevention may come to light. Keeping in mind that efficient vaccines were designed for CC prevention, on the one hand, and that BC is a predominantly male type of cancer, on the other hand, both girls and boys vaccination might become one of such prospects. It is noteworthy in this connection that when the item of reasonability of boys' vaccination is being discussed it is usually being done for the sake of CC prevention in their wives-to-be. Resolution is usually made in the negative in resource-constrained countries. As to the female BC, possibility to prevent women from urothelial carcinogenesis might become an additional convincing argument in favour of their vaccination.

Possible ways of HPV ingress into human urinary bladder lining should be thought over by both clinicians and experimenters. The idea of HPV-associated BC may form grounds for adding of some tests (aimed to detect anogenital HPV) to the currently accepted ways of preoperative check-up of BC patients. This idea may also become the reason to reconsider safety of cystoscope and catheter in treatment of BC patients infected with HPV in anogenital region.

Despite that HPV role in urothelial carcinogenesis is still open-ended question several research groups tried to find an answer to the related one: whether clinical course of BC is affected by HPV presence in urothelial cells.

Y. Andreeva and co-authors studied if papillomaviruses influence relapse incidence in BC patients (Andreeva et al., 2008). The authors preselected 44 BC specimens taken from patients with superficial tumors (stages Ta and T1) on the basis that there occurred koilocytes in these specimens (an indirect morphological sign of viral infection). The specimens were then subdivided into 3 groups: (1) 16 ones from patients with high relapse incidence, (2) 13 - from patients with moderate and (3) 15 - from patients with low relapse incidence. DNA of HPV16 and HPV18 was found by *in situ* hybridization in specimens from patients of the first and second groups only. Seven out of 16 specimens (44%) harboured HPV16 DNA in the first group. Three specimens (23%) were HPV18-positive while HPV16 genetic material was found in neither case in the second group. The authors concluded that HPV occurrence in urothelial cells increases the risk of a superficial BC relapse.

A. Lopes-Beltran and co-authors studied whether HPV DNA presence in cancer cells may influence BC patient survival (Lopes-Beltran et al., 1996). The group of 76 BC patients with transitional BC was formed without any preselection. In materials obtained at transurethral resections the authors detected DNA of HPV6, HPV11, HPV16 and HPV18 using PCR. Follow-up lasted for 5 years. The resultant survival among HPV-positive patients was found to be ~ 29 % (2 out of 7), while among negative ones - 75 % (52 out of 69). The authors concluded that HPV-DNA-positivity serves as a negative predictor of BC patient survival.

The results reported by C. De Gaetani and co-authors (De Gaetani et al., 1999) are in good agreement with those data. The authors found by *in situ* hybridization with the probes to viral types 16/18 and 31/33/35 HPV DNA in 17 out of 43 BC specimens. Follow-up lasted for 72 months. During this time 10 HPV-positive patients died (~59%). Meanwhile 5 out of 26 HPV-negative patients died (~20%).

If HPV contribution to urinary bladder carcinogenesis gains recognition current therapeutic methods might be supplemented in the near future with the administration to the bladder of HPV-positive BC patients of low molecular weight chemical substances inhibiting HPV oncogenes expression. Results of successful studies of such substances in experimental models were presented at the 25-th International papillomavirus conference (Hellner et al., 2009).

8. Conclusion

The problem of HPV involvement in urinary bladder carcinogenesis is still open. In a complex study performed on clinical specimens of dysplasia and carcinoma of urinary bladder from Russian patients with the use of several methods of HPV DNA detection (*in situ* hybridization, PCR with several types of primers) we registered up to 40-50 % of DNA HPV-positive cases. In many cases DNA HPV-positivity was accompanied with expression of viral oncogenes *E6* and *E7* at the levels of mRNA and/or protein. Thus we detected oncoprotein E7 HPV16 known for its ability to interfere with the normal pRb functioning (which leads to unchecked transition of a cell from G1 to S stage of the cell cycle) in every third BC specimen harbouring HPV16 DNA. Results reported by other research groups obtained both in clinical materials and in experimental models *in vivo* and *in vitro* confirm the idea of HPV as a possible causative agent of BC. There are certain signs that role of HPV in urinary bladder carcinogenesis may be somewhat different from their role in CC origination. Their most probable role in urothelial carcinogenesis seems to be partnership in initiation of the process jointly with other agents (such as parasitic helminths, components of cigarette smoke, chemical pollutants of industrial origin, etc.). The notion that HPV in some cases takes part in urinary bladder carcinogenesis may be helpful for BC prevention, prediction of its clinical course and, in prospect, for treatment of HPV-associated BC.

9. Acknowledgements

The authors are grateful to professors V.A. Kobliakov, B.P. Kopnin, B.P. Matveev and A.A. Shtil' for promoting discussions and critical reading of the manuscript and to Dr. V.A. Glazunova for patient assistance in technical work on the manuscript.

10. References

Adami, J., Gabel, H., Lindelof, B., Ekstrom, K., Rydh, B., Glimelius, B., Ekbom, A., Adami, H.O., & Granath, F. (2003). Cancer risk following organ transplantation: a nationwide cohort study in Sweden. *Br. J. Cancer*, Vol. 89, No 7, pp. 1221-1227.

Andreeva, Y.Y., Zavalishina, L.D., Morozov, A.A., Rusakov, I.G., & Frank, G.A. (2008). Localization of HPV DNA in superficial urothelial bladder carcinoma. *Oncourology*, No 1, pp. 34-35, ISSN 1726-9776. (In Russian).

Astori, G., Arzese, A., Pipan, C., de Villiers, E.-M.,& Botta, G.A. (1997). Characterization of a putative new HPV genomic sequence from a cervical lesion using L1 consensus primers and restriction fragment length polymorphism. *Virus Res.*, Vol. 50, No 1, pp. 57-63.

Aveyard, J.S., & Knowles, M.A. (2004). Measurement of relative copy number of CDKN2A/ARF and CDKN2B in bladder cancer by real-time quantitative PCR and multiplex ligation-dependent probe amplification. *J. Mol. Diagnostics*, Vol. 6, No 4, pp. 356-364.

Badawi, H., Ahmed, H., Ismail, A., Diab, M, Moubarak, M, Badawy, A, & Saber, M. (2008). Role of human papillomavirus types 16, 18 and 52 in recurrent cystitis and urinary bladder cancer among Egyptian patients. *Medscape J Med.*, Vol.10 (10), p. 232. Retrieved from: http://www.ncbi.nlm.nih.gov/pmc/articles/PMC2605136/.

Bailar, J.C. (1963). The incidence of independent tumors among uterine cancer patients. *Cancer*, Vol. 16 (Jul.), pp. 842-853.

Barghi, M.R., Hajimohammadmehdiarbab, A., Moghaddam, S.M., & Kazemi B. (2005). Correlation between human papillomavirus infection and bladder transitional cell carcinoma. *BMC Infect. Dis.*, Vol. 5: 102. Retrieved from: http://www.biomedcentral.com/1471-2334/5/102

Begum, S., Gillison, M.L., Nikol, T.L., & Westra W.H. (2007). Detection of human papillomavirus-16 in fine-needle aspirates to determine tumor origin in patients with metastatic squamous cell carcinoma of the head and neck. *Clin Cancer Res.* , Vol. 13, No 4, pp. 1186-1191.

Campo, M.S. (2002). Animal models of papillomavirus pathogenesis. *Virus Res.*, Vol. 89, No 2, pp. 249-261.

Campo, M.S., Jarrett, W.F., Barron, R., O'Neil, B.W., & Smith, K.T. (1992). Association of bovine papillomavirus type 2 and braken fern with bladder cancer in cattle. *Cancer Res.*, Vol. 52, No 24, pp. 6898-6904.

Cheng, S., Hsiao, L., Jung, S., & Volgareva, G.M. (2009). Detection of HPV E6 and E7 oncoproteins in bladder cancers. *Proceedings of the 25-th International Papillomavirus Conference*, Malmo, Sweden, May 2009, P-14.09.

Chissov, V.I, Starinsky, V.V., Petrova, G.V. (Eds.). (2010). *Malignant malformations in Russia (morbidity and mortality).*, P.A. Hertzen Moscow Research Oncological Institute. ISBN 5-85502-024-X, Moscow. (In Russian).

De Gaetani, C., Ferrari, G., Righi, E., Bettelli, S., Migaldi, M., Ferrari, P., & Trentini, G.P. (1999). Detection of human papillomavirus DNA in urinary bladder carcinoma by in situ hybridization. *J. Clin. Pathol.*, Vol. 52, No 2, pp. 103-106.

Del Mistro, A., Koss, L.G., Braunstein, J., Bennett, B., Saccomano, G., & Simons, K.M. (1988). Condyloma acuminata of the urinary bladder. Natural history, viral typing, and DNA content. *Am J Surg Path.*, Vol. 12, No 3, pp.205-212.

Dinney, C.P.N., McConcey, D.J., Millikan, R.E, Wu, X., Bar-Eli, M., Adam, L., Kamat, A.M., SiefkerRadtke, A.O., Tuziak, T., Sabichi, A.L., Grossman, H.B., Benedict, W.F., & Czerniak, B. (2004). Focus on bladder cancer. *Cancer Cell*, Vol.6, No 2, pp.111-116.

Durst, M., Gissmann, L., Ikenberg, H., & zur Hauzen, H. (1983). A papillomavirus DNA from a cervical carcinoma and its prevalence in cancer biopsy samples from different geographic regions. *Proc. Natl Acad. Sci USA*, Vol.80, No 12, pp. 3812-3815.

Fiedler, M., Muller-Holzner, E., Viertler, H.-P., Widschwendter, A., Laich, A., Pfister, G., Spoden, G.A., Jansen-Dürr, P., & Zwerschke, W. (2004). High level HPV-16 E7 oncoprotein expression correlates with reduced pRb-levels in cervical biopsies. *The FASEB Journal*, Vol. 18, No 10; pp 1120-1122. Retrieved from: http://www.fasebj.org/content/early/2004/06/29/fj.03-1332fje.long

Frank, G.A., Zavalishina, L.E., & Andreeva, Iu.Iu. (2002). Immunohistochemical characteristics and a degree of differentiation of urinary bladder cancer. *Arkhiv Patologii*, Vol. 64, No 6, pp. 16-18, ISSN 0004-1955. (In Russian).

Gallucci, M., Vico, E., Merola, R., Leonardo, C, Sperduti, I, Felici, A, Sentinelli, S, Cantiani, R, Orlandi, G, & Cianciulli, A. (2007). Adverse genetic prognostic profiles define a poor outcome for cystectomy in bladder cancer. *Exp. Mol. Pathol.*, Vol. 83, No 3, pp. 385-391.

Gillison, M.L., & Shah, K.V. (2003). Role of mucosal human papillomavirus in nongenital cancers. *J. Natl Cancer Inst. Monographs*, No 31, pp. 57-65.

Helal Tel, A., Fadel, M.T., & El-Sayed, N.K. Human papilloma virus and p53 expression in bladder cancer in Egypt: correlation to schistosomiasis and clinicopathologic factors. (2006). *Pathol. Oncol. Res.*, Vol. 12, No 3, pp. 173-178.

Hellner, K., Baldwin, A., Xian, J., Stein, R., Glicksman, M., & Munger, K. (2009). PAK3 inhibitors identified by high-throughput-screening as therapeutics for HPV-associated cancers. *Proceedings of the 25-th International Papillomavirus Conference*, Malmo, Sweden, May 2009, O-09.05.

IARC Monographs on the Evaluation of Carcinogenic Risks to Humans. Vol. 90. *Human Papillomaviruses*. ISBN 978-92-832-1290-4, Lyon, France, 2007. Retrieved from: http://monographs.iarc.fr/ENG/Monographs/vol90/index.php.

Kaneko, S., Nishioka, J., Tanaka, M., Nakashima, K., & Nobori, T. (1999). Transcriptional regulation of the CDK inhibitor p16[INK4a] gene by a novel pRb-associated repressor, RBAR1. *Biochem Mol Biol Int*. Vol. 47, No 2, pp.205- 215.

Khleif, S.N., DeGregori, J., Yee, C., Otterson G.A., Kaye F.J., Nevins J.R., & Howley P.M. (1996). Inhibition of cyclin D-CDK4/CDK6 activity is associated with an E2F-mediated induction of cyclin kinase inhibitor activity. *Proc Natl Acad Sci USA*. Vol. 93., No 9, pp. 4350-4354.

Kim, S.H., Koo, B.S., Kang, S., Park, K., Kim, H., Lee, M.J., Kim J.M., Choi, E.C., & Cho, N.H. (2007). HPV integration begins in the tonsillar crypt and leads to the alteration of p16, EGFR and c-myc during tumor formation. *Int J Cancer*, Vol. 120, No 7, pp. 1418-1425.

Kitamura, T., Yogo, Y., Ueki, T., Murakami, S, & Aso, Y. (1988). Presence of human papillomavirus type 16 genome in bladder carcinoma in situ of a patient with mild immunodeficiency. *Cancer Res.*, Vol. 48, No 24, pt.1, pp.7207-7211.

Klaes, R., Friedrich, T., Spitkovsky, D., Ridder, R, Rudy, W., Petry, U., Dallenbach-Hellweg, G., Schmidt, D., & von Knebel Doeberitz, M. (2001). Overexpression of p16(INK4a)

as a specific marker for dysplastic and neoplastic epithelial cells of the cervix uteri. *Int J Cancer.* Vol. 92, No 2, pp. 276-284.

Klaes, R., Benner, A., Friedrich, T., Ridder, R., Herrington, S., Jenkins, D., Kurman, R.J., Shmidt, D., Stoler, M., & von Knebel Doeberitz, M. (2002). p16INK4a immunohistochemistry improves interobserver agreement in the diagnosis of cervical intraepithelial neoplasia. *Am J Surg Pathol.*, Vol. 26, No 11, pp. 1389-1399.

Li, Y., Nichols, M.A., Shay, J.W., & Xiong Y. (1994). Transcriptional repression of the D-type cyclin-dependent kinase inhibitor p16 by the retinoblastoma susceptibility gene product pRb. *Cancer Res.*, Vol. 54, No 23, pp. 6078-6082.

Litlekalsoy, J., Vatne, V., Hostmark, J.G., & Laerum, O.D. (2007). Immunohistochemical markers in urinary bladder carcinomas from paraffin-embedded archival tissue after storage for 5-70 years. *Br J Urol Int*, Vol. 99, No 5, pp. 1013-1119.

Lopes-Beltran, A., Escudero, A.L., Vicioso, L., Munoz, E., & Carrasco, J.C. (1996). Human papillomavirus DNA as a factor determining the survival of bladder cancer patients. *Br. J. Cancer*, Vol. 73, No 1, pp. 124-127.

Maloney, K.E., Wiener, J.S., & Walther, P.J. (1994). Oncogenic human papillomaviruses are rarely associated with squamous cell carcinoma of the bladder: evaluation by differential polymerase chain reaction. *J Urol.*, Vol.151, No 2, pp. 360-364.

Milde-Langosch, K., Riethdorf, S., Kraus-Poppinghaus, A., Riethdorf, L., & Loning, T. (2001). Expression of cyclin-dependent kinase inhibitors p16MTS1, p21WAF1, and p27KIP1 in HPV-positive and HPV-negative cervical adenocarcinomas. *Virchows Arch.*, Vol. 439, No 1, pp. 55-61.

Morrison, C., Catania, F., Wakely, P., Jr., & Nuovo, G.J. (2001) Highly differentiated keratinizing squamous cell cancer of the cervix. A rare, locally aggressive tumor not associated with human papillomavirus or squamous intraepithelial lesions. *Am J Surg Path*, Vol. 25, No 10, pp. 1310-1315.

Moonen, P.M., Bakkers, J.M., Kiemeney, L.A. Schalken, JA, Melchers, WJ, & Witjes JA. (2007). Human papilloma virus DNA and p53 mutation analysis on bladder washes in relation to clinical outcome of bladder cancer. *Eur. Urol.*, Vol. 52, No 2, pp. 468-469.

Newell, G.R., Rawlings, W., Krementz, E.T., & Roberts, J.D. (1974). Multiple primary neoplasms in blacks compared to whites. III. Initial cancers at the female breast and uterus. *J. Natl Cancer Inst.*, Vol. 53, No 2, pp. 369-373.

Newell, G.R., Krementz, E.T., & Roberts, J.D. (1975). Exess occurrence of cancer of the oral cavity, lung, and bladder following cancer of the cervix. *Cancer*, Vol. 36, No 6, pp.2155-2158.

Nguyen, T.T., Nguyen, C.T., Gonsales, F.A., Nichols, P.W., Yu, M.C., & Jones, P.A. (2000). Analysis of cyclin-dependent kinase inhibitor expression and methylation pattern in human prostate cancers. *Prostate,* Vol. 43, No 3, pp. 233-242.

Parkin, D.M., Whelean, S.L., & Ferlai, J. (2003), IARC Press, Lyon, France, No 155.

Querci della Rovere, G., Oliver, R.T., McCance, D.J., & Castro, J.E. (1988). Development of bladder tumor containing HPV type 11 DNA after renal transplantation. *Br J Urol.*, Vol. 62, No 1, pp. 36-38.

Resnick, R.M., Cornekissen, M.T.E., Wright, D.K., Eichinger, G.H., Fox, H.T., ter Schegget, J, & Manos, M. (1990). Detection and typing of human papillomavirus in archival cervical cancer specimens by DNA amplification with consensus primers. *J. Natl Cancer Inst.*, Vol. 82, No 18, pp. 1477-1484.

Reznikoff, C.A., Belair, C., Savelieva, E., Zhai Y., Pfeifer, K., Yeager, T., Thompson, K.J., DeVries, S., Bindley, C., Newton, M.A., Sekhon, G., & Waldman., F. (1994). Long-term genome stability and minimal genotypic and phenotypic alterations in HPV16 E7-, but not E6-, immortalized human uroepithelial cells. *Genes and Dev.*, Vol. 8, No 18, pp. 2227-2240.

Ruas, M., & Peters, G. (1998). The p16INK4a/CDKN2A tumor suppressor and its relatives. *Biochim Biophys Acta*, Vol. 1378, No 2, pp.115- 177.

Sano, T., Oyama, T., Kashiwabara, K., Fukuda, T., & Nakajima, T. (1998). Expression status of p16 protein is associated with human papillomavirus oncogenic potential in cervical and genital lesions. *Am J Pathol.*, Vol.153, No 6, pp.1741- 1748.

Santin, A.D., Zhan, F., Bignotti, E., Siegel, E.R., Cane, S., Bellone, S., Palmieri, M., Anfossi, S., Thomas, M., Burnett, A., Kay, H.H., Roman, J.J., O'Brieb, T.J., Tian, E., Cannon, M.J., Shaughnessy, J. Jr. & Pecorelli, S. (2005). Gene expression profiles of primary HPV16- and HPV18-infected early stage cervical cancers and normal cervical epithelium: identification of novel candidate molecular markers for cervical cancer diagnosis and therapy. *Virology*, Vol. 331, No 2, pp. 269-291.

Serrano, M., Hannon, G. J. & Beach, D. (1993). A new regulatory motif in cell-cycle control causing specific inhibition of cyclin D/CDK4. *Nature*, Vol. 366, No 6456, pp. 704-707.

Trofimova, O., Kuevda, D., Shipulina, O., & Volgareva, G. (2009). Development of HPV genotyping and expression methods and validation on group of urinary bladder cancer. *Proceedings of the 25-th International Papillomavirus Conference*, Malmo, Sweden, May 2009, P-29.58.

van den Brule, A.J.C., Snijders, P.J.F., Gordijn, R.I.J., Bleker, O.P., Meijer, C.J.L.M., & Walboomers, J.M.M. (1990). General primer-mediated polymerase chain reaction permits the detection of sequenced and still unsequenced human papillomavirus genotypes in cervical scrapes and carcinomas. *Int. J. Cancer*, Vol. 45, No 4, pp. 644-649.

Volgareva, G.M., Zavalishina, L.E., Frank, G.A., Andreeva, Yu.Yu., Petrov, A.N., Kisseljov, F.L., & Spitkovsky, D.D. (2002). Expression of protein marker p16INK4a in uterine cervical cancer. *Arkhiv Patologii*; Vol. 64, N1, pp. 22-24, ISSN 0004-1955. (In Russian).

Volgareva, G., Zavalishina, L., Andreeva, Y., Frank, G., Krutikova, E., Golovina, D.,Bliev, A., Spitkovsky, D., Ermilova, V., & Kisseljov, F. (2004). Protein p16 as a marker of dysplastic and neoplastic alterations in cervical epithelial cells. *BMC Cancer*, Aug 31;4:58. Retrieved from: http://www.pubmedcentral.gov/articlerender.fcgi?tool=pubmed&pubmedid=153 39339

Volgareva, G.M., Zavalishina, L.E., Golovina, D.A., Andreeva, Y.Y., Petrov, A.N., Bateva, M.V., Petrenko, A.A., Ermilova, V.D., Kisseljova, N.P., & Frank, G.A. (2006). The protein p16[INK4a] as a reliable indicator of the HPV-induced carcinogenesis, In: *New Research on Cervical Cancer* (Rolland GZ, ed.). Nova Science Publishers, ISBN 13 978-1-60021-300-7 ISBN 10 1-60021−300-6, New York. pp. 129-147.

Volgareva, G., Zavalishina, L., Golovina, D., Andreeva, Y.Y., Cheban, N.L., Ermilova, V.D., Petrov, A.N., Bateva, M.V., Matveev, V.B., Shtil, A.A., & Frank, G.A. (2007). In search of bladder cancer markers: are human papillomaviruses and cellular *INK4a* expression associated? In: *Tumor Markers Research Perspectives* (G.A. Sinise, ed.). Nova Science Publishers, ISBN: 1-60021-423-1,New York, pp. 135-143.

Volgareva, G.M., Kuevda, D.A., Zavalishina, L.E., Shipulina, O.Y.,Trofimova, O.B., Golovina, D.A., Andreeva, Y.Y., Ermilova, V.D., Cheban, N.L., Glazunova, V.A., Bateva, M.V., Petrov, A.N., Matveev, V.B., Shtil, A.A., & Frank, G.A. (2008). Human papillomaviruses: is bladder urothelium a target of their carcinogenic action? *Proceedings of the World Cancer Congress*, UICC, Geneva, Switzerland, August 2008, P216.

Volgareva, G., Trofimova, O., Kuevda, D., Zavalishina, L., Golovina, D., Andreeva, Y., Ermilova, V., Cheban, N., Glazunova, V., Matvejev, V., Shipulina, O., & Frank, G. (2009). HPV and urinary bladder cancer. *Proceedings of the 25-th International Papillomavirus Conference*, Malmo, Sweden, May 2009, P-18.42.

Volgareva, G.M., Zavalishina, L.D., Golovina, D.A., Andreeva, Iu.Iu., Ermilova, V.D., Cheban, N.L., Kuevda, D.A., Trofimova, O.B., Shipulina, O.Iu., Pavlova, L.S., Petrov, A.N., Matveev, V.B., Shtil', A.A., & Frank, G.A. (2009). Detection of oncoprotein E7 HPV16 in the cancer and normal urinary bladder urothelium. *Arkhiv Patologii*, Vol. 71, No 1, pp. 29-30, ISSN 0004-1955. (In Russian).

Volgareva, G.M., Zavalishina, L.É., Trofimova, O.B., Korolenkova, L.I., Khachaturian, A.V., Andreeva, Iu.Iu., Ermilova, V.D., Cheban, N.L., Kuevda, D.A., Shipulina, O.Iu., Glazunova, V.A., Golovina, D.A., Petrov, A.N., Matveev, V.B., & Frank, G.A. (2010a). Are human papillomaviruses responsible for the occurrence of bladder cancer? *Arkhiv Patologii*, Vol.72, No 4, pp. 24-27, ISSN 0004-1955. (In Russian).

Volgareva, G.M., Zavalishina, L.E., Golovina, D.A., Andreeva, Y.Y., Ermilova, V.D., Trofimova, O.B., Kuevda, D.A., Shipulina, O.Y., Glazunova, V.A., Cheng, S., Pavlova, L.S., Cheban, N.L., Matveev, V.B., & Frank, G.A. (2010b). Cellular expression of *INK4a* gene in cells of bladder cancer associated with human papillomavirus-16. *Bulletin of Experimental Biology and Medicine*. Vol. 149, No 2, pp. 242-245, ISSN 0365-9615. (In English, Russian). May be purchased from SpringerLink:
http://www.springerlink.com/openurl.asp?genre=article&id=doi:10.1007/s10517-010-09

Yang, H., Yang, K., Khafagi, A., Tang, Y, Carey, T.E., Opipari, A.W., Lieberman, R., Oeth, P.A., Lancaster, W., Klinger, H.P., Kaseb, A.O., Metwally, A., Khaled, H., & Kurnit, D.M. (2005). Sensitive detection of human papillomavirus in cervical, head/neck, and schistosomiasis-associated bladder malignancies. *Proc. Natl Acad. Sci USA*, Vol. 102, No 21, pp. 7683-7688.

Zaridze, D.G. (2009). *Cancer prevention*. IMA-PRESS, ISBN 978-5-904356-05-7, Moscow. (In Russian).

Zaridze, D.G., Nekrasova, L.I., & Basieva, T.Kh. (1992). Increased risk factors for the occurrence of bladder cancer. *Voprosy. Onkologii (Problems in Oncology)*, Vol. 38, No 9, pp. 1066-1073, ISSN 0507-3558. (In Russian).

zur Hauzen, H. (2000) Papillomaviruses causing cancer: evasiom from host-cell control in early events in carcinogenesis. *J. Natl Cancer Inst.*, Vol. 92, No 9, pp. 690-698.

zur Hauzen, H. (2008) Papillomaviruses – to vaccination and beyond. *Biochemistry (Moscow)*, Vol.73, No 5, pp. 619-626, ISSN 0006-2979.

Permissions

The contributors of this book come from diverse backgrounds, making this book a truly international effort. This book will bring forth new frontiers with its revolutionizing research information and detailed analysis of the nascent developments around the world.

We would like to thank Dr. Abdullah Erdem Canda, for lending his expertise to make the book truly unique. He has played a crucial role in the development of this book. Without his invaluable contribution this book wouldn't have been possible. He has made vital efforts to compile up to date information on the varied aspects of this subject to make this book a valuable addition to the collection of many professionals and students.

This book was conceptualized with the vision of imparting up-to-date information and advanced data in this field. To ensure the same, a matchless editorial board was set up. Every individual on the board went through rigorous rounds of assessment to prove their worth. After which they invested a large part of their time researching and compiling the most relevant data for our readers. Conferences and sessions were held from time to time between the editorial board and the contributing authors to present the data in the most comprehensible form. The editorial team has worked tirelessly to provide valuable and valid information to help people across the globe.

Every chapter published in this book has been scrutinized by our experts. Their significance has been extensively debated. The topics covered herein carry significant findings which will fuel the growth of the discipline. They may even be implemented as practical applications or may be referred to as a beginning point for another development. Chapters in this book were first published by InTech; hereby published with permission under the Creative Commons Attribution License or equivalent.

The editorial board has been involved in producing this book since its inception. They have spent rigorous hours researching and exploring the diverse topics which have resulted in the successful publishing of this book. They have passed on their knowledge of decades through this book. To expedite this challenging task, the publisher supported the team at every step. A small team of assistant editors was also appointed to further simplify the editing procedure and attain best results for the readers.

Our editorial team has been hand-picked from every corner of the world. Their multi-ethnicity adds dynamic inputs to the discussions which result in innovative outcomes. These outcomes are then further discussed with the researchers and contributors who give their valuable feedback and opinion regarding the same. The feedback is then collaborated with the researches and they are edited in a comprehensive manner to aid the understanding of the subject.

Apart from the editorial board, the designing team has also invested a significant amount of their time in understanding the subject and creating the most relevant covers. They scrutinized every image to scout for the most suitable representation of the subject and create an appropriate cover for the book.

The publishing team has been involved in this book since its early stages. They were actively engaged in every process, be it collecting the data, connecting with the contributors or procuring relevant information. The team has been an ardent support to the editorial, designing and production team. Their endless efforts to recruit the best for this project, has resulted in the accomplishment of this book. They are a veteran in the field of academics and their pool of knowledge is as vast as their experience in printing. Their expertise and guidance has proved useful at every step. Their uncompromising quality standards have made this book an exceptional effort. Their encouragement from time to time has been an inspiration for everyone.

The publisher and the editorial board hope that this book will prove to be a valuable piece of knowledge for researchers, students, practitioners and scholars across the globe.

List of Contributors

Susanne Fuessel, Doreen Kunze and Manfred P. Wirth
Department of Urology, Technical University of Dresden , Germany

Daniela Zimbardi, Mariana Bisarro dos Reis, Érika da Costa Prando and Cláudia Aparecida Rainho
Department of Genetics, Institute of Biosciences, Sao Paulo State University - UNESP, Botucatu - SP, Brazil

Daben Dawam
Medway NHS Foundation Trust Medway Maritime Hospital Associate Teaching Hospital, University of London, United Kingdom

Yasuyoshi Miyata, Hideki Sakai and Shigeru Kanda
Nagasaki University Graduate School of Biomedical Sciences, Japan

Motoko Unoki
Division of Epigenomics, Department of Molecular Genetics, Medical Institute of Molecular Genetics, Kyushu University, Japan

Julieta Afonso
ICVS/3B's - PT Government Associate Laboratory, Portugal
Alto Ave Superior Institute of Health - ISAVE, Portugal

Lúcio Lara Santos
Portuguese Institute of Oncology - IPO, Portugal
University Fernando Pessoa - UFP, Portugal

Adhemar Longatto-Filho
Faculty of Medicine, São Paulo State University, Brazil
Alto Ave Superior Institute of Health - ISAVE, Portugal
Life and Health Sciences Research Institute - ICVS, University of Minho, Portugal

César Paz-y-Miño and María José Muñoz
Instituto de Investigaciones Biomédicas, Facultad de Ciencias de la Salud, Universidad de las Américas Quito, Ecuador

Samer Katmawi-Sabbagh
Kettering General Hospital NHS Trust, United Kingdom

Mohamed S. Zaghloul and Iman Gouda
Radiation Oncology and Pathology Departments,Children's Cancer Hospital and National Cancer Institute, Cairo University, Cairo, Egypt

G.M. Volgareva, V.B. Matveev and D.A. Golovina
N.N. Blokhin Cancer Research Center of the Russian Academy of Medical Sciences, Russia

Printed in the USA
CPSIA information can be obtained
at www.ICGtesting.com
JSHW011417221024
72173JS00004B/571